A Contemporary History of Alcohol in Russia

Introduction by
Denny Vågerö

Alexandr Nemtsov

Södertörns högskola
SE-141 89 Huddinge
2011

www.sh.se/publications

Translation: Howard M. Goldfinger

Cover: Jonathan Robson
Graphic Design: Per Lindblom & Jonathan Robson

Printed by E-print, Stockholm 2011

Södertörn Academic Studies 43
ISSN 1650-433X

ISBN 978-91-86069-24-7

For my daughter, my help, indeed

Russians believe that the main symbol of 20th century Russia was vodka. The Kalashnikov automatic rifle is in a distant second place.

All-Russia Center for the Study of Public Opinion (VTsIOM), 2002

Two thirds of the Russian population name alcoholism as the main problem in Russia. The majority of Russians look favorably on the alcohol campaign of the second half of the eighties.

All-Russia Center for the Study of Public Opinion (VTsIOM), 2006

Contents

Figures and tables (placement) 9

Alexandr Nemtsov's pioneering work on alcohol in
modern Soviet and Russian history *by Denny Vågerö* 13

Foreword (to the Russian original) 35
A contemporary history of alcohol in Russia 41

Part 1 47
Stages in the alcohol history of Russia 49
Chapter 1-1 Basic constituents of the alcohol situation 51
Chapter 1-2 The alcohol situation in other nations 65
Chapter 1-3 The alcohol situation in Russia before and after 1945 87
Chapter 1-4 The anti-alcohol campaign of 1985 99
Chapter 1-5 Consequences of the anti-alcohol campaign 109
Chapter 1-6 The alcohol situation 1987–1991 119
Chapter 1-7 The alcohol situation 1992–1994 127
Chapter 1-8 The alcohol situation 1995–1998 143
Chapter 1-9 The alcohol situation after 1998 159

Part 2 171
The alcohol history of Russia in the light of epidemiology 173
Chapter 2-1 Alcohol consumption as a human need 179
Chapter 2-2 The epidemiology of alcohol consumption in the World 189
Chapter 2-3 Epidemiological studies of Russian alcohol problems 205
Chapter 2-4 An estimate of actual alcohol consumption in Russia 235
Chapter 2-5 Alcohol aortality before, during and after the anti-alcohol campaign ... 261

Conclusion 303

Bibliography 327

Figures and tables (placement)

Figures

Fig. 1-1: Diagram of the constituent elements of the alcohol situation 51
Fig. 1-2a: Alcohol consumption in Great Britain (1900–1990) 59
Fig. 1-2b: Alcohol consumption in 6 nations of Europe,
    the United States and Japan (1895–1995) 60
Fig. 1-3 (a/b): Alcohol consumption in the European nations based on data from
    World Drink Trends and Leifman 71
Fig. 1-4: Alcohol consumption in Russia 1863–2006 90
Fig. 1-5: Number of registered drug addicts in Russia (1985–2000) 114
Fig. 1-6: Number registered with chronic alcoholism + alcohol psychosis
    + alcohol abuse (A), drug addiction + toxicomania + consumers of
    narcotic and psychoactive substances (D); (1991–1999) 114
Fig. 1-7: Age distribution of persons with drug addiction and toxicomania
    in 1985 and 1995 115
Fig. 1-8: Consolidated price indexes for alcoholic beverages and food
    products (1990–2005) 131
Fig. 1-9: Number of persons found to have committed crimes whilst sober
    or drunk from 1995 137
Fig. 1-10: Life expectancy for men and women and calorie and protein content
    of food consumed by Russian population (1992–1996) 151
Fig. 1-11: Age distribution of men's deaths in 1985–1986 in relation to 1984,
    and in 1992–1994 in relation to 1991 152
Fig. 1-12: Overall mortality and mortalities from alcohol poisoning (1965–2005) 153
Fig. 1-13: The production and sales of vodka and beer (1990–2000) 153
Fig. 1-14: Official figures and estimates of actual alcohol consmption
    in Russia (1990–2000) 164
Fig. 2-1: Alcohol consumption by regions of the World, age 15+ 191
Fig. 2-2: The theoretical distribution of consumers by alcohol use
    following Ledermann Hypothesis 197
Fig. 2-3: The relationship of average consumption in 21 groups of consumers 199
Fig. 2-4: The annual number of epidemiological publications on
    alcohol problems in Russia (1968–2002) 206
Fig. 2-5: Mortalities of "inexactly designated states" together with "from injuries
    (without specification)" (1965–2003) 220
Fig. 2-6: Figures from various authors on alcohol consumption, based on surveys 226
Fig. 2-7: Indexes of alcohol consumption in Russia (1970–2003) 236
Fig. 2-8: Monthly sales of sugar in Moscow (1984–1988) 237
Fig. 2-9: Monthly sales of alcoholic beverages in liters (Moscow, 1984–1987) 241
Fig. 2-10: Number of patients admitted per day with alcohol psychoses 241

Fig. 2-11: Mortality due to external causes, cirrhosis of the liver and morbidity by alcohol psychoses (1980–2002) 242
Fig. 2-12: Mortality by external causes (Moscow, 1981–1984). 243
Fig. 2-13: Official sales of alcohol in Moscow and Russia (1970–1993). Estimate of actual consumption and of unregistered alcohol in Moscow (1982–1993) 246
Fig. 2-14 (a/b): Deaths from external causes and their relationship with alcohol consumption (Moscow, 1984–1986). 248
Fig. 2-15: Sales of alcoholic beverages in Russia and 25 Russian regions (1981–1994) 252
Fig. 2-16: Relationship of registered alcohol and deaths from external causes 253
Fig. 2-17: Estimate of alcohol consumption and morbidity by alcohol psychoses in 25 Regions of Russia (1981–1994). 254
Fig. 2-18 (a/b): Number of criminals and number of murderers: overall number and number intoxicated by alcohol 259
Fig. 2-19: Number of deaths in Russia annually (1965–2005) 262
Fig. 2-20: Mortality from alcohol poisoning for men and women (Russia, 1965–2003). 263
Fig. 2-21: The overall number of deaths and cases with alcohol psychoses in Russia (1980–2003). 264
Fig. 2-22 a: The relationship of male and female mortality in Russia (1956–2003). 265
Fig. 2-22 b: The relationship of overall mortalities and mortality from alcohol poisoning (1975–2005) 265
Fig. 2-23: Number of male deaths per month in Russia (January 1983 to December 1988)...266
Fig. 2-24 (a/b): Change in the annual number of deaths for men and women (1965–2003) in relation to the line of regression (1965–1984) 269
Fig. 2-25: Mortality in men and women (1965–2003) (WHO new standard) 271
Fig. 2-26: Relationship of mortality of men and women who had consumed alcohol (1984–7 and 1992–2001) 272
Fig. 2-27: Alcohol consumption and mortalities from alcohol poisoning (1980–2001) in percentage terms with 1980 accepted as 100 % 277
Fig. 2-28 (a/b): Number of meaths of men and women (1965–1995) 280
Fig. 2-29 (a/b): Relationship between suicides and alcohol consumption (1980–2001) 283
Fig. 2-30: Averaged coefficients of correlation for 9 kinds of mortalities and alcohol consumption 286
Fig. 2-31: Diagram of calculations of alcohol-related mortality 287
Fig. 2-32 (a/b): Relationship of alcohol's contribution to various kinds of deaths for men and women in percent. Relationship of alcohol-related and overall Deaths in men and women. 289
Fig. 2-33 (a/b): Dynamics of basic types of deaths from external causes in men and women (1956–2003) (WHO new standard) 290/1
Fig. 2-34 (a/b): Dynamics of basic types of cardiovascular deaths in men and women (1970–2003) (WHO new standard) 292
Fig. 2-35 (a/b): Mortalities by homicide and suicide: sober and with alcohol in blood in 8 regions of Russia (1981–1990) 295
Fig. 2-36: Number of dead, registered homicides, murderers in state of intoxication or sober (1980–1999) 297
Fig. 2-37: Alcohol-related mortalities in 9 European countries and in Russia (1995) 299
Fig. 2-38: Alcohol consumption and life expectancy for men in Russia (1980–2002) 322

Tables

Table 1: Registered alcohol and an estimate of actual consumption in Russia (1960–2002) 53
Table 2: Change in consumption in several countries of Europe (1998 and 1988) 69
Table 3: Change in the level of consumption in 12 European countries and the U.S. 70
Table 4: Registered consumption in Western Europe and North America (2000/1) 74
Table 5: Registered alcohol consumption in Latin America (2000/1) 78
Table 6: Registered alcohol consumption in countries of Asia (2000/1) 79
Table 7: Registered and unrecorded alcohol consumption in African Countries (2000/1) 83
Table 8: Safe, dangerous and harmful daily consumption of alcohol 216
Table 9: Limits of episodic and regular alcohol consumption 217
Table 10: Examining the quantity and frequency of alcohol consumption in Russia 225
Table 11: Share of mortalities associated with alcohol 249
Table 12: Regions from which data are used 251
Table 13: Distribution of consumption of alcohol by regions of Russia 255
Table 14: Coefficients of linear regression for alcohol-related mortality (1980–2001) 274
Table 15: Correlation of various types of mortality with alcohol consumption 285
Table 16: Calculations and basic indexes of alcohol-related deaths in Russia (1980–2001) ... 288
Table 17: Share of mortalities associated with tobacco-, alcohol and drug use 293
Table 18: Loss of disability-adjusted life years ("DALYs") from in Russia (2002). 323

Alexandr Nemtsov's pioneering work on alcohol in modern Soviet and Russian history

by Denny Vågerö

> He wasn't a scoundrel, actually; he was an honest man. Maybe he could drink too much on occasion, but who didn't nowadays? The sick, possibly, or those who couldn't get hold of anything. Those who possessed nothing they could drink.

Vasil Bykau (1924– 2003), perhaps the greatest writer in Belarus ever, and widely read and loved in Russia also, describes Stupak Petrov in his book "The Veteran" ("Afganets"). The war in Afghanistan is over, the Soviet Union is gone. It is significant that Stupak, on returning from Afghanistan, loses his wife, and is left to himself and to the bottle.

As the Soviet Union collapsed and a new era emerged, the drinking of alcohol became a more serious problem. There were many Stupak Petrovs. Alexandr Nemtsov, in his pioneering work on alcohol in modern Russia, writes that in the 1990s Russian drinking was "taking more lives than crime, Afghanistan and the two Chechen wars". As research into Russian drinking has progressed, the severity of the problem has become much clearer. In 2010, a Russian boy aged 15 has just above a 50–50 chance of surviving to the age of 60; this is much worse than in many other so-called developing countries, such as Pakistan, India, Bangladesh and Kenya (Rajaratnam et al., 2010). Alcohol is a key contributor to this sorry state of affairs.

Södertörn University is now able to present, for the first time to western readers Alexandr Nemtsov's *Contemporary History of Alcohol in Russia*, an outstanding piece of scholarly work. Nemtsov's work on alcohol in Russia and the work which we have pursued at Södertörn University on health in Eastern Europe share many common themes. It has eventually brought together researchers in Moscow and Stockholm in a collaborative effort to make this publication possible. The material presented here constitutes a comprehensive and unique collection of information, much of which has not been known outside Russia before. The text is an edited translation of the Russian original, where Howard Goldfinger laid the ground work and Andrew Stickley with Erland Jansson and Jonathan Robson gave the text its final shape. The original text has been somewhat extended by Alexandr Nemtsov himself.

Russian drinking in the blurred mirror of history

The consumption of alcohol in Russia today is a cause for concern, but there is also a centuries-old mythology about its nature. The "Russian Primary Chronicle", or "A Tale From Times Gone By", recorded by the monk Nestor in the 1100s, is a prime source of myths about Russian drinking. Nemtsov points out that it was written more than a century after the events it describes. The chronicle tells of how Prince Vladimir of Rus', in agreeing to convert his people to Christianity rather than Islam or Judaism, also made it possible for them to go on drinking alcohol. Some modern writers have seen this as "sufficient reason for the whole country to embrace the faith", for instance Stephen White in his influential book "Russia goes dry" (1996). However, later historians have cast doubt on this popular idea. Geoffrey Hosking writes that it was geopolitics that decided the choice of religion. "The most important consideration was that he [Vladimir] wanted to maintain close links with Byzantium" (Hosking, 2001, p. 38). Segal, (1987, p. 6–7) writing about this period, explains that "a large body of historical documents shows that all the tribes of northern, eastern and central Europe had a tendency to indulge in periodic excessive drinking..." and asks further "whether the Slavs imitated the drinking customs of their Norman Masters [the Varangians] or developed the pattern of heavy drinking independently?" In other words, as the first Russian state took shape, Russian drinking habits may not have been unique at all, but common to many peoples in Northern, Central and Eastern Europe.

This book is important in that it gives a rich background of facts and evidence to the contemporary drinking problem. Nemtsov identifies and rejects some of the mythology. He points out that historical writings about Russian drinking habits in the past are often based on observations, not of the majority of the people and their actual drinking habits, but of smaller circles of people, often around the court, amongst the urban elite or in Moscow taverns. *Kabaki* (taverns) and royal and boyar feasts are the source of almost all the famous descriptions of Russian drinking in the medieval period", he explains. And furthermore: "Foreigners' descriptions of Russian drunkenness are almost exclusively based on observations of Moscow taverns, more rarely of Novgorod's and two or three other large cities to which foreigners were allowed access while traveling" (Nemtsov, p. 88). If this is indeed the case we should call on modern historians to help us establish a much clearer picture of early Russian drinking, at the court, and in towns and villages.

In the 1700s, Peter I, the great modernizer of Russia, helped to spread the practice of drinking vodka by introducing daily vodka rations for the navy and the army. Peter and his court were themselves often heavy drinkers, but their drinking was not representative of the population at large, as Nemtsov alludes to. Petrine drinking is reflected in world literature and has therefore colored our view of drinking in Russia, especially I presume from a vantage point outside Russia itself. Swedish author August Strindberg, who was a great admirer of Peter the Great, wrote a short play about him. He learnt about Peter from the biography by Waliszewsky (1899). Strindberg portrays Peter as someone who starts drinking vodka in the early morning, alone, and continues throughout the day, both on his own and in company (Strindberg, 1905). In Strindberg's mind the great man had to be a great drinker, a view that is common across many cultures.

George Munro, writing about the period of Catherine the Great, quotes a light-hearted set of rules which were pinned up on the wall in a St Petersburg Tavern: "Eat for sweetness and for taste, but pour moderately, so that everyone might always be able to find his legs as he goes out the door" (Munro, 1997). It indicates that, in the new capital on the Neva river, at least a modicum of caution had then emerged around drinking and its consequences.

Orlando Figes, in his "cultural history of Russia" (*Natasha's Dance*, 2002) also challenges some of the mythology: "contrary to the mythic image the overall consumption of vodka was not that great (in the year there were two hundred fasting days when drinking was prohibited)". He also maintains that "it was the test of a true Russian to be able to drink vodka by the bucketful..., drinking was a social thing – it was never done alone – and it was bound up with communal celebrations" (Figes, 2002, p. 167). Presumably, by "a true Russian" Figes refers to the male variant, since a true Russian woman would have hardly fit such a description.

Smith and Christian estimate the annual consumption of alcohol at around 5 liters for every adult male in 1790 (Smith & Christian, 1984). Nemtsov notes that in the European part of tsarist Russia alcohol consumption during the 1800s reached its peak, at 6.2 liters per person in 1863 (Nemtsov, p. 89). This peak, interestingly enough, followed on from the abolishment of serfdom in 1861, another great transition in Russia, and on a subsequent lowering of alcohol prices in 1863. Nevertheless, average levels of alcohol consumption in the 1700s and 1800s were not remarkably high. In fact they were often lower than in other European countries. In Sweden, in 1863, per capita consumption of alcohol was 9.6 liters in the adult (15+ years) population (CAN, 2008).

The pattern of drinking heavily at each drinking session was well established in Russia at this time and upheld by the cultural norms of the elite, including the court. Rural (village) drinking traditions, which were focused around important social occasions, could also include excessive drinking, but they were originally not based on vodka, but on weaker kinds of fermented drinks, such as *kvas*, *braga*, beer or wine. Engelgardt, a prominent St Petersburg chemist who was exiled to rural Russia (Smolensk region) in 1872 observed the habits of "the Russian village": "They drink, they begin to get rowdy, the conversation livens up, but never does it take an immodest turn" (quoted from Frierson, 1997). Engelgardt contrasts this with the excesses of the St Petersburg aristocracy. In fact, as Frierson points out, Engelgardt sees Russia as caught in a binary lock, with the St Petersburg aristocracy and the village constituting the two contrasting poles and, indeed, two drinking cultures.

With Nemtsov, we may conclude that drinking in Russia during the tsarist era was not greater than in many other European countries in terms of the amount of alcohol that was consumed. What was different was rather the style of drinking. One must also admit that we know very little about the variation in amounts and styles of drinking in the Russian population during this era. Such differences could have been very large between geographical areas, ethnic groups and social classes. Gender differences were certainly significant. The social, religious and ethnic division of Russia must to some extent have been mirrored in different, relatively distinct, drinking traditions (Segal, 1987). Unfortunately, here too occur weaknesses in our knowledge of the subject. Thus, in spite of the low average consumption of alcohol in Russia as a whole there may well have been segments of the population whose per capita consumption was very high, while in others people hardly drank alcohol at all. Christian, for instance, gives per capita consumption of vodka per annum in St Petersburg in 1858 as 23.1 liters (Christian, 1990, p. 73). Such pockets of extreme alcohol consumption are likely to have had a disproportionate influence on population health and life expectancy, but similar patterns would have been found over much of Europe at this time.

As Russia mobilized for World War I, a ban on alcohol sales in cities was introduced. In August 1914 it was extended "to the end of the war" by an "imperial decree" from Nicholas II. One of the first acts of the new Provisional Government under Kerenski, in March 1917, was to introduce the permanent prohibition of alcohol. In November 1917, the new Soviet power took the decision to destroy all existing stocks of alcohol. The Soviet Union was born in the midst of war and civil war. The three governments that succeeded each other, from that of the tsar to that of Kerenski to that of Lenin, were all trying to keep the country "dry". Not until 1921–22 were wine and beer sold freely again. Vodka (40 percent ABV) was not sold freely again until 1925.

From this dry beginning of the new Soviet state, alcohol consumption could only increase, and so it did. The 1917–1945 period is especially interesting, particularly the conflict between the state deriving tax revenue from high levels of vodka consumption and the issue of maintained social and public health through the curtailment of excessive drinking. The former turned out to be the stronger. However, Nemtsov gives evidence that the increase in alcohol consumption in the inter-war period was modest. This is consistent with the rapid increase in life expectancy during this period, when Russia moved out of poverty and illiteracy.

In spite of revolution, civil war, famines and repression the health of the population improved markedly during the first decades of Soviet power. Stephen

Wheatcroft has shown that historical traumas, like the civil war and the Volga famine of 1921–1922 or the Ukrainian famine of 1932–1933 certainly interrupted the underlying long term trend of improved population health, but never steered it off course. There was a long-term trend towards rapid secular improvement in welfare and life expectancy, which was accompanied by massive short-term welfare and mortality crises (Wheatcroft, 1999). The latter were closely linked to, indeed driven by, political changes, but unlike for post-war mortality fluctuations, alcohol did not play a major role in pre-war mortality fluctuations.

The full consequences for population health of Russia's tormented history still remain to be worked out. Today we know that those individuals who experienced and survived such hardship and trauma may have been scarred for life in a number of ways, especially if they were young when it happened. Children born during the Ukrainian famine, for instance, have been found to be more prone to diabetes in adult life (Khalangot, 2008) and people growing up in St Petersburg during the siege 1941–44 are more likely to suffer from hypertension, circulatory disease and breast cancer decades later (Sparen et al., 2004; Koupil et al., 2009). Whether hardship in childhood makes people more likely to take up drinking in later life, perhaps in particular at times of new hardship, is a very relevant, but still unanswered, question.

It is the period following World War II, 1950–2000, which is in focus in this book. And, Nemtsov writes, this is a period when the modern problem of excessive drinking takes shape and, finally, gets out of hand totally, thereby contributing to the long term stagnation and deterioration of the health of the population.

Post-war developments trigger massive increases in alcohol consumption and stagnation in the population's health

The substantial increase in alcohol consumption during the Soviet era took place primarily after World War II. "A particularly coarse culture of alcohol consumption formed in Russia in the post-war period", Nemtsov writes (p. 92). Therefore, he maintains, it is during this period that alcohol becomes of major importance as a driver of health developments and as a factor behind stagnating or falling life expectancy. In spite of the "Iron Curtain", Soviet drinking trends reflected international trends of rising alcohol consumption as people had more money. This is not the whole picture however. Is the increase in purchasing power sufficient explanation, Nemtsov asks? Or are there also long term political and social forces driving this development? Alcohol consumption rose steadily through the period of "thaw" and the period of "stagnation", he observes, with levels of consumption being twice as high in 1980 as in 1960. To me, it seems likely that the stagnation period is a key factor. As early as 1970 Andrei Sakharov had warned that Soviet Union was in danger of "stagnation" or "*zastoy*":

> In the course of the past decade it has been possible to discern worrying signs of discord and stagnation in the national economy of our country. ... The real income of the population has scarcely risen at all, food, medical care and everyday services have improved extremely slowly, and differently from region to region. The shortage of goods is becoming more common. ...What is particularly worrying for the future is the stagnation in education... Alcoholism is tragically on the increase and drug addiction is beginning to make its presence felt. In many parts of the country, criminality is rising systematically. In many areas there are increasing symptoms of corruption... There is no way out of the difficulties that the country is facing other than to set off on a path towards democratization. We still have the opportunity to set the right course and to carry out the right reforms. In a few years it could well be too late.

The latter conclusion was prophetic. Sakharov, with Valentin Turchin and Roy Medvedev, wrote their letter of appeal in March 1970. It was addressed to Brezhnev, Kosygin and Podgorny, who then headed the Communist party, the Soviet Council of Ministers and the Presidium of the Supreme Soviet, respectively. Their outspoken warning that inactivity might have "disastrous consequences" was ignored, as was the letter as a whole. In fact it became classified information. Not until 1990, under Gorbachev, was the letter published (Sakharov et al., 1990). Turchin, after Sakharov's death, claimed that this letter was the beginning of *glasnost*, the first attempt to end the period of stagnation (Turchin, 1991). Indeed, many of the demands in this letter became part of *glasnost* and *perestroika* (Brown, 1997).

Stagnation, collapse and transition: negative mortality trends

The fate of stagnation of Soviet society can perhaps be said to have been sealed in the aftermath of the events of 1968. The five-country occupation of Czechoslovakia and the resistance to it across Europe threw Soviet and East European leadership into something of a bunker mentality. Repression increased in Eastern Europe. The Sakharov letter had claimed that any attempt "to put the screws on would not only fail to solve our problems, but would aggravate them and finally lead the country into a tragic road of no return" (Brown, 1997). But the screws were put on for the next fifteen years.

Stagnation is an appropriate characterization of the whole period from 1968 to 1984 also in terms of life expectancy and health. This contrasts with the 1945 to 1965 period when both adult and child mortality fell. In terms of health, I believe we can distinguish between two periods, the first two post-war decades with positive life expectancy trends (partly driven by control of infectious disease mortality among children) and stagnation from 1968 to 1984. In contrast to the falling infant and child mortality rates, mortality among adult men was rising slowly and there was a rise or a standstill among adult women over the whole stagnation period in almost all the communist-led countries in Europe and in each of the republics of the Soviet Union, including the largest, Russia (Mezentseva & Rimachevskaya, 1990). It was a system-inherent problem, tied to the way the system was managed. Men were hit harder than women, adults more than children and working-age men most of all. The disease was eating its way into the heart of the Soviet power structure. The system could not deliver health improvements to its people.

The whole stagnation period was also characterized by a fairly steady increase in alcohol consumption. Perhaps as a response to this, statistics about alcohol consumption and alcohol-related deaths were suppressed during this period. This is a matter well documented in this book. To me, it seems likely that the successive and long term increases in alcohol consumption, at least up to 1985, were partly determined by the desperate hopelessness of a stagnating society.

But Alexandr Nemtsov also shows that this increase in alcohol consumption starts as early as the aftermath of World War II and continues into the first decade of the third millennium. In fact, the present very high levels of alcohol consumption are historically unprecedented. They represent the highest point of a several decade-long rising trend, admittedly with sharp temporary fluctuations. About these fluctuations Nemtsov writes, "that the sharp, often contradictory, changes in alcohol consumption ... often coincide with changes in other historically important aspects of Russian life, in particular the political" (p. 49). What is also true is that these sharp changes are mirrored in changes in mortality and life expectancy. Nemtsov's book, in a convincing fashion, brings this out. As Nemtsov as well as other observers have noted, the synchronicity of these changes suggests a causal relation.

Perhaps, we can identify two major drivers behind the post-war development of alcohol consumption. First there is the fact that people are getting more money and can better afford to drink. Secondly, there are a number of fundamental political and social developments that can be summarized as thaw, stagnation, *perestroika*, system collapse and transition to market economy, the latter with several ups and downs. These changes obviously have a huge impact on the ability, willingness or need to drink, to cope with grief, give comfort, to do business or simply for the enjoyment. The increase in drinking during periods when poverty increases rapidly, as in 1991–94, is unexpected from a conventional point of view. Jukkala et al. (2008), analysing Moscow data, have suggested that among men poverty increases the likelihood of excessive drinking, while among women poverty is more clearly linked to abstention. Rojas et al. (2008), analysing data from Taganrog in Southern Russia noted that among men poverty and economic strain made both extremes on the drinking continuum (abstention and heavy drinking) more likely. The net balance of these contradictory influences during recession can obviously be quite different from what is predicted by a simple economic model of drinking, based on price elasticity of alcohol as the main factor.

Furthermore, alcohol drinking habits are transmitted culturally through friendship networks and families in such a way that a drinking father is more likely to have a drinking son than is a non-drinking father (Velleman, 1993; Velleman & Orford, 1990) while a friend who drinks is more likely to make you yourself drink (Rosenqvist et al., 2010). Skog (1985) makes a distinction between wet and dry cultures. The implication is that friends and acquaintances, as well as social norms in general, are more likely to encourage you to drink in a wet culture than in a dry one. Thus the web of social contacts can help reinforce and multiply changes in drinking habits that are triggered by social and political events, thereby creating large fluctuations over time, much like the ups and downs of a contagious disease. In a wet culture, in particular, the magnitude of such fluctuations can be considerable, as the case of Russia proves.

Alcohol is not the only cause of alcohol-related mortality (Nemtsov, 2008). There is much work to be done if we are ever to answer the question: "Why does Ivan drink?" Such work would benefit from sociological surveys in this field, in close collaboration with epidemiologists (Carlson, 2009). This has been the approach taken by the Stockholm Centre of Health of Societies in Transition (SCOHOST) at Södertörn University which I led from 1997 to 2007 and which has been working together with the Institute for socioeconomic studies of the population (ISESP) in Moscow (Carlson, 2001; Carlson & Vågerö, 1998; Ferlander et al., 2009; Jukkala et al., 2008; Leinsalu, 2004; Mäkinen & Reitan, 2006; Rojas & Carlsson, 2006; Rojas et al., 2008; Stickley, 2006; Stickley et al., 2008, 2009a; Stickley & Carlsson, 2009; Vågerö & Kislitsyna, 2005).

Extremes of alcohol policy: 1985 and 1992

In May 1985, as one of the first measures under the new general secretary of the Communist party, Michael Gorbachev, the last big Soviet-style campaign was set in motion, a campaign to curb alcohol consumption. It was a forceful and ruthless campaign, which included a variety of measures from the promotion of fruit juice drinking to price rises on vodka, the closing of vodka distilleries and the up-rooting of century-old vines in Georgia, amounting in fact to semi-prohibition. Soon afterwards, Gorbachev launched two further campaigns which were, however, different from what had been seen in most previous Soviet-style campaigns. They became known as *perestroika* and *glasnost*. Perestroika meant it was possible to challenge party views in all fields and glasnost meant that it was possible to report more honestly what was going on in the country. These changes electrified the country and broke the long period of stagnation. The impact was great across the whole of Eastern Europe and beyond.

The vitalisation of the system resulted in a rapid improvement in life expectancy. The combination of the anti-alcohol campaign, perestroika and glasnost, was in my view a powerful factor behind the surge in life expectancy that took place from 1985. In 1987 life expectancy in Russia was 65 for men and 74 for women. It has never in Russian history, before or after, been higher. Alcohol consumption in 1987 was back to the level of the 1950s.

Gorbachev's anti-alcohol campaign, as Therese Reitan (2001) emphasized in her account of its reception, was generally seen as successful by the medical profession, which was looking at the decreasing mortality rates. Political scientists, on the other hand, saw the campaign as a failure, as the last Soviet-type campaign, and as one which undermined confidence in the political leadership among the people. In fact, some observers claimed that the anti-alcohol campaign helped to undermine the system and thus contributed to its later downfall. One intriguing aspect of Nemtsov's book is that it reveals what happened behind the scenes during the Gorbachev-era anti-alcohol campaign. It is clear that it was used as a tool in the internal battle in the Central Committee, finally helping to undermine Gorbachev.

The suppression of alcohol markets during the anti-alcohol campaign also gave rise to a wider clandestine illegal or semi-legal production, first as home-brewed alcohol (*samogon*) but later as organised production and distribution on a larger scale. This is one negative consequence of the anti-alcohol campaign that Nemtsov discusses at length. He points out that the embryo of an illegal production and distribution network, covering the whole of the Soviet Union, was being formed during this period.

The collapse of the Soviet system between 1989 and 1991 was followed by an almost unprecedented fall in life expectancy for men in Russia, by seven years between 1987 and 1994. In Russia, as well as in the 14 other republics of the former Soviet Union, mass poverty, uncertainty about the future and excess drinking were driving forces in this development. Drinking was facilitated by the market reforms of 1992, when the alcohol market was deregulated in ways which would have been unthinkable in any West European country. For those who could not afford vodka at its market price, cheap surrogate alcohols were widely available, usually in the form of technical alcohol. They could also be presented as medical tinctures or eau-de-colognes, but were in fact concentrated ethanol (Leon et al., 2009).

World War I semi-prohibition and the rise of samogon

In 1905, when the war with Japan broke out, mobilisation of Russian soldiers failed, due to wide-spread binge drinking, triggered by the order to mobilise. In 1914, and in order to guarantee the mobilisation of soldiers for the war effort, the sale of vodka was banned in cities. The ban was intended to last for the entire war, but in 1914 no one expected the war to be drawn out over several years.

This early prohibition episode has been studied by several scholars (Vvedensky, 1915; Karlgren, 1916; Christian, 1995; Stickley et al., 2009b). What were its consequences? There is some evidence that alcohol consumption fell quite sharply. But it is also true that the consumption of illegal alcohol (homebrewed) and surrogates increased. David Christian, in his analysis of this episode (1995) suggests that

> from the point of view of the Russian government it must be counted as a total, even a disastrous failure. From the point of view of Russian drinkers it must be counted an unexpected though difficult victory, and one whose consequences endured well after the conclusion of the formal ending of prohibition in 1925.

The "victory for drinkers" referred to by Christian was "the emergence and spread of samogon" (brewed alcohol).

The monopoly over liquor successfully built up by consecutive tsarist governments was destroyed by the emergence of wide-spread domestic production of samogon. Christian maintains that "post-Soviet Society continues to pay the price today for the failures of earlier attempts to control alcohol consumption". This is a conclusion that is exactly in line with Nemtsov's analysis of the 1985 campaign.

A close observer of these events was Anton Karlgren, professor of Slavonic studies in Copenhagen and a journalist at the Swedish daily newspaper, *Dagens Nyheter*, who travelled in Russia during the first period of World War I. In his book (1916), about the prohibition episode, he took a different and more positive view. He concluded that alcohol consumption had gone down, but he was concerned that the drinking of surrogates like eau-de-colognes, medical tinctures and varnishes etcetera had risen. Karlgren observed that in St Petersburg the number of people admitted to alcohol abuse clinics had fallen, indicating a fall of excessive drinking. At the same time the number of pharmaceutical outlets in St Petersburg had increased, indicating a rise in the drinking of surrogates. Karlgren's conclusions were partly based on his own observations and interviews in Russia. But he also studied a number of interview surveys, undertaken in the *guvernements* of Moscow, Penza, Poltava, Kharkov and Kostroma. The validity of these surveys is doubtful, however. Although the number of respondents was large (2,000 in Penza), these constituted only a fraction of the number of questionnaires sent out (around 20,000 in Penza) (Nemtsov, personal communication). There must be a large amount of uncertainty about any conclusions based on these surveys, which are however still quoted in the scientific literature.

Karlgren, of course, was writing for a Swedish audience, where a similar discussion to that in Russia about the evils of alcohol drinking was taking place, resulting six years later in a (Swedish) referendum on the prohibition of alcohol, a proposal which was rejected with the smallest possible margin.

Vvedensky was one of the leading contemporary researchers of the 1914 anti-alcohol law in Russia (Vvedensky, 1915). He pointed out that there was in fact rather limited support for the restrictive policies. There were only seven Russian medical societies and medical services which publically supported this law. He wrote: "One can't deny that this list is short or at least shorter than we wished or hoped it could be". And "without vodka there appeared a kind of emptiness in the structure of the common people's life ... adjustment to new conditions assumes painful and even dangerous forms".

In conclusion, the evaluation of the 1914–18 prohibition was as controversial as was the verdict on Gorbachev's anti-alcohol campaign 70 years later. Both campaigns also became part of the battle for power inside government. According to Karlgren, the proponents of prohibition during World War I found in this reform a useful weapon to undermine Kokotsev, president of the Tsar's council and finance minister. Nemtsov, similarly, points to the efforts to use Gorbachev's campaign to undermine his position (Nemtsov, p. 102-104).

We can conclude, from these two experiments in prohibition or semi-prohibition, that a reduction of alcohol drinking, especially binge drinking, does indeed reduce illness and premature death. At the same time, however, alcohol drinking can only be reduced in the long run if the means used to reduce the problem are accepted by the large majority of the population.

Scramble for control of alcohol markets – legal and illegal

SCOHOST at Södertörn University followed the Russian media systematically during the 1990s. This was reported in a newsletter, called "The Alcohol issue in Russia and the Baltic Sea Region" (www.scohost.se/alcohol_issue). Looking at these newspaper articles again one is met by stories of how those who were trying to take control of the alcohol market operated on the limit of what was legal and sometimes beyond it, for instance taking over legal brands by violent means. The terms "alco-mafia" or "alco-barons" are used. One of the most intriguing aspects of Nemtsov's book is the insight it gives into how the "alco-mafia" grows in Russia by operating both legally and illegally and in the grey area in-between. Nemtsov gives an account of how the early criminal structures, operating the clandestine alcohol market, grew and helped to establish the new market actors in the 1990s. This was perhaps the first structure that was ready to operate on a national scale in the new market economy of 1992.

The 1992 reforms to liberalise alcohol markets had managed to deprive the Russian state of the very substantial tax revenue from alcohol, which it always enjoyed previously, at the very moment when alcohol sales increased sharply. The state had resigned from its responsibilities and the profitable alcohol trade produced a fierce battle for control across Russia. Nemtsov describes how North Ossetia emerged as a key region in terms of both illegal and legal production of alcohol in the 1990s. The illegal import of untaxed wine or spirits from outside Russia, usually through South Ossetia, played a key role in this. The unknown "vodka war" between Russia and Georgia in 1997 is described in some detail by Nemtsov. It gives additional background to the 2008 war between the two countries.

Another observer, BBC journalist Misha Glenny, writes the following in his book about global organised crime.

> Between 1991 and 1996, the Russian state effectively absented itself from the policing of society, and the distinctions between legality and illegality, morality and immorality barely existed. In any event, there were no hard-and-fast definitions of organised crime, money-laundering or extortion and by implication all commercial transactions were illegal and legal at the same time. This applied as much to drugs and women as it did to cars, cigarettes and oil. Had the rule of law prevailed at the time, then there is no question that the oligarchs' behaviour would have warranted severe punishment. (Glenny, 2009)

Glenny did not discuss alcohol in his book. It would have been a natural extension to his theme about global organised crime, and in the case of Russia it amounts to a grave omission. Nemtsov, in contrast, highlights the issue. He demonstrates that alcohol was deeply embedded in the birth of the criminal or semi-criminal oligarchical system of that decade. Further, it is clear that this system reached out beyond the borders of Russia.

Today, the Russian state has managed to regulate alcohol markets to a certain extent. There is again substantial tax revenue from the trade, but there has been very little success in controlling and reducing drinking. However, the first signs of a change are there. President Putin, raised some concerns in his speech to the nation in 2005 (Putin, 2006), and his successor Dmitri Medvedev in 2009 acknowledged that Russian alcohol drinking is a serious problem, indeed "a threat to national security". Medvedev also commented positively on Gorbachev's anti-alcohol campaign, but at the same time opposed demands for a ban on sales of alcohol (*Ria Novosti*, 19 January 2010).

Russia and Europe – is there a need for a common agenda of alcohol control?

The 53 countries which form the European Region of the World Health Organisation are all found in the region of the world where the level of alcohol drinking is highest, and probably also where it takes the highest death toll

(WHO, 2005). Furthermore, mortality variation across Europe is great and is in no small part influenced by European alcohol consumption patterns.

European mortality trends started to diverge from the late 1960s, mainly because of the long period (1968–1984) of health stagnation in the countries that then made up communist Europe. Glasnost, perestroika and the anti-alcohol policies of Gorbachev broke this stalemate in the East, but the collapse of the system in 1989–91 lead to an immediate widening of health differences between Eastern and Western Europe. This has been referred to as the European Health Divide (Vågerö & Illsley, 1992) or the European Mortality Divide (Bobak & Marmot, 1996). In 2005 life expectancy for men differs by around 16 years between the old EU (15 old members) and Russia, but the 12 new members of EU have eventually begun to catch up with the old. The European Health Divide has grown, and at the same time moved eastwards, leaving countries like Russia, Ukraine, Belarus and Moldova at an increasing health disadvantage (Vågerö, 2010).

Jürgen Rehm, a leading European alcohol researcher, makes a convincing case for alcohol being an important factor in the health differentiation between countries in the European Union as well as across Europe as a whole. In particular, alcohol contributes to the large (and increasing) life expectancy gap between Russia and the countries of Central and Western Europe (Rehm et al., 2004; Rehm et al., 2007b).

Rehm (Rehm et al., 2007a) estimated the alcohol-attributable fraction of mortality in Russia to be 18 percent for men aged 20–64, for women in the same age group it was estimated to be 9 percent. The authors suspect that this estimate may be biased downwards. A previous study by Rehm et al. (2006) covering European Russia and men in age groups 15–59 estimated this fraction to be 27 percent for men. The underestimation of the death toll attributable to alcoholic beverages which Rehm and co-authors worry about in their study may only be part of the problem. Western epidemiology, until very recently, has long missed out the fact that large quantities of alcohol in Russia are drunk as surrogate liquids of very high alcohol content, which allows fast and potentially lethal intoxication. Surrogate liquids are discussed by Nemtsov. Some of the studies quoted in this introduction were not published until after the Russian original of Nemtsov's book was already finalised, but in most ways they tend to support or reinforce the conclusions drawn by Nemtsov. Leon et al. (2007) in their study of mortality in Izhevsk, Russia, focused on the contribution of surrogate alcohol, estimated by them to be drunk by around 8 percent of men in this region. Surrogate drinking or other types of extreme alcohol drinking were estimated to account for 43 percent of mortality among men aged 25–54 in Izhevsk. A later study published in the Lancet, suggests that more than one in two deaths among Russian men in that age group, and a third of deaths among women, may be attributable to excessive alcohol drinking, including surrogates (Zaridze et al., 2009). The latter study therefore concluded that alcohol is of even greater importance than tobacco for premature death in Russia.

There is no doubt today that a very considerable fraction of male working-age mortality in Russia is attributable to alcohol (Shkolnikov et al., 2002; Leon et al., 2010). This is also one of the major points addressed in Nemtsov's book.

Female mortality is linked to women's alcohol consumption to a much smaller extent. Male/female differences in drinking are in general greater in the eastern than in the western parts of Europe. Consequently, the drinking habits of women in Central and Eastern Europe differ much less from women in the West, than do the drinking habits of the men in the same comparison. Among women in the UK, in fact, heavy drinking is slightly more common and abstention less common than among women in both Poland and Russia, an unexpected finding reported in a European collaborative study (Rehm et al., 2007b).

We may conclude that alcohol consumption patterns in Europe have a considerable impact on health differences within Europe at large, both between countries and within them (Norström, 2002). They also contribute hugely to gender differences in life expectancy across Europe – but most notably in Russia.

Further, the politics and economics of alcohol in the old and new member states of the EU, in the Balkans, Russia and Ukraine as well as in all the other post-Soviet republics are connected in a myriad of direct and indirect ways. Policies in one country are obviously influenced by the situation in neighbouring countries. States adjust their taxes and policies in relation to what neighbouring countries do and in particular to the legal, semi-legal and illegal trade in alcoholic beverages across the continent and beyond.

Some countries have felt themselves forced into a negative spiral of reducing taxes on alcohol and relaxing alcohol control policies. The smuggling of vodka from Russia to Estonia played a part in setting low taxes in Estonia. When Estonia joined the EU in 2004, Finland lowered taxes to deter Finns from going to Tallinn and buying large quantities of cheap alcohol. Swedish alcohol taxes were lowered as a response to the growing illegal and semi-legal import of alcohol from Germany and other countries. The alcohol trade in Europe, including that in Russia and Ukraine, feeds on the very large differences in prices and policies between countries and regions in Europe. The net result of such regional dynamics in Europe has been a reduction in taxes on alcohol, the deregulation of alcohol markets, increasing levels of alcohol consumption and a growing concern about alcohol-related problems across the European region at large.

The implications of these facts are far-reaching, yet not recognised at the highest level in Russia, nor elsewhere in Europe. Is there then cause for concern in the European region? Yes, indeed there is.

The World Health Organisation (WHO) in Europe, European governments and in particular the EU should now take a much more proactive role. EU policies which previously looked upon alcohol as just another commodity to be traded in the single market have had a negative impact. These policies represented the traders' view, rather than that of public health. Similarly, Russian and Ukrainian polices have paid very little attention to the public health consequences of the legal, semi-legal and illegal alcohol trade. In these countries, too, the traders' view has been dominant, complemented by that of local or central governments who want to maximise their tax revenue from alcohol sales. Both these perspectives are in fact short-sighted. It has been shown many times, and in many countries, that the long term costs of alcohol-related disease, accidents, suicides and violence far exceeds the revenue that governments can make from taxes on alcohol.

Alcohol related problems in Europe are so closely interwoven that they could be seen to constitute one common problem (Vågerö, 2007). Maybe, therefore, European countries, including Russia and Ukraine, should look for a common solution, or at least make it a common concern and work together. The WHO Regional Office in Europe, with its new and dynamic leadership under Zsuzsanna Jakab, could play a leading role in this effort. There are new developments within the World Health Organisation that could be helpful. Its supreme body, the World Health Assembly, decided in May 2008 to call for a discussion of the means to reduce alcohol-related harm globally. The 2010 World Health Assembly decided to implement a global strategy to combat alcohol-related harm on every continent. I hope Europe will lead the way and show how this can be done in practice.

These are some steps that European governments can take immediately: European governments could pronounce as their common view that alcohol is not just another commodity to be traded in the single market, or across European borders, but rather one that gives rise to public health concern all over Europe as well as globally. European governments could aim to reduce excessive alcohol consumption across the whole continent, rather than encouraging the expansion of alcohol businesses in each other's backyards.

The EU is another important player. It should encourage, rather than discourage, member states who want to pursue a policy of limiting alcohol consumption and alcohol-related harm at home and abroad. The EU and Russia, as well as the EU and Ukraine, should also work together to formulate their common interest in this field. It is time to start a dialogue within the framework of the EU-Russia and EU-Ukraine long term collaborative agreements about ways to reduce alcohol-related harm across Europe. This dialogue could be facilitated by the WHO-Europe. It is of pan-European interest to limit illegal alcohol production in Russia, Ukraine or anywhere else, so that Russia, Ukraine and others succeed in raising alcohol price levels in the long term. The EU, Russia and Ukraine should agree on how to limit and combat illegal alcohol production and trade across Europe as well as support each other in efforts to reduce excessive alcohol consumption.

I hope also that European governments will support the idea of a legally binding Global Framework Convention on the Control of Alcohol. The example set by the adoption of a Framework Convention on Tobacco Control shows what can be done. Many international public health bodies have already embraced this idea, for instance the American Public Health Association and the World Medical Association, as well as medical journals, such as the Lancet (Editorial, 2007).

In developing a global strategy we can learn from the Russian experience. We should listen to the voice of Alexandr Nemtsov. He has spent nearly three decades studying this experience. It is particularly valuable that Nemtsov has followed the story of Russian alcohol from the inside and at the same time has been able to build his conclusions on both western and Russian research. It has given him a unique insight, which he shares with us in his *Contemporary History of Alcohol in Russia*. He is fully aware of the human costs and suffering that are caused by excessive alcohol drinking. But his pioneering work on alcohol in modern Russian history also brings with it a warning: a strategy to control alcohol that is not accepted by the majority of the population will not succeed.

References

Bobak M, Marmot M (1996) East-West mortality divide and its potential explanations: proposed research agenda. *BMJ* 312. 421–425.
Brown A. (1997) *The Gorbachev Factor.* Oxford: Oxford University Press
Bykov V. (1999) *Afganets.* Moskva: Izdatel'stvo Vremya
CAN (2008) *Drogutvecklingen i Sverige 2008.* Rapport 113,. Stockholm
Carlson P. (2001). Risk behaviours and self-rated health in Russia 1998. *Journal of Epidemiology and Community Health.* 55. 806–817.
Carlson P. (2009) Commentary: Russia's mortality crisis, alcohol and social transformation. *International Journal of Epidemiology.* 38. 156–157. doi:10.1093/ije/dyn202.
Carlson P., Vågerö D. (1998) The social pattern of heavy drinking during transition in Russia. Evidence from Taganrog 1993. *European Journal of Public Health.* 8. 280–285.
Christian D. (1990) *Living water. Vodka and Russian society on the eve of emancipation.* Oxford, New York: Oxford University Press
Christian D. (1995) Prohibition in Russia 1914–1925. *Australian Slavonic and East European Studies.* 9. 89–108.
Editorial (2007) A framework convention on alcohol control. *The Lancet.* Vol 370. September 29.
Ferlander S., Makinen IH (2009) Social capital, gender and self-rated health. Evidence from the Moscow Health Survey 2004. *Social Science & Medicine.* 69. 1323-1332.
Figes O. (2002) *Natasha's dance. A cultural history of Russia.* St Ives: The Penguin Press
Frierson C. (1997) Food, hunger and rational restraint in the Russian peasant diet: One populist's vision. In: M. Glantsand J. Toomre (eds.) *Food in Russian history and culture.* Indiana University Press
Glenny M. (2009) *McMafia. Seriously organised crime.* London: Vintage Books
Hosking G. (2001) *Russia and the Russians. A history from Rus to the Russian Federation.* Bath: Allen Lane Penguin Press
Jukkala T., Mäkinen IH, Kislitsyna O., Ferlander S., Vågerö D. (2008) Economic strain, social relations, gender, and binge drinking in Moscow. *Social Science and Medicine.* 66. 663–74.
Karlgren A. (1916) *Ryssland utan vodka. Studier av det ryska spritförbundet.* Stockholm: Åhlen o Åkerlund Förlag
Khalangot M. (2008) *Type 2 diabetes in Ukraine in cohorts during the famine 1932–1933.* www.lorentzcenter.nl/lc/web/2008/319/CD%20LORENTZ%20CENTER%20WORKSHOP/Poster%20Ukraine.pdf. Accessed on July 22nd, 2010.
Koupil I., Plavinskaja S., Parfenova N., Shestov D., Danziger P., Vågerö D. (2009) Cancer mortality in women and men who survived the siege of Leningrad (1941–1944). *International Journal of Cancer.* 124(6). 1416–21.
Leinsalu M. (2004) *Troubled transitions. Social variation and long-term trends in health and mortality in Estonia.* Stockholm University: Health Equity Studies no 2.
Leon D., Saburova L., Tomkins S., Andreev E., Kiryanov N., McKee M., Shkolnikov V. (2007) Hazardous alcohol drinking and premature mortality in Russia: a population based case-control study. *The Lancet.* 369. 2001–2009.Leon D., Shkolnikov V., McKee M. (2009) Alcohol and Russian mortality: a continuing crisis. *Addiction.*104.1630-1636.

Leon D., Shkolnikov V., McKee M., Kiryanov N., Andreev E. (2010) Alcohol increases circulatory disease mortality in Russia: acute and chronic effects or misattribution of cause? *International Journal of Epidemiology.* 39. 1279-1290.

Mäkinen I., Reitan. T. (2006) Continuity and change in Russian alcohol consumption from the tsars to transition. *Social History.* 31 (2). 160–179.

Mezentseva E., Rimachevskaya N. (1990) The Soviet country profile: health of the USSR population in the 1970s and 80s - an approach to a comprehensive analysis. *Social Science and Medicine.* 31(8). 867–77.

Munro G. (1997) Food in Catherinian St Petersburg. In: M.Glants and J.Toomre (eds.). *Food in Russian history and culture.* Indiana University Press

Nemtsov A. (2008) Is alcohol the only cause of alcohol-related mortality? *Addiction.* 103. 1754–1755.

Norström T. (ed.) (2002) Alcohol in post-war Europe. Consumption, drinking patterns, consequences and policy responses in 15 European countries. Stockholm: Almqvist & Wiksell International

Putin V. (2006) Annual address to the Federal Assembly of the Russian Federation, April 25, 2005. Moscow: Government of the Russian Federation.

Rajaratnam J., Marcus J., Levin-Rector A., Chalupka A., Wang H., Dwyer L., Costa M., Lopez A., Murray C. (2010) World wide mortality in men and women aged 15–59 from 1970–2010: a systematic analysis. *The Lancet.* 375. 1704-1720.

Rehm J., Room R., Monteiro M. et al (2004) Alcohol use: In: M. Ezzati, A. Lopez, A. Rodgers, C. Murray (eds.). *Comparative quantification of Health Risks; Global and regional burden of disease attributable to selected major risk factors.* Geneva: WHO. p 959–1108.

Rehm J., Taylor B., Patra J. (2006) Volume of alcohol consumption, patterns of drinking and burden of disease in the European region 2002. *Addiction.* 101. 1086-95.

Rehm J., Klotsche J., Patra J. (2007a) Comparative quantification of alcohol exposure as risk factor for global burden of disease. *International Journal of Methods in Psychiatric Research.* 16. 66–76.

Rehm J., Sulkowska U., Manczuk M., Boffetta P., Powles J., Popova S., Zatonski W. (2007b). Alcohol accounts for a high proportion of premature mortality in central and eastern Europe. *International Journal of Epidemiology.* 36 (2). 458–67.

Reitan T. (2001). The operation failed, but the patient survived. Varying assessments of the Soviet Union's last anti-alcohol campaign. *Communist and Post-Communist Studies.* 34 (2). 241–260.

RIA Novosti, January 19, 2010; accessed at: http://en.rian.ru/russia/20100119/157613922.html

Rojas Y., Carlson P. (2006) The stratification of social capital and its consequences for self-rated health in Taganrog, Russia. *Social Science and Medicine.* 62. 2732–2741.

Rojas Y., Stickley A., Carlson P. (2008) Too poor to binge? An examination of economic hardship and its relation to alcohol consumption patterns in Taganrog Russia. *Scandinavian Journal of Public Health.* 36. 330-331.

Rosenquist N., Murabito J., Fowler J., Christakis N. (2010) The spread of alcohol consumption behavior in a large social network. *Annals of Internal Medicine.* 152. 426–433.

Sakharov A.D., Turchin V.F., Medvedev R.A. (1990) Letter. *Izvestiya TsK KPSS.* 11.150–159.

Segal B. (1987) *Russian drinking. Use and abuse of alcohol in pre-revolutionary Russia.* New Brunswick, NJ: Rutgers Centre of Alcohol Studies.

Shkolnikov V., Mesle F., Leon D. (2002) Premature circulatory disease mortality in Russia. Population and individual level evidence. In: Weinder et al. (eds.). *Heart disease: Environment, stress and gender"*. Amsterdam: IOS Press
Skog O.J. (1985) The collectivity of drinking cultures: a theory of the distribution of alcohol consumption. *British Journal of Addiction.* 80 (1). 83-99.
Smith R., Christian D. (1984) *Bread and salt. A social and economic history of food and drink in Russia.* Cambridge: Cambridge University Press
Sparén P., Vågerö D., Shestov D., Plavinskaja S., Parfenova N., Hoptiar V., Paturot D., Galanti M. (2004) Long term mortality after severe starvation during the siege of Leningrad: prospective cohort study. *BMJ.* 328 (7430). 11-15.
Stickley A. (2006) *On interpersonal violence in Russia in the present and the past: a sociological study.* Södertörn doctoral dissertations no 7. Stockholm.
Stickley A., Carlson P. (2009) The social and economic determinants of smoking in Moscow, Russia. *Scandinavian Journal of Public Health.* 37. 632-639.
Stickley A., Kislitsyna O., Timofeeva I., Vågerö D. (2008). Attitudes toward intimate partner violence against women in Moscow, Russia. *Journal of Family Violence.* 23. 447-456.
Stickley A., Ferlander S., Jukkala T., Carlson P., Kislitsyna O., Mäkinen IH (2009a) Institutional trust in contemporary Moscow. *Europe-Asia Studies.* 61. 779-796.
Stickley A., Razvodovsky Y., McKee M. (2009b). Alcohol mortality in Russia: A historical perspective. *Public Health.* 123. 20-26.
Strindberg A. (1905) Den store (The great one). In: *Historiska miniatyrer.* Stockholm: Albert Bonniers förlag.
Turchin V.F. (1991) Scientist and prophet. In: Than Van (ed.). *Andrei Sakharov. Facets of a life.* Editions Frontiere and P. N. Lebedev Physics Institute. Cedex, France.
Zaridze D., Brennan P., Boreham J., Boroda A., Karpov R., Lazarev A., Konobeevskaya I., Igitov V., Terechova T., Bof etta P., Peto R. (2009) Alcohol and cause-specific mortality in Russia: a retrospective case–control study of 48 557 adult deaths. *Lancet.* 373. 2201-14.
Vågerö D. (2007) Commentary. The role of alcohol in mortality differences between European countries. *International Journal of Epidemiology.* 36. 46–469.
Vågerö D. (2010) The East-West health divide in Europe: growing and shifting eastwards. *European Review.* 18 (1). 23-4.
Vågerö D., Illsley R. (1992) Inequality, health and policy in East and West Europe. *International Journal of Health Sciences.* 3 (3/4). 225-239.
Vågerö D., Kislitsyna O. (2005) Self-reported heart symptoms are strongly linked to past and present poverty in Russia – evidence from the 1998 Taganrog interview survey. *European Journal of Public Health.* 15. 418-423.
Vvedensky I.N. (1915) *Opyt prinuditel'noĭ trezvosti.* (In English. An experience of enforced abstinence). Moskva: Izdanie moskovskogo stolichnogo popechitel'stva o narodnoĭ trezvosti.
Velleman R. (1993) *Alcohol and the family,* London, Institute of Alcohol Studies.
Velleman R., Orford. J. (1990) Young adult offspring of parents with drinking problems: recollections of parents' drinking and its immediate effects. *British Journal of Clinical Psychology.* 29. 297–317.
Waliszewsky K. (1899) *Peter der Grosse.* Deutsche ausgabe von Wilhelm Bolin. Berlin: E Hofmann.
Wheatcroft S. (1999) The great leap upwards: anthropometric data and indicators of crises and secular change in Soviet welfare levels, 1880–1960. *Slavic Review.* 58 (1). 27–60.

White S. (1996) Russia goes dry: Alcohol, state and society. New York: Cambridge University Press.
World Health Organisation (WHO) (2005) Alcohol policy in the WHO European Region: current status and the way forward. Fact sheet EURO/10/05. Copenhagen, Bucharest. http://www.euro.who.int/document/mediacentre/fs1005e.pdf (Accessed on 11 May 2010).

Foreword
(to the Russian original)

My heightened interest in the problem of heavy drinking in Russia was triggered by a trip that I took with a friend in 1971 to Kostromsk Region. We were to visit the village of Zaborye, where my friend grew up. As we approached the village, we came to a small cemetery. There my friend learned, from the headstones, that four of his boyhood friends, whom he could recall from the age of 12, were dead. In the village we were told that all four had died from excessive drinking. My friend was at that time just a little over 30 years old.

I began my studies of alcoholism in 1982. As 1985 was ending I came to realize that the recently declared anti-alcohol campaign was going to be a gift for me. It opened the door to studying a wide range of phenomena that had hitherto been off-limits. Within a year or two, the epidemiology of Russia's alcohol problem was my major research focus. Since then I have published three small books on the subject and more than 40 articles in Russian and English. The time has now come for a summing up, one more attempt to think through my work and to see it in relation to the evidence accumulated by other researchers.

My first book, *The Alcohol Situation in Russia* (Alkogolnaya Situatsiya v Rossii; 1995) took events up to 1992. Publication, as it happened, coincided with a new, abrupt and mistaken shift in alcohol policy. In other words, a new and very important stage in the history of alcohol, in Russia was underway. During it, the negative consequences of alcohol consumption in Russia reached world-record heights. The new circumstances helped widen the appreciation of the country's alcohol problem and made clear the need for further analysis. Moreover, the change showed the need to bring the various stages of alcohol use in Russia into a historical perspective and see them in their historical contexts; most importantly, the contemporary context.

I could not avoid at least a brief look at the many centuries of alcohol use in Russia, a story usually rendered in the darkest of colors. I believe there is another way of looking at this history, a different way of distributing the usual dark tones by place and time. It is important to balance historical descriptions of Russian drunkenness in its capitals with a look at the country as a whole, that is, to look at the whole population of the country and its conditions. In fact, I see little connection between the historical consumption of alcohol in Russia and contemporary problems related to alcohol.

Alcohol consumption has grown dramatically in Russia in the past 50 years, and the end is not in sight. But, unlike history, a book about history must end somewhere. In this instance, the main cut-off is 2000, although some things are traced through to later than 2000 because, while set in motion earlier, they intensified in the 2000–2003 period, during the writing of this book. Thus, the period 2000–2003 is the last to be dealt with. The starting point is, essentially, the first post-war decade. The alcohol-related events framed by these endpoints make up the first part of the book.

Hardly any work of modern history would be complete without quantitative data. However, in this case, official statistics are unreliable. Approximate accuracy can be attained only by reworking the official numbers, and that is the task in the second part of the book, in which the constituent elements of the history are viewed in epidemiological terms. Some of the results of the calculations made in the second part of the book appear as "events" in the first. In addition, because of their importance, the data on alcohol mortality have their own separate volumes: Alcohol Mortality in Russia, 1980–1990 (*Alkogolnaya smertnost' v Rossii, 1980–1990-e gody*; 2001a) and Alcohol Losses by Region in Russia (*Alkogolny uron regionov Rossii*; 2003b). Those statistics are presented here in a condensed and significantly supplemented and reworked form.

Such is the book's overall structure. At the same time, one can only regret that the epidemiological understanding of alcohol consumption in Russia, a matter so vital in such a large and heavy-drinking country, is far from complete. Many aspects of the Russian alcohol picture have been neglected in this work because they have yet to be dealt with scientifically or resist analysis, as is the case with the quantification of alcohol-related illnesses, because of the imprecision of the relevant statistics.

For vital assistance of many kinds at various stages in the preparation of this work, the author is indebted to V. Shkolnikov (now of the Max Planck Institute for Demographic Research), B. Brui (of the Russian Bureau of Statistics), T. Gryukova (of the Moscow Bureau of Statistics), V. Plaksin and L. Krasavin (of the Russian Ministry of Health) and A. Demin (of the Russian Association of Public Health). The author is deeply grateful for their support. Thanks also to A. Vishnevsky (of the Demography Institute of the State University-Higher School of Economics) and E. Andreev (of the Max Planck Institute for Demographic Research) for valuable comments and assistance on the problem of alcohol-related deaths. The final calculations on alcohol-related death rates were performed with hands-on help from the mathematician A. Terekhin, to whom the author is indebted not only for help with the calculations, but also for his "science". A significant amount of the documentary material used here is from the website of the National Alcohol Association, for the use of which the author is grateful to its director, P. Shapkin.

I also wish to acknowledge the importance of the many publications by D. Lvov and N. Petrakov of the Russian Academy of Sciences, by the publicist V. Kostikov. The sociologists Yu. Levada and O. Krishtanovskaia in bolstering my understanding of the effects of economic and social trends on sales of alcohol also deserve acknowledgment. My thanks go out to all of them for the steadfastness of their positions, the directness and detail of their comments and, most important, their grasp of the essence of these very complex phenomena.

I wish to pay special tribute to Alexander Nechaev (1955–2004). The idea for my epidemiological studies arose in discussions with him in October–November 1985 about the anti-alcohol campaign. Shortly thereafter, in December 1985, the studies on alcoholic psychoses and alcohol poisoning began in Moscow with Dr Nechaev as an active collaborator.

The section of the book on alcohol mortality was supported by the John D. and Catherine T. MacArthur Foundation, without whose aid this project could not have been completed.

I am grateful as well to the leadership of the Moscow Psychiatric Research Institute for recognizing the importance of the alcohol problem, for supporting my research and for allowing me to concentrate on the subject and work on it in an uninterrupted manner.

* * *

We all know that people tend to make their views about society and sometimes their scientific findings conform to their personal biases. So it is only fair that, writers who take up social problems and especially problems directly tied to our daily lives, make clear their own positions. All the more is this true of so emotionally fraught and personally colored a topic as alcohol consumption. It would be ideal if discussions of alcohol problems could be restricted to non-using, independent observers. While all very well, it is too much to ask in this case. I will, instead, offer this alcohol self-portrait.

I have not drunk any vodka for 10 to 15 years, indulging rarely, and only in company, in a small amount of red wine or beer. But even this occurs increasingly seldom now, both because I am busy more than ever before and because "Some are present to my mind only, others are farther away" (*Evgeniy Onegin*, Alexander Pushkin). I have imposed no bans or limitations on myself as regards the consumption of alcohol. Nor do I take credit for my moderation in alcohol consumption; that moderation reflects the absence of any wish to drink, probably inherited from my parents and forebears.

I have had friends who are, or were, "mild" alcoholics. I have no severely alcoholic friends, a fact perhaps "abetted" sometimes by the drinkers themselves.

We are more likely to feel revulsion than sympathy for heavy drinkers. One does feel sympathy and want to help those who have reached the end of the line though. For life, even in so reduced a form, is a value in itself.

Amen, meaning "truly so"

Alexandr Nemtsov

Note to the English language edition: Howard M. Goldfinger translated the book from Russian. This translation was made possible with the support of Patricio V. Marquez, lead health specialist of the World Bank. Södertörn University, and its publication department, gave invaluable editorial and linguistic support and CHESS at Stockholm University helped to finance the translation. The English language edition contains some material that was not included in the original Russian version.

A contemporary history of alcohol in Russia

Russia has in the past few decades seen a succession of enormous changes, the latest obscuring the one before and soon rendering it forgotten. These have been large events, indeed. What else can one call the breakup of the Soviet Union, the disintegration not only of the Soviet empire, but of the Russian Empire, a structure built up over centuries? Against such a background, the coup of October 1917 is merely a milestone. In such a context, the anti-alcohol campaign of 1985 is hardly visible.

At the same time, the anti-alcohol campaign was the only one of its kind in the past half-century in the entire world. And, as it turned out, it was a unique event in the long history of alcohol in Russia: the authorities not only substantially and very rapidly cut consumption of alcohol, but for the first time significantly reduced government receipts from sales of alcohol, a steady source of state funds across the course of the 1900s.

The anti-alcohol campaign was the first widely publicized action of the leadership that came to power in March 1985 and the last experiment that the Soviet system carried out on its citizens. One cannot claim that the experiment had only negative results; over a period of six or seven years, the campaign saved approximately one million Russian lives. However, by its nature, as a top-down administrative action, the campaign simply could not achieve its main objective – a long-term reduction in alcohol consumption. The extreme nature of the anti-alcohol measures led to a unanimity never before seen in Soviet popular resistance, at the heart of which was a soaring rise in the unlicensed production of alcoholic beverages, despite the heightened severity of punishment.

As a result of the anti-alcohol campaign, Russia initially experienced a very rapid and significant reduction in alcohol consumption (1985–1986) and then an almost equally rapid rise in consumption. This perhaps first massive victory for the Soviet people over the authorities came thanks to the underground production of liquor as alcohol consumption returned to near pre-campaign levels by 1991. The trend continued, abetted by more illegal alcohol products and the circumstances surrounding the market reforms. The victory was a Pyrrhic one, though. Russian drinking was again taking more lives than were criminals, Afghanistan and the two Chechen wars. Alcohol deaths did not become fewer, but Russians may have grown inured to them.

The almost experimental conditions created by the anti-alcohol campaign brought to light many of the ugliest connections between alcohol and the Russian social order, making them more accessible for study. The anti-alcohol campaign once again showed the variety and complexity of the effects of ethyl alcohol, a simple chemical agent. The campaign also again brought into focus the social and, more significantly, the cultural role of alcohol, making clear that the "anti-culture" of the world around alcohol was itself an important part of Russian culture.

That the Soviet system collapsed soon after the Soviet leadership attacked the country's alcohol traditions, which from the outset of Soviet rule had been deeply rooted in the culture and daily routines of the population, is worth thinking about. Although "after this" is not the equivalent of "because of this", the anti-alcohol campaign did contribute to public anger towards the authorities. In organizing the campaign, the authorities were hardly motivated by health concerns – the Soviet system, defeated in the Cold War, facing collapse and bereft of former resources, was looking for new means of surviving. It turned to the "human factor". It would raise productivity by sobering up the population. However, throughout Soviet history whenever the leaders turned to the "human factor", it was almost always a signal of dwindling reserves and of uncertainty about the solidity of their power. The decision by the Soviet leadership to crack down hard on alcohol also reflected the leadership's simplistic understanding of the alcohol situation, an inability to see it in its full dimensions with all its Russian particularities and looming consequences. In other words, it showed incompetence.

The administrative-command approach to solving the country's alcohol problems was the campaign's undoing. But the Soviet Union's successor country, Russia, soon found itself facing an alcohol situation even more troubled than that faced by the previous Soviet government, again due in part to incompetence. Its liberal transformation of the economy, the so-called market reforms, led to a redistribution of property and an end to the government monopoly on alcohol production. This opened the door to the alcohol mafia, which had grown significantly stronger in the twilight of Soviet rule from the underground production of illegal liquor, during the anti-alcohol campaign. Thanks to the campaign, the alcohol mafia was ahead of all other mafia groups in developing nationwide economic ties. It was well prepared for market-type relationships.

The lives saved by the anti-alcohol campaign were more than matched by the deaths at the height of the market reforms, when the illegally produced alcohol products that replaced *samogon* (homebrew) flooded the country. A war over the redistribution of property was underway, crime was rising, homicides were a daily event, and contract murders, a media favorite, became all the rage. Yet the loss of life from these causes was, and still is, immeasurably smaller than the lives lost to alcohol, which go almost unreported by the media.

One cannot help but be astonished at the dynamism of the last two decades (1980–2000) of Russian history, including its alcohol history: a three-year-long (1992–1994) "surge of drunkenness" followed by a reduction in the consumption of alcohol beginning in 1995, and a decline in the negative consequences of heavy drinking. Was this not a cause for celebration? But what lay behind these dramatic changes? What was the alcohol situation in Russia? And what do we mean when we talk of an alcohol situation? What are its constituent elements and what kind of judgments can we make about it? Is judgment even possible when the official statistics on alcohol and related matters are so fragmentary? Can epidemiology come close to revealing a full picture of actual alcohol consumption and its consequences? What is the alcohol fate of Russia?

These are the questions to which this book is directed. Their difficulty is obvious – the alcohol problem is but one of many, old and new, that confront the government in an acute form. But this does not reduce the relevance of coming to a judgment about the alcohol situation, and of drawing conclusions about the human losses which resulted. These losses must be given their rightful place in the hierarchy of losses that the nation has experienced in this time of socioeconomic shock and uncertainty.

An axiom of government is that effective rule is possible only when the initial situation in a policy area is understood and the goal sought is clear. In the case of the alcohol situation, neither is known in Russia, which means that there cannot be effective control. The author's personal experience of public affairs in the field of alcohol policy-making, and his acquaintance with the history of decision-making on alcohol-related matters (1985, 1992 and beyond) have made it clear to him that such decisions often stem from immediate political concerns and may be made without concern about – and often with contempt for – the final results and the national interest.

The desirable aim of alcohol policy though is perfectly obvious – Russia needs a slow but steady reduction in alcohol consumption to an acceptable level. Such a level may be roughly defined as the level of consumption that provides substantially more profit from alcohol sales than the costs incurred by those sales, including the human costs. But neither the public nor the nation's leaders currently understand this. The government has primarily, and with little success, been concerned with problems of the alcohol market rather than with lowering alcohol consumption and improving the nation's health.

The nation does not have a truly national leadership, i.e. a leadership closely tied to it. The abyss between the ruling structures and the public, traditionally vast in Russia, seems to have grown larger, and there may be no one who is ready to work systematically towards making the nation healthy.

It is nevertheless possible to describe the basic events in the nation's alcohol history and, insofar as possible, make clear the driving forces behind them. This book focuses on analyzing the problem, on diagnosing the "illness" and is addressed primarily to a public audience. How to "cure" these problems, even theoretically, is far beyond the capacity of the author, because "treating" these vital – but in the government's eyes merely personal – problems is impossible without "treating" and curing the wider socioeconomic "illnesses" of Russia.

All attempts by the author to draw the attention of those in power to the vast burden created by the alcohol situation in the country have been fruitless. And there have been numerous attempts. The first was made in 1992, and came in the form of an appeal to I. V. Nit, the leader of a group of experts advising the president. In 1993–1994 there were meetings with A. V. Yablokov, assistant to the president for ecology and health, and E. V. Lakhova, an assistant on questions of women, families and children. Moreover, there have been detailed submissions made to the government and a report to a session of the Interagency Commission of the National Security Council of the Russian Federation. I have also made my concerns known in many newspaper articles since 1992.

Of course, these efforts cannot be described as titanic. But such as they were, they revealed the increasing disregard shown by the power structures for information coming from below. The resulting "sobering-up" of the author led to my decision to focus on scientific work and scholarly publications. The most recent of these are two small books about alcohol-related mortality in Russia – in the country as a whole (2001a) and by region (2003b). The books include calculations of the vast human losses caused by alcohol. Almost 4,000 copies were distributed to hundreds of persons in responsible government positions, including members of the presidential administration. But only three or four unusual readers and the wonderful "demoscope.ru" showed interest in the books and the problems they addressed.

Admittedly, there has been no visible result. And yet the recent alcohol history of Russia is a dramatic story. This book seeks to tell it.

Part 1

Stages in the alcohol history of Russia

Many things make it difficult to describe the alcohol situation in Russia. For one, since the late 1950s, the admission of alcohol problems would have seemed to fly in the face of claims to be the nation building communism. Instead of trying to solve the nation's alcohol problems, and informing society about the growing burden of alcohol, from the mid-1960s the leaders of the country consigned to secrecy all data on the production, sale, consumption and effects of alcohol.

This long period of secrecy regarding the alcohol situation in Russia and the total ban on epidemiological studies of alcohol-related problems wiped out Russian 'alcohology', a field that had come into being in the 1860s and was active through to the mid-1930s. Thereafter, until 1987–1988, what little available information there was on the Russian alcohol situation was concerned with alcoholism. Foreign publications (including, for example, Treml's *Alcohol in the USSR*, 1982) were kept in the secure sections of a few libraries and were virtually off-limits.

As part of Gorbachev's reforms and glasnost, this secrecy ended. However, the subject was now ideologized to serve the interests of the anti-alcohol campaign. This ideologization ended with the end of the campaign, but by then the country was too poor to support science, especially such relatively costly science as the epidemiological studies that would have made it possible to paint an accurate picture of the Russian alcohol situation. And such research is particularly important because of the absence of reliable government statistics, long kept secret in the Soviet era and now – sometimes deliberately and sometimes not – corrupted in the very process of recording them.

These limitations notwithstanding, it is absolutely necessary to get a full picture of the alcohol situation, its dynamics and essentials. Because of the underdeveloped state of Russian alcohology, however, completeness is out of the question. One must work with the data available and draw attention to what is lacking.

Every history, including this history of alcohol, requires a division into time-periods. I have taken as the basis for my periodization the sharp, sometimes opposite, changes in levels of alcohol consumption. The points of transition, it may be noted, often coincide with changes in other historically important aspects of Russian life, in particular, the political.

Chapter 1–1
Basic constituents of the alcohol situation

By "alcohol situation", we refer to the whole range of phenomena associated with the consumption of alcohol globally, in a particular country or in a particular region. The alcohol situation is conceived as a four-part structure (Fig. 1-1). The basic elements of the alcohol situation function constantly, but some may be active in varying degrees at various times. This chapter will discuss the main structural elements. The details will be considered in later chapters in connection with changes in the alcohol history of Russia.

Fig. 1-1: Diagram of the constituent elements of the alcohol situation.

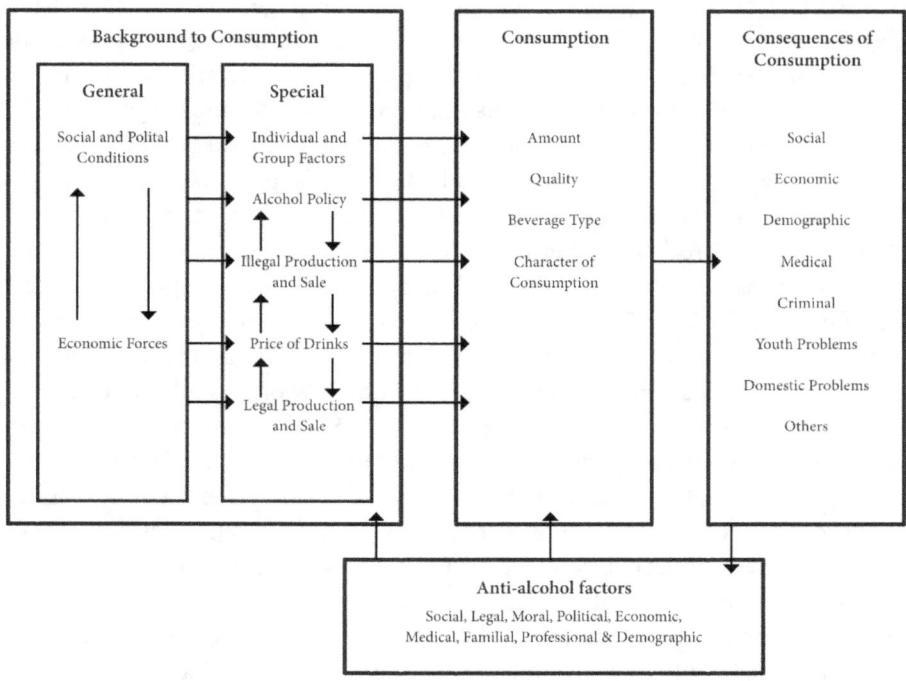

The central position in the structure is alcohol consumption or, in Russian, *vypivka*, which is the link between the prerequisites of consumption and its consequences. In relation to the other elements of the alcohol situation, consumption is structurally simple and relatively easy to describe and measure. It is, essentially, the overall amount of alcohol consumed by the population of a country.

Data on alcohol consumption can be presented in terms of the overall quantities of particular beverages consumed (in liters, half-liters, barrels, and bottles) or as the amount consumed per capita. Usually, the quantity of consumed alcohol is expressed in terms of the quantity of 100 percent ethyl alcohol contained in all the beverages consumed by a single individual per year (average per capita per annum consumption). However, a more exact figure is obtained by calculating the average consumption per person for individuals aged 15-years-old and older. Alcohol is seldom consumed by younger persons, so their share of consumption is negligible (with respect to total consumption). Unfortunately, the "15 plus" figure, widely used around the world, is not used in Russia.

Moreover, the measure published annually by the USSR and RSFSR State Statistical Committee until 1961 and then again after 1988 was further deficient in including only "consumption from state sources". In other words, the figure included only alcohol reaching the population through state and cooperative sources. The figure did not take into account that scourge of Russia, *samogon* (homebrew) or, more generally, illegal alcohol beverage production or, later, illegally imported alcohol products. It is true, however, that in the depths of the USSR and RSFSR State Statistical Committee secret calculations were made, beginning in 1980, of samogon consumption, based on family spending and retail purchases of sugar. These findings are no longer secret (Table 1), but they have not been officially recognized, studied or widely publicized. Further, it is likely that the official calculations of samogon production are extremely unreliable after 1988, when breakdowns began to occur in the supply of sugar to the population. Indeed, as a result of this, these calculations were stopped after 1990 (Table 1). After 1994 the State Statistical Committee of the Russian Federation discontinued the old method for estimating consumption and began taking account of some unregistered alcohol in measures of the quantity of alcohol sold (Table 1). Besides these statistics, there are a number of other estimates of actual consumption of alcohol in Russia made by Russian and foreign researchers (Chapter 2-3).

Consumption of unregistered alcohol is by no means an exclusively Russian phenomenon. It is a fact of life in many countries. Consumption of illegally manufactured or imported alcoholic drinks as a percentage of total consumption ranges from 12 percent (Finland, 1984) to 30 percent (Denmark, 1984) (Österberg, 1987). In wine-producing countries the consumption of unregistered alcohol is common, e.g., Italy in Europe and Chile in South America (Chapter 1-2). Overall, the trend in consumption of illegal alcohol has been downward in Europe and is

Table 1: Registered alcohol and an estimate of actual alcohol consumption in Russia (1960–2002), in liters of pure alcohol per capita per year ("volume of sales", calculated by a new method, is given in parentheses in the first column).

Year	Russian State Statistics Committee		Estimations of Alcohol Consumption Per Capita Per Year				
	Recorded Alcohol	Samogon + (1)	Treml, 1997	Nemtsov, 2000	Nemtsov, 2002	Nemtsov, Ch. 2–4	Average 2, 3, 4
	1	2	3	4	5	6	7
1960	4,60		9.8				
...							
1970	8.30		12.0				
1971	8.44						
1972	8.63						
1973	8.82						
1974	9.52						
1975	9.88		13.10				
1976	10.17						
1977	10.36						
1978	10.57						
1979	10.60						
1980	10.51	13.5	14.00				13.8
1981	10.20	13.3		14.88			14.1
1982	10.13	13.1		14.75			13.9
1983	10.26	13.3		14.83			14.1
1984	10.45	13.8	14.25	14.63			14.2
1985	8.80	12.3	13.30	13.31			13.0
1986	5.17	10.2	10.57	10.77			10.5
1987	3.90	10.0	10.70	10.96			10.6
1988	4.40	8.3	11.20	11.57			11.4
1989	5.29	8.7	11.66	12.04			11.9
1990	5.56		11.76	12.29			12.0
1991	5.57		12.27	12.67			12.5
1992	5.01		13.81	13.23			13.5
1993	5.00		14.43	13.90			14.2
1994	6.80 (6.8)			14.60	14.6	14.6	
1995	6.50 (9.3)				14.1	13.9	
1996	(7.2)				13.2	12.9	
1997	(7.5)				12.3	12.1	
1998	(7.3)				12.2	11.7	
1999	(7.6)				13.3	12.9	
2000	(8.1)				14.1	13.9	
2001	(8.3)				15.0	15.0	
2002	(8.7)						
2003	(9.1)						

now about 10 percent of total consumption, excluding Finland (20 percent) and Sweden (25 percent) (Lindberg, 1999).

Illegal alcohol and unregistered alcohol are not the same thing. The former is produced "underground", illegally and without payment of license fees or excise taxes. All illegal alcohol is unregistered. But unregistered alcohol also includes alcoholic beverages produced by legal enterprises that make their way into the domestic market without the payment of excise taxes. Unregistered alcohol also includes alcohol consumed outside one's own country, by tourists, for example. As an example, and without meaning offense to Finland, it can be said that the negative consequences for the alcohol-abusing Finn who goes to Russia to drink happen and are counted in Finland, but the alcohol consumed in Russia counts toward the Russian total.

The WHO's Global Status Report on Alcohol 2004 gives a detailed classification of the sources of unregistered alcohol that goes uncounted in tallies of alcohol consumption:

1. Home production, which is legal in many countries for the production of wine and beer, but not for hard liquor;
2. Sales by stores involved in international trade and the illegal importation of alcohol by tourists;
3. Contraband alcoholic beverages brought into a country by organized criminal groups or by tourists carrying in more alcohol than allowed;
4. Alcohol intended for industrial, technical or medical purposes;
5. Consumption of alcohol by tourists while visiting other countries;
6. Beverages containing levels of alcohol lower than that recognized by law as constituting an alcoholic beverage.

This classification covers the basic part of the unregistered alcohol consumption in Russia. Some refinements are in order though, especially with regard to No. 4, which is prominent as a source in Russia. It includes significant quantities of alcohol stolen in Russia while being moved by rail. In addition, large quantities of illegal alcoholic beverages are produced by small, short lived, "underground workshops", which can hardly be classed as industrial production and yet, cannot be categorized as domestic production either, even though the production or sale to consumers often takes place in private homes and apartments. Finally, one must include liquids designed for technical and domestic purposes, such as glass-washing mixtures that contain ethyl alcohol along with denatured additives.

For Russia, the WHO classification would need a seventh category for unregistered alcohol produced in significant quantities by legal, licensed enterprises in the form of "above-the-plan", illegal and untaxed output ("third-shift vodka").

Crucial to the picture of Russian alcohol consumption (Fig. 1-1), aside from overall quantity, is the type of consumption – the specification of beverages by strength and quality, the distribution of drinking over time and whether consumption is accompanied by food, as well as particular regional and ethnic attributes. The type of consumption concerns what the population drinks and how it drinks, in a country as a whole and by region. This very important category is poorly represented in Russian alcohology.

Information on the variety of beverages is important because the social and medical effects of particular beverages differ greatly. By far the most serious effects arise from consuming strong drinks, especially in the heavy doses that quickly lead to high concentrations of alcohol in the blood. The result of this kind of consumption is a more profound and more prolonged form of inebriation, a greater loss of self-control and a significantly greater metabolic burden on the organism. In turn, this leads to more serious social (for example, criminal) and medical effects in terms of a greater risk of disease and death (for example, from road traffic accidents). Unfortunately, this type of consumption is typical in Russia. According to the official data on registered spirits, hard liquor predominates (accounting for 53 percent of the total alcohol consumed in 1984, 66 percent in 1990, 82 percent in 1993 and 78 percent in 2000). In fact, the actual share of hard liquor in the overall consumption figure is higher than this, because a major portion of illegally produced alcohol is hard liquor. Studies using population samples also show that consumption in the form of heavy, or "shock" doses is predominant – i.e. great quantities of alcohol, very often the entire amount consumed in the day, are consumed in a very short period of time (Chapter 2-3). In other words, the most undesirable, or "northern", way of alcohol consumption predominates in Russia.

An essential feature of the alcoholic beverages consumed in Russia is their low quality in terms of the toxic presence of methanol (monovalent alcohol), polyvalent alcohols, aldehyde, essential oils, ethylene glycol and acetone (Nuzhny, 1995).

We should note here, though, that these substances are equal or only slightly more toxic than ethyl or grape (diatomic) alcohol. Even though they are toxic, their concentration is lower and therefore less toxic than the ethyl alcohol in 40 percent ABV liquor. It is reasonable, then, to suggest that the toxicity of the additives listed above does not exceed the 0.01 toxicity of grape alcohol and, generally, is significantly lower (Nuzhny, 1995). That means that the basic toxin in vodka is ethyl alcohol.

Russian public opinion mistakenly thinks that illegal alcoholic beverages are harmful because of their low quality. While quality is a factor, it is a relatively minor one in comparison with the extraordinary quantity consumed. This is not an endorsement of poor-quality alcohol, but rather a plea for rethinking the priorities and emphases of alcohol policy.

Russians also consume such surrogate beverages as colognes, lotions, deodorants, antistatic agents and BF glue (industrial/medical adhesive), the toxicity of which stems from substances added to serve the products' original purposes. In some regions, the dominant surrogates are medicines, which may be as much as 90 percent alcohol (Leon et al., 2007).

In the past, low quality was associated with some of the vodka, fruit and berry wines (*bormotukha*) and cheap alcohol-fortified wines that consumers bought at state stores or drank as samogon (Filatov, 1986). There are two kinds of samogon: *dlya sebya* ("made for oneself") and *na prodazhu* ("made for sale"). The former might well be of significantly better quality than several varieties of the vodka sold through state agencies. A sharp decline in the quality of alcoholic beverages occurred in 1992–1994 in connection with the market reforms and the appearance of new types of illegal liquor (Chapter 1-7).

In discussing quality, one should bear in mind that the quality of alcoholic beverages depends on the taste, color, smell, clarity and several other characteristics, not just on toxic substances.

The last of the important factors to be emphasized is the nature of consumption, which includes breaking consumers down by size of typical dosage, sex, age, social position, etc. Of special interest here are children, adolescents, young people and women. These groups have the most direct connection to the future physical, psychological and social health of the nation. In addition, groups that face a higher risk of alcoholism (certain kinds of male work-groups, e.g. sailors) and workers in professions whose drinking poses particularly high risks (drivers and others in transportation, for example) demand greater attention. Unfortunately, it is very difficult to get an accurate picture of the nature of alcohol consumption in Russia; existing research is selective and sheds light only on a few elements, and does so, most often poorly (Chapter 2-3).

After this very general characterization of the core of the alcohol situation – large-dose drinking – we can turn to the consequences, both positive and negative. The former – and for which, essentially, alcohol is consumed – have been studied in only a handful of works, all of them non-Russian (Chapter 2-2). The question of positive social consequences resulting from alcohol consumption has not even been raised. Apparently, moral considerations or perhaps the preconceptions of the "cultured" part of society, aware of the obvious heavy burden caused by alcohol consumption and the ephemeral quality of positive consequences, are at work in this neglect. But the absence of such studies makes it impossible for us to imagine what would have happened to Russia during the social and economic shocks of the period 1980–2000 without alcohol. The sanctimoniousness of part of Russian society forces me to add this qualification: this is not a call for drunkenness but one for realism in assessing the alcohol situation. Population studies of the relationship between the positive and negative consequences of alcohol consumption and determining the level of consumption at which the negative consequences begin to dominate would provide a reliable criterion for an optimal level of consumption and for a realistic alcohol policy – a policy that takes into account the real needs that encourage alcohol consumption (Chapter 2-1).

The negatives of alcohol consumption are also difficult to quantify if large-dose consumption is excluded. Yet it is clear that alcohol is a risk-factor for health (Lisitsyn, 1985; Ogurtsov, 1997; Anderson, 1995) and cause of death, especially violent death, the likelihood of which is 10.4 times greater for drinkers than for non-drinkers (Nemtsov & Nechaev, 1991). For chronic drinkers the risk of death from falls is 16 times greater, from burns or in fires 10 times greater, and from industrial accidents 2-3 times greater than for others (Smith & Kraus, 1988).

In the most general terms, alcohol's negative effects can be divided into those linked to the chronic abuse of alcohol and those linked with drunkenness itself. Inebriation raises the likelihood of a wide range of negative medical and social phenomena, including, for example, accidents that involve trauma or death. Thus, in one of Russia's biggest cities, 83 percent of those killed in fires, 63 percent of drowning victims and 62 percent of those killed in falls were found to have been inebriated (Polyakov & Petrov, 1989). Alcohol is a frequent cause of public disturbances, violations of work discipline, and acts of vandalism, domestic conflicts and fights. Many crimes are committed by people who are inebriated (Chapter 2-5). Importantly, a rise in alcohol consumption is associated with a worsening of such problems, while declines in consumption are associated with an improvement (Plant, 1991). This was clearly confirmed in Russia during and after the anti-alcohol campaign.

Naturally, the negative consequences of alcohol occur especially often among alcohol abusers. But one cluster of negative phenomena is restricted to heavy drinkers and alcoholics – the health effects resulting from frequent and massive alcoholization. These include liver failure, acute alcohol pancreatitis, alcohol miocardiodystrophy, cancer of the interior of the mouth, larynx and esophagus, which are substantially more frequent among heavy drinkers than among moderate drinkers (Anderson, 1995). A frequent problem for heavy drinkers is alcohol dependency, or alcoholism, which always leads to a coarsening of the individual's human qualities and a degeneration of the personality and sometimes to alcohol psychosis. The most serious consequence of chronic drinking is early death.

Besides medical problems, heavy drinkers and alcoholics often experience domestic and work-related conflicts that can entail a loss of social status and family breakdown, professional demotion and with that the increased likelihood of financial problems. All this tends to force alcohol abusers to the very lowest rungs of the social ladder. One of these "rungs" is typified in Russia by the so-called *bomzh* (economically and socially marginalized individuals or outcasts), who are now appearing on a massive scale.

It is difficult to put a value on the whole range of consequences of alcohol consumption. Many of these phenomena are socially unacceptable as well as morally and legally censored and are largely hidden. The alcohol problem is an iceberg, the visible portion of which is only a small part of the whole.

The unseen portion of the "alcohol iceberg" includes more than half of all alcoholics who never appear at the special narcological clinics (Krasik & Moskvitin, 1988; Entin & Dineeva, 1996). It is only in connection with anti-social behaviour and law violation that they face any sort of social correction.

Not wishing to discount the heavy burden of the problems of alcoholics, the percentage of alcoholics in national populations is relatively small, ranging from the minute (Iran, Saudi Arabia) up to 5–6 percent of the adult population (U.S., Canada, Cuba; Babor et al., 2003). Studies suggest that alcoholics in Russia are a relatively modest 4.8 percent of the adult population.

It is now well established that, overall, alcoholics cause fewer problems than heavy-drinking non-alcoholics, who in Russia make up approximately one-half of the adult male population (Petrov & Dovgy, 1989; Zaigraev, 2004b). It is this cohort of heavy-drinking non-alcoholics whose behavior under the influence of alcohol causes the biggest proportion of work-days lost in Russia (Chapter 1-6).

To put a price tag on the full extent of the damage to Russia from alcohol consumption is very difficult, especially the losses in recent years, where the economic, social and spiritual life of the nation has been in systemic crisis. The government shows little concern for the ordinary everyday lives of the population. This indifference, together with the failure of the anti-alcohol campaign, has sharply reduced the interest in alcohol problems. Today such problems are mentioned, but they can be "weighed" only with difficulty. Only a few, generally the most serious alcohol problems come to the surface ("corpses can't be hidden") and can be more or less exactly quantified with respect to alcohol consumption (Chapter 2-5). However, in recent years, as a result of the criminalization and general social degeneration of Russian life, corpses sometimes stay "hidden" forever or at least for a long time. Indeed, actual corpses, in fact, now sometimes come to autopsy already too decomposed to tell the age of the deceased, let alone their identity. It is thus impossible to determine the degree of alcoholization that preceded the death and its role as a cause of the death.

The situation concerning the third constituent element of the alcohol situation – the preconditions for consumption, which are always dominant in these situations – is even trickier. This element was studied least of all in Russia because of the strict ideological givens: in the Land of Developed Socialism there could be no reasons for drunkenness. However, there were, are, and will continue to be such reasons. This is the crux not only of the problem of alcohol consumption but of people's lives, whether in Russia or anywhere else. For a great number of people, alcohol is a solution to problems that arise in daily life or is a way to avoid having to deal with them (Chapter 2-1).

The preconditions for alcohol consumption can be divided into the general and the special. The former are related more obliquely and indirectly to alcohol problems. These general preconditions – political, economic, social and spiritual – are usually slow to affect the level of alcohol consumption. But this was not the case with the anti-alcohol campaign of 1985, a political action. And we know that wars always reduce the level of alcoholization of the population, despite increases in everyday difficulties. This was particularly evident during World War I, which was preceded by quite a high level of alcohol consumption in Europe: during the war, alcohol consumption dropped in every country involved – in England, for example, by two thirds (Fig. 1-2a; Plant, 1992). It also fell in Russia both during the World War I (Mendelson, 1916) and World War II (Zaigraev, 1992).

Fig 1-2 (a/b): Alcohol Consumption in Great Britain (Fig 1-2a) (1900–1990; source: Plant, 1992) and in 6 Nations of Europe (Fr – France, It – Italy, Sp – Spain, Ger – Germany, Sw – Sweden, Fin – Finland), the United States – USA, and Japan – Jap (Fig 1-2b), 1895–1995 (for Japan from 1965). Source: The National Alcoholic Association www.naacnt.ru

Fig 1-2a

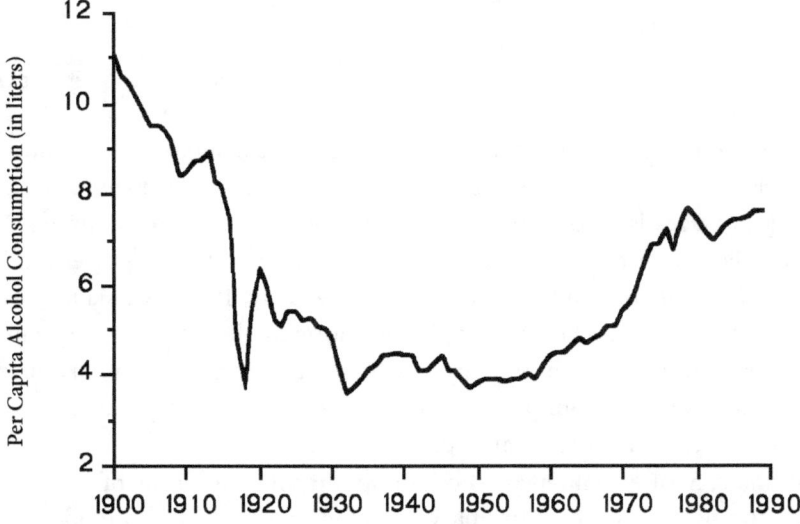

However, rapid changes in alcohol consumption under the influence of general factors are rather exceptions to the rule. More typical was the slow, post-war rise in alcohol consumption that occurred in most of the countries of Europe and North America, which reflected a general growth in the economic well-being of the populations of these continents (Simpura, 1995). On the other hand, the slow decrease in alcohol consumption recorded in France in this period has been linked, among other things, to a massive movement of the rural population to the cities, a change that affected the eating and drinking habits of a large segment of the population.

Fig 1-2b: Alcohol consumption in Great Britain (Fig 1-2a) (1900–1990; source: Plant, 1992) and in 6 nations in Europe (Fr – France, It – Italy, Sp – Spain, Ger – Germany, Sw – Sweden, Fin – Finland), the United States – USA, and Japan – Jap (Fig 1-2b), 1895–1995 (for Japan from 1965). Source: The National Alcoholic Association www.naacnt.ru

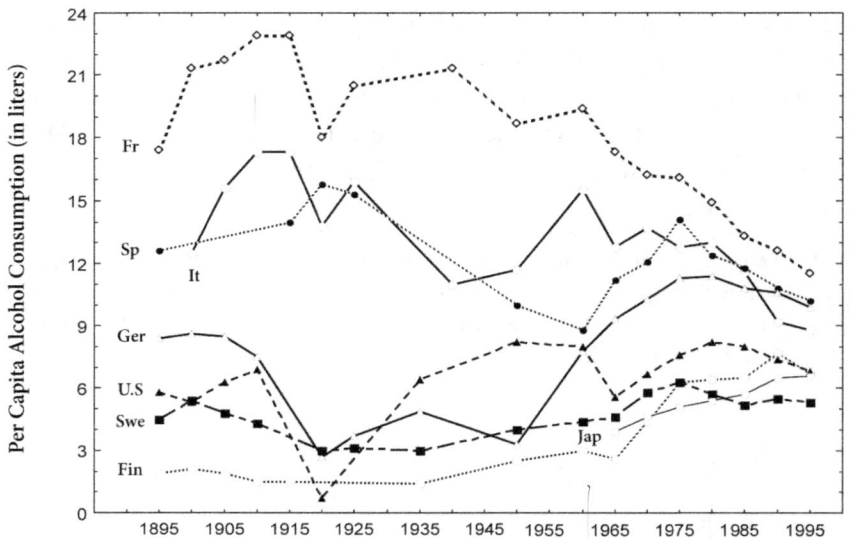

Among the economic factors that influence alcohol consumption, the most important is the income of the population – every economic downturn and/or lowering of wages is accompanied by a decrease in alcohol consumption. Even mild recessions affect the level of alcoholization, as was the case, for example, at the time of the oil crisis in the 1970s (Smart & Murray, 1983). Russia may be the sole exception to this. The catastrophic economic collapse and sharp curtailment of industrial output in the early 1990s went hand-in-hand with a marked increase in alcohol consumption in Russia. This important paradox deserves special consideration and is examined in Chapter 1-7.

But one cannot explain alcohol consumption solely in terms of market economics, for alcohol is not an ordinary commodity, i.e. it is a commodity whose availability governments limit by the imposition of high taxes, restrictions on where and when it may be sold or drunk and the age of buyers (Babor, 1995). In recent years, Russia has also been an exception to this rule: alcoholic beverages in Russia are virtually ordinary merchandise. The government has lost control of the alcohol market, restrictions on sales are often ignored, and untaxed illegal alcoholic products abound.

The second, special, group of preconditions for alcohol consumption (Fig. 1-1) are more closely related to alcohol consumption, and show up more readily as changes in consumption and are tightly related to each other. Quite conservative drinking traditions exert a stabilizing influence; traditions of this kind determine the dominant beverages, their strength, the character of the drinking episode, what constitutes socially acceptable dosages and the tolerance or intolerance shown towards drunkenness, in particular, to heavy drinking by women and young people.

Drinking in Russia, as in the rest of the world, is almost always a group or collective undertaking. "Company" is one of the key words when considering the problem of alcohol consumption. Company acts as a spur to drinking and brings in new users. It can be very difficult to resist the "collective wisdom" of drinking or drunken company. However, the reasons for drinking and the motivations for alcohol consumption are profoundly personal. Despite the similarity in the behavior of people in building up to and then fully engaging in drinking, the fact remains that in the friendly company of drunks, everyone "solves" the great issues of his/her individual life – even if they cannot solve them in reality.

The relationship between the price of alcoholic beverages and other commodities is important. It determines whether the population considers alcoholic beverages, especially hard liquor, luxury items or not (Plant, 1992).

The Marxist idea of poverty as a seedbed of drunkenness has not stood the test of time. We now know, for example, that poor peasants used more alcohol after moving to the city and improving their living standards as industrial workers than they did before the change occurred. Moreover, recent decades have shown that there is a strong relationship between alcohol consumption (unlike tobacco use) and income, consumption rising with increases in income (Godfrey & Maynard, 1995).

This short list of special preconditions for alcohol consumption should include the volume of alcoholic beverages produced and the volume sold (Fig. 1-1). Production and sales, which are dependent on demand, in turn, can themselves spur demand. And this goes beyond what we ordinarily think of as advertising, the influence of which on the level of alcohol consumption has yet to be rigorously assessed (Plant, 1991). Of far greater significance for the growth of alcohol consumption are the variety of beverages and the range of prices, which are determined by the volume of output. Also important are the reach of the sales network (in other words, the proximity of the product to the consumer), their hours and locations as well as the age at which, legally, persons are permitted to purchase alcohol, and whether alcohol may be purchased by persons already inebriated (Chapter 2-2). The place of sale is also significant (for example, whether the possibility exists for making purchases in the street, without entering a place of sale) as well as the exterior aspect of the store, which itself can be a powerful form of advertising, as it can present the passer-by with the whole range of available beverages (as is permissible in Russia).

For Russia, a matter of special interest is the production and sale of unregistered alcoholic beverages, a significant part of which is samogon (Zaigraev, 2004b). In essence, the producers of samogon were in competition with the state in Soviet times, supplying the population with specific goods that the state trading sector was unable to supply at particular times and places or could only provide at prices unattractive to consumers. The last decade has seen the supplementation of samogon with illegal (unlicensed) semi-industrial and industrial production (at licensed plants) as well as by illegal imports of alcohol and alcoholic beverages (Chapters 1-7 and 1-8).

Finally, the last but very important precondition of alcohol consumption is the alcohol policy of the state, which has at its command ways to regulate consumption of alcohol by the general population or by particular groups in it (drivers, for example). By cracking down on illegal production and by imposing excise and customs taxes, the state can affect the price of beverages and thus alter their availability and, consequently, their level of consumption. The excise tax system makes it possible to shift demand from hard liquor to lower-proof liquors, wines and beer, and this can help lower the general level of alcohol consumption.

A systematic and unremitting lowering of the consumption level of alcoholic beverages and, consequently, of the negative effects of such consumption should be the main function of a state's alcohol policy, especially when the consumption level is high. Many factors work against such policies. The major one in Russia, as elsewhere in the world, is people's desire for alcohol (Chapter 2-1).

However, the government has an obligation to regulate this felt need by decreasing the social pressures on the population and easing its economic burdens. Such obligations have an independent and long-term character. Lowering the level of alcohol consumption will follow on from them. Conversely, a high level of consumption is a sure indication that something is wrong in the relations between the state and its citizens. The state also has more specific tasks – controlling the quality of alcoholic beverages and protecting the public from illegal alcoholic beverages.

There are two simple, interrelated principles for the setting of excise taxes and thus the prices of alcoholic beverages. The first is that the taxes generated should compensate in full for the economic losses that accompany alcohol consumption. The second is that the excise taxes should be proportional to the alcoholic strength of the beverage, as the harm caused by alcohol is proportional to its strength.

This seems a suitable place for a caveat: the stipulations just described apply to an ideal government alcohol policy, and Russian realities, the subject of chapters to follow, are far from ideal. Put more bluntly, the current Russian alcohol policy takes no account of the health of the nation.

The fourth and final constituent of the alcohol situation are the anti-alcohol factors (Fig. 1-1). These relate not only to anti-alcohol propaganda or a sobriety movement; they are, rather, the sum of all the phenomena that contribute to lowering the consumption of alcohol products or lessening the risk of alcohol's negative consequences. Essentially, anti-alcohol factors, both the obvious and less obvious, function at the level of all three main constituents of the alcohol situation (Fig. 1-1), however great the level of consumption may be. Moreover, many of these factors are stimulated when the level of consumption is high.

The anti-alcohol factor that deserves to be mentioned first is a sensible alcohol policy, one that balances the needs of the budget and the preservation of the health of the nation. Other factors include laws aiming to restrict consumption, for example, by minors or vehicle drivers, and the prices of alcoholic beverages, which are always much higher than the cost of production. No matter how low prices may be, there will always be a cohort of the population for whom even very low prices will be unacceptable.

Anti-alcohol factors also include the treatment of all the medical consequences arising from alcohol consumption, not only those of the victims of alcoholism. The latter do require special focus for they are the propagandists of drunkenness and active recruiters of new consumers of spirits. Finally, consumption can be restrained by family and work-related factors, for example, in the form of a strict wife or strict supervisor. Currently, social life in Russia has been degraded to the point where strict wives are perhaps the country's most effective anti-alcohol device.

There is still one more factor that can, if only conditionally, be included as anti-alcohol. This is a limit on the increase in consumption. As has been established in law, three times in recent decades, the growth in consumption has not been permitted to exceed a level of 18–20 liters per capita per year.

The existence of this "anti-alcohol law" is no reason for complacency: In the opinion of the experts at the WHO, a level of alcohol consumption that exceeds 8 liters per capita on an annual basis represents a national danger (Mäkelä et al., 1981; Single et al., 1981), and the WHO is now considering if even this amount might be unsafe at the national level. In the view of the WHO's experts and other specialists (Walsh, 1985; Plant, 1991), problems arising from alcohol consumption are inseparable from the overall average individual consumption of alcohol (Chapter 2-2). Where a high level of consumption exists, the main objective should be a gradual but steady reduction in the consumption of alcoholic beverages to an acceptable level, which has been defined by the experts of the WHO's European Regional Bureau as 8 liters per capita per year (Mäkelä et al., 1981; Single et al., 1981).

Chapter 1-2
The alcohol situation in other nations

Russia was for a long time cut off from the world by the "Iron Curtain". The Soviet people knew practically nothing about contemporary life beyond their borders. One result was a loss of guidelines with which to make judgments about themselves and people outside the cordon. This gave rise to a national egocentricity, which often took the form of robust cheerleading for the home side or meek deference to outsiders, or to a cocktail of these contradictory moods. On the one hand, there was Soviet propaganda, and on the other the bits of information about life in the West that came through movies and the occasional Western gadget. An unrealistic view of the world can be harmful and sometimes even destructive. A minor example: many Russians believe that Finns are alcoholics. This belief is based on the fact that a few alcoholic Finns travel to St Petersburg with one aim: to drink their fill. They do so because their homeland makes it very difficult for them to drink in similar manner there.

In response to the great Russian poet Tyutchev's "Umom Rossiyu ne ponyat'" (Russia is not to be understood intellectually), another Russian poet, Igor Guberman, more than 100 years later, asserted: "Davno pora, … Umom Rossiyu ponimat'" (It is long overdue that Russia be understood intellectually). In order to do so it is not only necessary to be realistic about one's self and one's own nation, but it is also necessary to know about how other people live, how people drink beyond Russia's borders and what kinds of alcohol problems they face.

First of all, one must note that alcohol consumption in the nations of the world is marked by great diversity, both in the quantities of alcohol consumed, in the kinds of beverages preferred and in the distribution of preferences among hard liquors, wines and beer. The second important characteristic of the world alcohol situation is that drinking habits have changed over time and often quite differently in different countries. Thus, there cannot be a general description of the alcohol situation across the world. It must be described in terms of time and country, although there are some general trends (Chapter 2-2).

This chapter will use the level of alcohol consumption as the main measure of the alcohol situation in the countries of the world. It has been chosen for purposes of brevity of exposition, although the alcohol situation cannot simply be reduced to it. The level of consumption of spirits is the leading but not the only factor in weighing the seriousness of an alcohol situation.

At the same time it is necessary to bear in mind that the level of consumption and, thus, the seriousness of the situation can be calculated in various ways. We have used average individual consumption for individuals aged 15 and above. But nations vary not only in terms of the proportion of children and adolescents in their populations but also in the proportion of the population that drinks alcoholic beverages; for example, the proportion of drinkers is 93 percent in Peru and Denmark, 65 percent in the United States and 40 percent in Costa Rica (Babor et al., 2003; WHO, 2004). This means that the alcohol load borne by individual drinkers is higher in the U.S. than, for example, in Denmark, although average individual consumption is higher in Denmark. However, these important details must be left aside, for the concern here is with the general national problems connected with the use of alcohol. With this in mind, the statistics that follow reflect the average consumption for those aged 15 years and older, the standard accepted throughout the world, while average individual consumption measures as recalculated by the author will be specially stipulated.

One further characteristic of the data on alcohol should be noted: the accessibility and completeness of information varies among countries, especially the exactness of data on consumption. The most reliable data are those for the industrially developed countries of Europe and North America.

Western Europe, the United States and Canada

Since the start of record keeping on alcohol consumption in Western Europe, the nations from this part of the continent have experienced two peaks in consumption. The first was in the last decades of the 1800s (Negrete, 1980; Room, 1991). It was associated with many factors but, of primary importance was the movement of large masses of people towards work in factories and plants, the growth of cities and the industrial production of cheap spirits.

However, as early as the beginning of the 1900s, several wealthy countries in Europe – England (Fig. 1-2a) and Germany (Fig. 1-2b), for example – began to see a gradual decrease in alcohol consumption, especially of hard liquor. This was thanks to the industrial revolution that brought with it an increase in the quantity, quality and variety of industrial products and a decrease in their price. Commodities became accessible to broad sections of the population. By the same token, alternatives were being created to alcoholic beverages; commodities began to compete with drinking (Plant, 1991). It would be an oversimplification to link the drop in consumption at this time with this factor alone: this, indeed, was also the time when taxes and, consequently, the price of alcoholic products started to rise. In other words, in the late 1800s–early 1900s, in several European countries and North America, governmental regulation of the alcohol market began and, simultaneously, there was a slow decrease in alcohol consumption that continued right up to the beginning of World War I (Fig. 1-2a). This change in the alcohol situation at the start of the 1900s can be seen as the most general trend for Europe and North America. The wine-making countries stood apart. France, for example, experienced an unprecedentedly high level of consumption in the late 1800s (more than 20 liters of pure alcohol per person per year) and, with the exception of the periods of the two world wars, maintained that high level of alcohol consumption up to the early 1960s (18 liters per person per year in 1963).

The sharp drop in alcohol consumption during World War I occurred not only in France. It took place in almost all countries in Europe. This indicates that the breakdown of the world economy, as a result of the war, had a greater effect on the consumption of spirits than physical and psychological tensions, which were also sharply raised at this time and which might have been expected to increase consumption. In the 1920s and 1930s, a relatively low level of consumption was maintained through the period of post-war economic ruin. Consumption again dropped during World War II.

However, with the healing of the deepest wounds from World War II, from the middle of the 1950s, a new round of growth in alcohol consumption took place in the countries of Europe and North America. The first to experience the trend were the industrially developed countries. The exception in Europe was France, where, from the late 1950s through to the early 1960s, a decline in consumption occurred (Fig. 1-2b). From the start of the 1970s, a decline in this index took place in Italy and, somewhat later, in Spain and Portugal (Simpura, 1995; Gual & Colom, 1997), that is, in almost all of Europe's wine-producing countries with high levels of alcohol consumption: Italy (13.9 liters in 1973), Spain (14.2 liters in 1975) and Portugal (14.1 liters in 1976; World Drink Trends, 1994). The decline in the overall consumption of alcohol in these countries was, to a significant extent, the result of an almost 50 percent decline in the consumption of wine.

A number of factors were responsible for these changes. Their relative roll varied by country, although the principal one may be considered as the increase in the relative proportion of beer and hard liquors being consumed (Gual & Colom, 1997) as well as the appearance of new, non-alcoholic drinks (soda, mineral water, juices) in Europe, where they had been little known in the preceding 30–40 years.

The displacement of wine, the traditional drink of the Mediterranean countries, was helped by the marketing pressure applied by a small number of very powerful international brewery companies, who produced beer and hard liquors, while the wine market was dominated by small and medium-sized firms incapable of resistance. Moreover, much wider advertising of beer was allowed, in view of its relatively low alcohol content. Another factor was the post-war urbanization and the consequent alteration in the previously rural population's way of life, in particular. There was a decline in the practice of whole families sitting down to eat together and, in the course of their meals, consuming large quantities of wine. Eating away from the family began increasingly to be accompanied by the consumption of beer, which also became the preferred beverage on weekends (Sulkunen, 1989). Nonetheless, France, Italy and Spain remain among the leading consumers of wine, now joined by Luxembourg, Switzerland, Denmark and Austria, countries far from the Mediterranean. In the latter countries, the alcohol from wine now makes up almost half of all the alcohol consumed.

Another factor encouraging the decrease in alcohol consumption, in several countries of Europe and North America, is the increased understanding in society of the harmfulness and danger of alcohol, especially hard liquors, and, most importantly, their connection with road traffic accidents, especially for children, adolescents and young people. Along with this understanding came the emergence in Europe and America of many social organizations with active anti-alcohol programs. One such organization became particularly well known. In the United States in 1996, on the initiative of the Mothers Against Drunk Driving (MADD), 724 pairs of shoes were displayed at the capitol of the state of Florida. All the shoes belonged to victims killed by drunk drivers in the same state in 1995. Many actions of this kind encouraged politicians to act in regard to the minimum permissible age for alcohol consumption, on where and when spirits could be sold and on banning drinking at work.

Economic reasons also played a role in the decline in consumption, specifically the alcohol policy of the European Economic Community (the Common Market or EES), which made the entry of Spain and Portugal into the community conditional on a sharp reduction in wine production. As a result, the price of wine rose quickly in these countries in relation to the price of other beverages.

Many of these same factors were at work in bringing about a decrease in alcohol consumption in other countries, yet in most of the countries of Europe and North America, consumption increased until the late 1970s–early 1980s (Fig. 1-6). Overall, for the 15 years from 1965 until 1980, per capita consumption of alcohol rose worldwide by 15 percent (Walsh and Grant, 1985) and, for the 25 years from 1960 through to 1985, by 50 percent (Robinson, 1986).

Alcohol consumption increased particularly quickly in those European countries that had very low rates of consumption (2–4 liters per person per year) in the immediate post-war period (the Federal Republic of Germany, Finland, Iceland, Norway and Sweden). Thus, from 1950 through to 1980 the rise was 320 percent in Germany, while for Finland, it was 240 percent. In contrast, in those countries where consumption had been high at the war's end (for example, in neutral Sweden – 10.4 liters), the increase was relatively moderate (30 percent).

In a number of countries, the level of alcohol consumption remained unchanged through the 1980s and 1990s (e.g. Great Britain and Denmark), but in Finland the rise continued through to the onset of the 2000s.

However, as already mentioned, in the European countries with especially high consumption levels (France, Spain, Italy), the post-war years saw a notable decline in consumption. These contrary tendencies brought the consumption rates in the indicated countries closer to each other (Fig. 1-2b).

But the heart of the matter lies not only in the overall rise in the quantity of alcohol consumed in the immediate post-war period; qualitative changes were also underway in alcohol consumption, trends that became increasingly universal. Thus, wine-producing regions saw an increase in the proportion of alcohol consumed in the form of beer and hard liquor, a pattern that had earlier predominated in the northern countries, which in turn, were now drinking more wine. Thus, the increasing similarities among the European countries were also reflected in the realm of drink preferences.

The overall tendency can be described as follows: where there had been a clear domination by one kind of traditional alcoholic beverage (hard liquor, wine, or beer), the dominant beverage lost some of its share of consumption to "foreign" types of alcoholic beverages, but remained dominant. Overall, amongst the countries of the EEC, the general trend in the period from 1970 through the 1990s was toward the following distribution in the shares of consumption: 50 percent beer, 35 percent wine and 15 percent hard liquor. It is now recognized that this division is optimal for minimizing the negative consequences of alcohol consumption (Edwards et al., 1994).

To illustrate the point, consider the country-by-country data for Europe (Table 2) and for Russia (these figures are based on official data for 1988 however, when the anti-alcohol campaign was still underway in Russia).

Table 2: Change in consumption of basic alcoholic beverages in several countries of Europe (1998 as a percentage of 1988).

Country	Spirits	Beer	Wine
Belgium	-28	-17	+8
United Kingdom	-27	-13	+27
Germany	-5	-11	-12
Spain	-11	-3	-12
Italy	-50	+15	-18
Poland	-26	+33	-23
Portugal	-3	+22	-1
France	-3	-2	-22
Czech Republic	-52	+23	+30
Switzerland	-27	-13	-13
Average	-23.2	+3.4	-3.6
Russia	+233	+31	-6

Source: *World Drink Trends 1999, Global Status Report on Alcohol 2004*

The struggle to lower alcohol consumption has not been without setbacks; on occasion new types of beverages managed to complement rather than replace earlier traditional preferences. This was particularly evident in those countries experiencing very rapid rises in overall alcohol consumption such as Finland, whose experience of a failed alcohol policy is instructive. The government, disturbed by the high level and rapid rise in alcohol consumption (2.5 liters in 1965 and 3.1 liters in 1968), began enforcing a new law on alcohol on 1 January, 1969. The major part of the law involved the easing of restrictions on production and a significant widening of sales of beer and light wines, which, the legislators felt, would "crowd out" strong liquors. The result was that, one year later, consumption of beer had risen sharply (by 135 percent), while wine consumption had also risen by 14 percent. Although the level of consumption of hard liquor declined, it did so only slightly. Consequently, there was an overall increase in alcohol consumption (from 4.3 liters in 1969 to 6.5 liters in 1974), which later stabilized (Lyalikov, 1987) at 6.6–7.1 liters (1995–1998).

The growing similarity in the levels, types and character of alcohol consumption in the industrially developed countries, known as the homogenization of consumption, is closely connected to the increasing uniformity in lifestyles in these countries. Data from 12 countries of Europe and the United States show how these processes are reflected in the increasing similarity in their levels of alcohol consumption. Indeed, what stands out is the substantial reduction in the differences between these countries' levels of consumption (standard deviation), despite the decline in consumption up to 1950 and its rise in the 1950–1980 period (Table 3, the standard deviation calculated by the author).

Table 3: Change in the average level of consumption and its variations (standard deviation; liters of pure alcohol per capita per year) in 12 European* countries and the United States.

	1905	1950	1960	1970	1980	1990
Per Capita Consumption	9.4	6.9	7.6	8.4	9.6	8.7
Standard Deviation	6.2	5.0	5.1	3.8	3.2	2.4

* *Belgium, United Kingdom, Germany, Denmark, Spain, Italy, Netherlands, Norway, Finland, France, Switzerland, Sweden. Sources: The National Alcoholic Association http://www.naa.cnt.ru*

Almost all the data are from official tallies and reflect the consumption of registered alcohol. For most Western European countries, consumption of unregistered alcohol comprises 5–20 percent of total consumption, but this figure is 24 percent for Poland, 28 percent for Finland and 33 percent for Norway (Rehn et al., 2001). The same authors give significantly higher indexes for unregistered alcohol consumption in Russia (95 percent), the Baltic countries that were formerly a part of the Soviet Union and for the latter's former European satellites. It should be noted,

1-2: THE SITUATION IN OTHER NATIONS

however, that defining registered and especially unregistered alcohol presents major problems. This is a source of disagreement among various writers who use a variety of methodologies to calculate their figures for alcohol consumption (Figs. 1-3a and 1-3b).

Fig. 1-3 (a/b): Alcohol consumption in the European nations based on data from two sources: World Drink Trends (1999; 1-3a) and Leifman (2001, 1-3b), for 1997–1998 (1-3a) and 1996–1998 (1-3b). Fig. 1-3a includes no information on unrecorded alcohol in nine countries only. Russia is represented by the author's data recalculated to age 15 +.

Fig. 1-3a

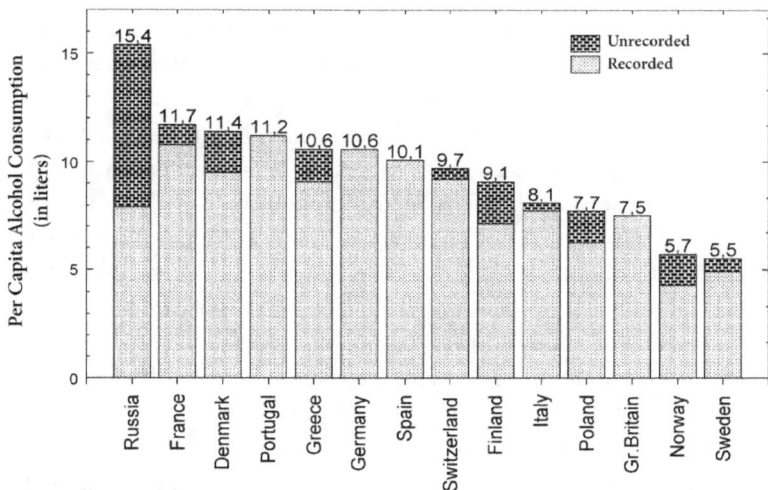

Fig. 1-3b

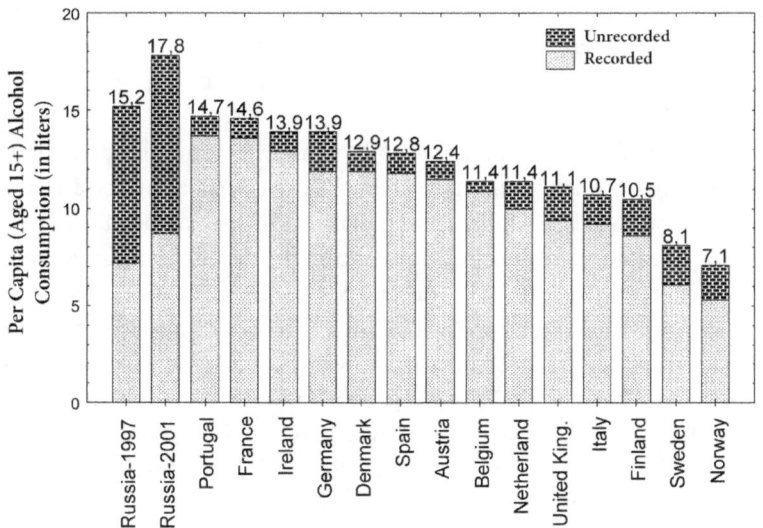

This "linear" presentation of the alcohol situation in Europe and the United States requires the addition of, at least, an analysis of two further factors that play an important role in alcohol consumption – the price of alcoholic beverages and the level of personal income of the subject populations. These are factors that can substantially affect consumption: consumption of hard liquor rises in times of economic prosperity and declines during economic downturns. At the same time, high prices on strong spirits have, in several countries (e.g. Denmark and Ireland) transformed such beverages into luxury items, in contrast to beer, which is usually perceived as an everyday commodity and, by many people, as a food product.

Overall, the rise in consumption in Western Europe and North America in the immediate post-war period reflects a rise in real incomes and a decline in the actual price of beverages made with spirits. From the 1960s, the price of alcohol began to drop, sometimes substantially. Thus, the average earnings of an industrial worker in Europe for one hour's work could then buy the same quantity of spirits that would have required a day's wages 10 years earlier (Walsh, 1985). The situation was somewhat different in the United States, which has experienced a steady rise in prices of hard liquor over the last 40 years. However, the income of the population has risen even faster. As a result, since 1960 the actual price of hard liquor is 48 percent lower, while the price of beer is down 27 percent, and the price of wine is down 20 percent (Mocher, 1988). Spending by American families for alcoholic beverages has thus subsequently declined from 5 percent to 1.4 percent of family income (Treml, 1982). At the same time, consumption has increased from 5.6 liters in 1961 to 8.2 liters in 1980.

The dependence of consumption on income was evident during the economic downturn of 1974–1975 caused by the oil crisis. This was a time when many European countries witnessed a halt to the rise in alcohol consumption, while in Britain consumption of hard liquor even declined for a short period of time. The end of the recession saw the return of the former trend of rising alcohol consumption (Plant, 1992).

The increase in real incomes in the period from 1950 through to the 1980s affected various social groups in the industrially developed countries differently. The greatest changes were possibly in the social and economic position of women, giving them greater all-round independence. One aspect associated with the latter change was the lowering of moral and social limitations on alcohol consumption by women and their appearance in public places under the influence of alcohol. The results of such emancipation were quickly reflected in a rise in female alcoholism: in the early 1900s, the proportion of female to male alcoholics in Europe stood at 1 to 10; in the 1980s, it was 1 to 5 and, in certain countries, it had risen even higher (to 1:3.4, for the Federal Republic of Germany in 1985).

The social view of drinkers also changed. For the first half of the century, abuse of alcohol was thought mainly to be characteristic of the poorer classes.

However, it was later demonstrated that high consumption is characteristic both for those experiencing material hardship (who are, incidentally, more easily observed) and for those with high incomes whose work was associated with great responsibility and great mobility and, who were thus, less accessible to narcological research (Chapter 1-1 and 2-2).

In the 1960s and 1970s the first generation of the post-war baby boom reached drinking age. Its size, and the social effects on it of weakened family relationships, seriously affected the post-war rise in alcohol consumption. In several European countries (Finland and others), the age associated with the highest level of alcohol consumption dropped down towards 30. Early alcoholism, affecting those under 18 years of age, became a serious problem.

The increase in the number of alcoholics was a clear indicator and result of the rise in alcoholization. It is difficult to describe this problem in its full dimensions as a great number of alcoholics are never recorded as such. Moreover, the diagnostic definition of alcoholism has changed over the years. With this in mind and using estimates for the United States in the 1980s, the number of alcoholics can be put at 10–15 million, or 4–6 percent of the population. The literature, however, includes an even higher estimate of 8 percent (Nace, 1984).

It is important to underline the fact that, during the boom time for drugs and drug dependency in the U.S., "alcohol remained the most widely used narcotic" (Seixas & Eggleston, 1976). This continued to be the case even later. Thus, in 1987, the number of deaths associated with drug use (mainly opiates, cocaine and marijuana) in the U.S. was 6,750, as compared with 125,000 associated with alcohol consumption (Fahrenkrug, 1990). The same sort of ratio is also characteristic for the other industrially developed countries, despite the widening trend of lowered alcohol consumption in many regions of the world.

A new tendency in accordance with the factors I indicated above mirrors a change in profound values in post-industrial society, a change that is partially connected with new technologies, computerization and the internet. But the most important thing, in the world, was the new mobilization of conservative forces under the banner of other ideas brought on by postmodernism which were accompanied by a greater number of "ecological niches", greater tolerance for those who think differently and for new forms of behavior and, finally, the rejection of absolutes. This led to greater freedom and a widened menu of acceptable lifestyles. However, not all conflicts disappear even in free and materially well-off societies; there will always be psychologically unfree people, who are unsure of themselves, alone, subject to mood swings and sensitive to external circumstances. For some of these people, psychological support will suffice. Others will need the "crutch" of pharmacology. And another group will turn to the "comforts" of alcohol or drugs.

There is an increasing value being placed on health, both personal and of the population. A healthy way of life is becoming an ethical category and is acquiring an almost material value. The West is investing ever greater resources in health services. The health of the population seems to have become the national idea in the U.S. and some countries of Europe. In terms of income, the poor are approaching the rich, young workers are approaching mature workers and, increasingly, people are being united in a single new class – the class of consumers. The "consumption of things" is crowding out the consumption of alcohol, and Western society is becoming increasingly negative towards the abuse of spirits.

A new piece of jargon has appeared, "thingism" in English and *veshchizm* in Russian, signifying an increasing interest in consumer goods that verges on an addiction to things and their acquisition. Many people in Russia equate this kind of dependency with spiritual and intellectual emptiness, as if poverty and spirituality were sisters. For our purposes, it is important to point out that "thingism" has in the past, as now, operated as a powerful anti-alcohol factor. Examples have already been given at the national level. At the individual level, the acquisition of property (a car, for example) by an alcoholic in remission often keeps him from returning to drinking. To put it more generally, the decrease in alcohol consumption in the U.S. and Canada, the countries best analyzed in this respect, is the result of profound cultural changes (Smart, 1989; Clark & Hilton, 1991; Room, 1991).

Table 4: Registered alcohol consumption in countries of Western Europe and North America (2000–2001; liters of pure alcohol per person aged 15+; average consumption, as calculated by the author, is given in parentheses).

Country	Consumption	Country	Consumption
Luxembourg	17.5 (14.2)	United Kingdom	10.4 (8.4)
Ireland	14.5 (11.5)	Belgium	10.1 (8.3)
France	13.5 (10.9)	Netherlands	9.7 (7.9)
Germany	12.9 (10.9)	Greece	9.3 (8.0)
Austria	12.6 (10.6)	Italy	9.1 (7.8)
Portugal	12.5 (10.5)	USA	8.5 (6.7)
Spain	12.3 (10.5)	Sweden	6.9 (5.7)
Denmark	11.9 (9.6)	Slovenia	6.6 (5.5)
Switzerland	11.5 (9.5)	Norway	5.8 (4.6)
Finland	10.4 (8.5)	Iceland	5.7 (4.4)

Source: Food and Agriculture Organization of the United Nations, World Drink Trends 2003, Global Status Report on Alcohol 2004.

To conclude this section, I present the WHO data on the registered consumption of alcohol for the nations of Western Europe and North America for 2000–2001 (Table 4). In analyzing this material, one should not forget that it is based on those aged 15 and above and that the proportion of adolescents in the national populations ranges from 14 percent (Greece, Italy) to 23 percent (Iceland). Moreover, as it is only statistics relating to the consumption of registered alcohol that are being used they are therefore incomplete. The statistics in the table are thus somewhat approximate. However, it is clear that Western Europe and North America show the highest levels of alcohol consumption of all among the regions of the world.

Eastern Europe

Unlike the statistics for Western Europe and North America, the statistics for Eastern Europe must be interpreted with great caution. This is especially true with regard to the official information from the new countries formed after the disintegration of the Soviet Union. It is clear that the consumption of alcohol in the former Baltic Soviet republics (Lithuania, Latvia and Estonia) approached Russian levels during the Soviet period, i.e. it was very high and hard liquor predominated. Thus, for example, the official figure for Latvia in 1984 is 10.5 liters of alcohol per person per year (the same as for Russia), but actual consumption exceeded 13 liters, a little less than the actual consumption in Russia (Nemtsov, 1992c).

Thereafter, the three Baltic republics, along with the rest of the Soviet Union, conducted the anti-alcohol campaign and saw a lowering (Latvia 9.8 liters in 1987) and then a rise in alcohol consumption (Latvia 13.4 liters in 1991; Nemtsov, 1992c). However, Strzdins (1994) and Strzdins et al. (1995a) calculate that the figures for Latvia in the first half of the 1990s range from 16 to 20 liters and even to 27.3 liters (Strzdins et al., 1995b). At the same time consumption in Estonia and Lithuania was calculated to be 9–12 liters (Kariis, 1994; Subata & Grimaluskienne, 1994). The similarity in the dynamics of alcohol consumption among the Baltic states in the preceding years makes this difference in the 1990s seem very unlikely, and the figures produced by the Latvian authors for Latvia, which are based on models, appear to be exaggerated. Figures for consumption in Belarus, Ukraine and Moldova are closer to 9–12 liters (WHO, 2004; Rehn et al., 2001).

Unlike the situation in the former republics of the Soviet Union, where a lessening of alcohol consumption took place as a result of the anti-alcohol campaign and powerful repressive pressures from above, the decline experienced in Poland in the 1980s happened as a result of political pressure from below: the newly active Solidarity movement accused the government of making the nation drunk. The heated national debate was accompanied by a reduction in the production of alcoholic beverages, the rationing of purchases, limitations on hours of sale and increases in the prices of alcoholic drinks (Moskalewicz et al., 1997). The result was a decline in alcohol consumption (using official figures) from 8.7 liters in 1980 to 6.4 liters in 1982–1983, which later stabilized at 7.0–7.2 liters, of which approximately 6.0 liters was vodka. From 1990, Polish statistics have taken into account only beverages produced in Poland, ignoring imports. Furthermore, no attempts are made to quantify the amount of illegal samogon, which, according to the WHO, came to 1.5 liters in Poland in the late 1990s (World Drink Trends 1999). New economic conditions and the liberalization of the trade in alcohol led to a steep rise, possibly as high as 50 percent, in alcohol consumption in Poland between 1989 and 1992, a fact confirmed by the steep rise in the number of cases of alcoholic psychoses. The same period saw similar increases in alcohol consumption in Slovakia and Bulgaria (Moskalewicz et al., 1997).

The consumption of vodka in Czechoslovakia in the post-war years was low and relatively stable (3.5–4.4 liters of alcohol; Moskalewicz et al., 1997; WHO, 2004). However, the overall consumption of alcohol was steadily rising, reaching 10.1 liters per person per year in 1995, largely as a result of a steady rise in the consumption of beer. By the end of the 1900s, Czechoslovakia had caught up and passed Germany in beer consumption and had become the world leader in this regard: 9.4 liters of alcohol consumed in the form of beer (2000); Germany (7.3 liters) – in fourth place behind Ireland (9.2 liters) and Switzerland (7.5 liters; WHO, 2004). For purposes of comparison, in Russia the alcohol consumption attributable to beer was 1.5 liters in 2000.

It is important to bear in mind that Czechoslovakia, unlike Poland, took up Gorbachev's anti-alcohol campaign in the Soviet period and, for a short time, brought alcohol consumption down from 9.2 liters in 1984 to 8.0 liters in 1987. Following the breakup of Czechoslovakia, it was revealed that the Czech portion of alcohol consumption exceeded the Slovak. For the year 2000, the comparative figures were 13.6 liters for the Czech Republic and 11.6 liters for the Slovakia.

Hungary is noted for having a high level of alcohol consumption: the figure was 11.8 liters per person per year in 1980. According to official figures, the country experienced a decline in consumption (to 10.2 liters in 1995 and 9.4 liters in 1998). However, it is assumed that Hungary has a very high level of illegal alcohol production and consumption, no less than 4 liters per capita (1995; Rehm & Gmel, 2001) and possibly more (1998, Rehn et al., 2001).

Bulgaria and Romania have similar levels of alcohol consumption (7.13 liters and 7.63 liters, respectively, and 3–4 liters of unregistered alcohol; 2001) and a similar overall pattern of consumption, i.e. there is a slight domination by wine against a background of a general lowering of alcohol consumption since the early 1980s, when it stood at 11.5–12.5 liters.

Latin America

The economic difficulties experienced by many countries on this continent have long hampered the compilation of reliable statistics, including those on alcohol. But a general impression of the region has taken shape which shows that unlike in the advanced industrial countries, a rapid increase in alcohol consumption was underway (Smart, 1991). This is attested to by the rise noted in cases of cirrhosis of the liver (between 1952 and 1982, the increase was 70 percent in Chile; Naveillan & Vargas, 1989).

Today, as a result of a major effort carried out under the aegis of the World Health Organization (Babor et al., 2003; WHO, 2004), the alcohol situation in the South American countries is somewhat clearer. Major differences in the levels of consumption and their trends have been documented for various countries in the region. This, together with the presence of so many countries with small populations in this region, makes a brief exposition difficult. In connection with this, it is worth looking at the alcohol consumption in the largest South American countries (Table 5), which shows a difference of 4–5 times between the countries with the highest and lowest consumption. In analyzing the material that follows, it should be borne in mind that many of these countries are active tourist destinations, especially Brazil, Cuba and Paraguay and that tourism accounts for a significant portion of these nations' alcohol consumption.

Latin American countries also differ in their drink preferences. In much of the continent, in recent years, beer has dominated alcohol consumption, accompanied by a low (Bolivia, Mexico, Ecuador) or significant level of consumption of hard liquor (Brazil, Venezuela, Colombia). Moreover, in some of these countries, beer has been predominant for decades (Venezuela, Colombia, Mexico, Ecuador), but in others only during the last 5, 10 or 15 years (Bolivia, Brazil, Paraguay, Peru), before which hard liquor prevailed along with some small or even negligible consumption of wine. Hard liquor continues to be dominant in Cuba, Haiti and El Salvador.

In the countries in the southern part of the continent, where wine-production is well developed, the consumption of wine is most prevalent (Argentina, Uruguay, Chile) and defines the general level of alcohol consumption. However, unlike in Uruguay, where wine consumption, with some fluctuations, has remained stable, Argentina and Chile have experienced a steady and significant reduction in alcohol consumption in the past two or three decades, from 15–18 liters at the start of the 1960s to 5–6 liters in recent years. This has occurred exclusively due to a fall in the consumption of wine, although all three countries have experienced a rise in beer consumption in the last decade to the point where it now accounts for one-quarter, or more, of all alcohol consumed.

Bolivia, Guatemala, Colombia and Ecuador, like Argentina and Chile, have experienced a drop in alcohol consumption in the last 15 to 25 years. In Paraguay, despite a significant rise in beer consumption having taken place in the past15 years, the overall level of alcohol consumption is sharply down because of a reduction in the consumption of hard liquor. In contrast, consumption in Brazil has risen steadily from 2 liters (1961) to 5.5 liters in 1997, reflecting the

Table 5: Registered alcohol consumption in Latin America (2000–2001; liters of pure alcohol per person per year for persons aged 15+; average individual consumption, as calculated by the author, is given in parentheses).

Country	Consumption	Country	Consumption
Venezuela	8.8 (5.8)	Peru	4.7
Argentina	8.6 (5.9)	Mexico	4.6
Grenada	7.4 (4.8)	Belize	4.5
Uruguay	7.0	Cuba	3.7
Paraguay	6.7	El Salvador	3.5
Haiti	6.5	Bolivia	3.4
Dominican Republic	6.1	Jamaica	3.4
Panama	6.0	Nicaragua	2.5
Chile	6.0	Honduras	2.3
Colombia	5.9	Ecuador	2.0
Costa Rica	5.5	Guatemala	1.6
Brazil	5.3		

Source: *Food and Agriculture Organization of the United Nations, World Drink Trends 2003, Global Status Report on Alcohol 2004*

increased consumption of hard liquor and beer, which have contributed in equal measure to the rise. In addition, Brazil's consumption includes quite a large amount of unregistered alcohol – 3 liters (in 1995). The latter is made up largely of home-produced hard liquor. Approximately the same amount of unregistered alcohol is consumed in Mexico, but it consists of low-proof (6–7 percent ABV) beverages of agave-based local production. The consumption of unregistered alcohol in the other countries in the region is lower – between 1 and 2 liters.

This short account should make it clear that most of the countries in Latin America have been in step with the worldwide trends towards the lowering of alcohol consumption with a rise in beer consumption. The result is that alcohol consumption in the region may be considered as being moderate, at least in comparison with the nations of Europe, the United States and Canada.

Asia

To keep this review short, attention will be focused on the most populous countries of the continent or to states that are politically active on the world stage. Neither Afghanistan nor Taiwan are among the countries selected (Table 6), because of an absence of data, arising from several causes. However, it is known that alcohol consumption in Afghanistan used to be moderate, but that in the most recent years, in connection with a rise in social tensions and the return of refugees, consumption has risen, especially in Kabul.

Among the Asian countries, the leader in terms of consumption is probably is the Republic of Korea (South Korea), as it is the Asian country with the highest level of unregistered alcohol (about 7 liters). In recent decades, in connection with socioeconomic changes in the country and consequent changes in the style of life, including a sharp increase in the urban population, there has not only been a substantial increase in the consumption of spirits (which comprised 1 liter per capita in 1960), but also a shift from the consumption of low-proof alcoholic beverages like beer consumed during meals, to hard liquor often consumed on their own. As a result, adult men consume 18.4 liters of alcohol per year and suffer the most pronounced consequences (about 12 percent of South Korean men are alcoholics). Despite the seriousness of its alcohol problems, the general trends of the developed countries are also reflected in South Korea: since the 1970s (16 liters of alcohol) there has been a decline in overall consumption in conjunction with a rise in the consumption of wine (about 3 liters of alcohol) and beer (2 liters).

Table 6: Registered alcohol consumption in countries of Asia (2000–2001; liters of pure alcohol per person per year for persons aged 15+; average individual consumption, as calculated by the author, is given in parentheses).

Country	Consumption	Country	Consumption
Thailand	8.47 (6.5)	India	0.82
Republic of Korea	7.71 (6.1)	Syria	0.62
Japan	7.38 (6.3)	Bhutan	0.57
Laos	6.72 (3.8)	Brunei	0.49
Cyprus	6.67 (5.2)	Qatar	0.44
Democratic People's Republic of Korea	5.68 (4.1)	Burma	0.36
China	4.45 (3.5)	Cambodia	0.36
Lebanon	4.13 (3.0)	Iraq	0.20
Philippines	3.75	Sri Lanka	0.18
United Arab Emirates	2.75	Jordan	0.11
Singapore	2.73	Indonesia	0.10
Bahrain	2.63	Nepal	0.08
Israel	1.99	Yemen	0.08
Mongolia	1.96	Pakistan	0.02
Maldives	1.72	Iran	0.00
Turkey	1.48	Kuwait	0.00
Vietnam	1.35	Bangladesh	0.00
Oman	1.32	Saudi Arabia	0.00
Malaysia	1.06		

Source: Food and Agriculture Organization of the United Nations, World Drink Trends 2003

The picture is quite different for Thailand, with a predominantly (80 percent) rural population, which accounts for the core consumers of alcohol and the principal source of alcoholics. Hard liquor dominates consumption here (7.1

liters) while the consumption of unregistered alcohol is estimated to comprise 2 liters per capita per year.

Japan began the post-war period with a very low level of alcohol consumption (under 2 liters per person) but has seen a slow and steady increase in consumption up to the present (6.6 liters in 1995, Fig. 1-3; and 7.4 liters in 2000). The trend was abetted by the post-war occupation of Japan by American troops, who brought with them aspects of the American lifestyle, including a relatively high level of alcohol consumption.

The increase in per capita alcohol consumption in Japan has been accompanied by an increase in the consumption of all types of alcoholic beverages, but the relation among them has changed. Whereas earlier hard liquor of local origin, for example rice wine (*sake*), dominated, in recent years the share of beer consumed has begun to outpace other beverages (up to 68.5 percent). However, sake remains traditional for holidays. Japan is a model of how old wine-drinking traditions have been preserved while new forms of alcohol consumption have been added during the process of Westernization (Simpura, 1995). The result has been a general rise in consumption and, consequently, a rise in its negative effects. Thus, more than 20,000 persons were hospitalized in connection with alcoholism in Japan in 1987 (Sumida, 1990), while there are some 2.2 million alcoholics, or 1.8 percent of the country's population (Takagi et al., 1986). Unregistered alcohol consumption in Japan is estimated at 2 liters per capita per year.

Over the last 40 years, alcohol consumption in China has risen by 10 times (it was 0.5 liters in 1960). The country is notable for its wide regional and gender-based differences in alcohol consumption. Consumption is higher in the northern areas than in the southern, in rural areas than in urban and among men than among women (men consume 10–13 times more than women).

Consumption is also higher among certain ethnic groups, including the Tibetans and Mongolians. For the continent of Asia, China also stands out as regards the variety of alcoholic beverages consumed both in terms of their strength (sorghum-based vodka can contain 50–60 percent alcohol) and type (distilled or fermented liquors using a wide variety of grains, fruit and berry wines of many kinds, medicinal liquors made from medicinal grasses). It should be said that many consumers of alcohol in China view alcoholic beverages as sacramental, while others hold the view found in traditional Chinese medicine that alcohol "is the pilot of medicines that can lead medicines to the location of the ailment". Experts have estimated the consumption of unregistered alcohol in China at 1 liter per capita per year.

Besides Japan and South Korea in Asia, Israel also maintains good statistics on alcohol. However, this is a country without acute alcohol problems. As in the countries of Europe, consumption in Israel declined until the beginning of the 1980s (about 5 liters in 1975). To the official statistics on consumption (Table 6), one should add 1.0 liter of unregistered alcohol. Russian immigrants of the past

10–15 years are particularly evident among the heavy users of alcohol in Israel (Hasin et al., 1999; Rahav et al., 1999).

Unfortunately, information on the other Asian countries is limited. It should be noted that the majority of these countries have a relatively low level of alcohol consumption (Table 6) along with a low level of consumption of unregistered alcohol (not higher than 0.5 liters). The Philippines is an exception in the latter regard (about 3.0 liters of alcohol, mostly wine made from sugarcane), as is Turkey (2.7 liters of alcohol, mostly in the form of hard liquors like *chachi*) and India (1.7 liters of alcohol and possibly more, judging by the relatively severe alcohol-related consequences seen in road traffic accidents and poisonings).

Analysis of the data in Table 6 might suggest that alcohol consumption rises with an increase in Gross National Product, but this correlation is insignificant. One can more meaningfully state that alcohol consumption in Asia increases from the west to south and southeast and that the first eight or nine countries on the list, all of which "top" the 4-liter average per capita per year rate of consumption, would fit well in this regard in the list for Europe (Table 4), especially if unregistered alcohol is taken into account. Overall, then, consumption in Asia remains moderate in comparison with Western countries.

Africa

This is the poorest continent on the planet with the lowest life expectancy for the population, the largest portion of [who are] rural people and minors under the age of 15.

Information about the alcohol situation in many African countries remains very limited, despite the considerable efforts of many researchers during the 1980s and 1990s and, most recently, by a large group of scientists working under the aegis of the World Health Organization (Babor et al., 2003; WHO, 2004). Thus, for Algeria, Angola, Guinea, Congo, Liberia, Libya, Niger, Togo and Chad, there are only official statistics on consumption (Table 7). There are however African countries for which such statistics do not even exist (e.g. the Ivory Coast).

Those states which have been studied in more detail have revealed that there is great variety in terms of both the production and consumption of alcoholic beverages in Africa. For the other continents, significant differences appear in particular countries or regions. In Africa, such differences can be manifest in neighboring villages, which may be, it is true, tens of kilometers apart. Because of the limited data on the continent, all known quantitative data on alcohol consumption in the countries of Africa are considered here (Table 7). It is important to bear in mind that the statistics given in the table are for persons aged 15 and older, although, for example, in Uganda minors under the age of 15 comprise approximately 50 percent of the population.

The 1900s, especially the period from 1930 through to the 1950s, brought much that was new into the production of alcoholic beverages in Africa (Willis, 2001). Until then distillation had been unknown, and almost all alcoholic drinks were produced by fermentation. The development of distilling was spurred by the introduction of new varieties of corn, bamboo and rice with higher sugar contents as well as by the development of the sugar industry, which made sugar more accessible to the populace.

Despite these changes, much in the production of spirits in Africa remains at the level of handicraft and is often very outdated. In Gabon, for example, in production of a type of beer, rye berries are introduced, supposedly to speed fermentation and increase the "strength" of the beverage. In Namibia sulfur dioxide is used in producing the most popular wine from a local fruit (berkhemi). It is thought to give the wine clarity and a pleasant color and aroma. In a region of Botswana and in Uganda, acid from automotive batteries is added to a beverage similar to beer. Many African alcoholic drinks contain toxic concentrations of methanol, complex ethers, acids and other by-products of distillation.

Alcohol consumption in Africa is not the highest in the world, but the consequences of alcohol consumption are extraordinarily destructive because of the low levels of development e.g. the almost complete absence of medical care in many areas, terrible poverty, very poor nutrition and the many diseases that accompany these conditions. This applies to the continent as a whole, but there are African countries with very high levels of alcohol consumption attributable to legal production (Uganda) and illegal home production (Uganda, Zimbabwe). The special feature of the alcohol situation in Africa, in the view of specialists, is that the consumption of illegal alcohol accounts for more than half (about 60 percent) of the alcohol consumed. This is the highest such measure in the world. Moreover, in Kenya only 1 percent of alcohol consumption is of legally produced beverages (Partanen, 1991). This makes controlling the quality of such beverages very difficult which in part, explains another African problem: people often consume highly toxic beverages containing large amounts of zinc, manganese, formaldehyde, carcinogens and other substances.

Consumption of beer or similar beverages which are produced using malt, yeast and hops is dominant in Africa. The base items used may be grains (sorghum, proso, corn, barley, wheat, rice), manioc, lentils, various fruits (often bananas or oranges, more rarely coconuts), berries and flowers (anise). The choice of the base ingredient usually has a seasonal character. Some localities prepare sour beer (0.5 percent acid; Benin), while others use spices in their beers – pepper, leaves of aromatic plants, tobacco. Such beer usually has a strength of 2–5 percent ABV, but it can be as high as 11 percent ABV. A beer made in Nigeria is so thick and firm that it is used directly as a food product. Home-made beer is

Table 7: Registered and unrecorded/illegal (estimate) alcohol consumption in African Countries (2000–2001; liters of pure alcohol per person per year for persons aged 15+; average individual use, as calculated by author, is given in parentheses).

Country	Recorded Alcohol	Unrecorded Alcohol	Country	Recorded Alcohol	Unrecorded Alcohol
Uganda	19.17 (9.58)	10.7 (5.4)	Central African Republic	1.66	1.7
Reunion	13.39 (9.77)	–	Ghana	1.54	3.6
Nigeria	10.04 (5.62)	3.5 (2.0)	Eritrea	1.54	1.0
Swaziland	9.51 (5.40)	4.1 (2.3)	Malawi	1.44	–
Burundi	9.33 (5.04)	4.7 (2.5)	Lesotho	1.38	1.5
Gabon	7.93 (4.68)	–	Madagascar	1.38	–
South Africa	7.81 (5.23)	2.2 (1.5)	Benin	1.22	–
Rwanda	6.80 (3.74)	4.3 (2.4)	Djibouti	1.08	–
Sierra Leone	6.64 (3.72)	2.4 (1.3)	Togo	0.95	–
São Tomé and Principe	6.07 (3.16)	–	Ethiopia	0.91	1.0
Botswana	5.38 (3.23)	3.0 (1.8)	Equatorial Guinea	0.90	–
Tanzania	5.20 (2.86)	2.0 (1.1)	Tunisia	0.65	0.5
Zimbabwe	5.08 (2.9)	9.0 (5.1)	Mali	0.49	–
Cape Verde	3.72 (2.19)	–	Senegal	0.48	0.8
Cameroon	3.66 (2.08)	2.6 (1.5)	Morocco	0.41	–
Seychelles	3.61 (2.56)	5.2 (3.7)	Sudan	0.27	1.0
Mauritius	3.16	–	Chad	0.23	–
Liberia	3.12	–	Guinea	0.14	–
Zambia	3.02	1.0	Niger	0.11	–
Angola	2.91	–	Egypt	0.10	0.5
Guinea-Bissau	2.76	–	Comoros	0.08	–
Namibia	2.39	–	Algeria	0.03	0.3
Congo	2.36	–	Mauritania	0.01	–
Gambia	2.27	–	Libya	0.00	–
Dem. Rep. Congo	2.01	–	Somalia	0.00	–
Kenya	1.74 (1.03)	5.0 (3.0)	Ivory Coast	–	–
Mozambique	1.67	–	Western Sahara	–	–

Source: Food and Agriculture Organization of the United Nations, World Drink Trends 2003, Global Status Report on Alcohol 2004.

five or six times cheaper than industrially produced bottled beer, which, as a result, is drunk comparatively rarely (as little as 0.5 percent of the total amount of beer consumed in Tanzania). In other countries, such as Kenya for example, industrially produced beer makes up 16 percent of beer consumption (Partanen, 1991).

Wine made from the juices of palms, coconuts, young bamboo or fruit (e.g. cashew fruit and banana) is widely consumed, especially in coastal regions. For Africans, as for the rest of mankind, spirit beverages often fulfil many social functions, specifically religious and ritualistic. For these, palm wine and coconut wine are preferred. They are also used in medical treatments and in some other traditional applications.

Wine here is fermented using a variety of methods: in its own shell (coconuts) and in containers made from pumpkins, bamboo or clay. The strength of such beverages ranges from 3–5 percent ABV through to 8–15 percent ABV, but sometimes sugarcane juice, sugar or molasses is added to raise the alcohol content. The preparation of wine in many areas takes quite unusual forms. For example, the coconuts may be left on the tree, with a hole pierced in the shell. When the wine begins to mature and its aroma seeps into the surrounding area, residents spend a week guarding the palms around the clock and beating the trunks with sticks to drive off monkeys and elephants attracted by the scent of the wine.

Following the distillation of the fermented juice of palm, sugarcane or grain-based beer, and sometimes with the addition of sugar or molasses, strong drinks usually contain 30–40 percent ABV. However, double distilling is also sometimes undertaken (for example, in Botswana), bringing the strength up to 80 percent ABV. At the same time, the technology used is very basic, with the machinery consisting of gasoline canisters or oil barrels. In Uganda, where *waragi*, a strong beverage, is the chief item of alcohol consumption, there is widespread distortion of its strength by adding, for example, battery acid.

There are no reliable statistics on the incidence of alcohol psychoses in Africa, but separate observations indicate that instances of psychosis (Botswana) are not rare, nor are poisonings (Kenya) from poor-quality alcohol. Alcohol is also an important factor in traumas, but in Africa this is more often the result of mutual aggression and fighting with sticks, knives and other objects. Serious cases of the beating of women and children by drunken husbands, previously not observed (Botswana), are now more common. In many countries there is a high percentage of drunk-driving (up to 60 percent of those tested in Kenya), and there is a high incidence of serious injury on the roads. Recent years have also seen the spread of alcoholism among young men in conjunction with growing unemployment.

Production of spirits in domestic conditions is chiefly the work of women, for whom sales of alcohol have become a substantial source of family income. At the same time, consumption of alcohol by married women is strongly disapproved of, and the principal consumers continue to be men (up to 18–20 liters per adult male in Tanzania). With the complications in family life caused by the husband's heavy drinking, women are also beginning to abuse alcohol.

Alcohol is playing an important role as a stimulator of chance sexual encounters, and so aggravating Africa's dramatic HIV infection problem. In Uganda, HIV is twice as common among drinkers as among non-drinkers (10 percent versus 5 percent), and in Zambia it is one of the main causes of the spread of HIV, especially among married women.

In many African countries (Kenya and Uganda, for example), illegal production of alcoholic beverages for sale, and even sales themselves, are against the law. Nonetheless, this activity is widespread because of the corruption among officials (Partanen, 1991; Haugerud, 1995), especially in Kenya and Tanzania. Corruption where strong spirits are concerned was virtually official in Uganda (Obbo, 1980). It has since been replaced by a disregard for the problem, by the authorities, and the free production and trade in distilled beverages (Willis, 2000).

When analyzing the issue of alcohol in Africa, R. Smart (1991) came to the conclusion that there was a relationship between low levels of alcohol consumption and low levels of economic development. At the same time, this continent has potential as a market for alcoholic beverages. But it is difficult to speak at all concretely about the future of alcohol consumption in Africa. One can only suppose that poverty will long continue to restrain any significant increase in alcohol consumption, especially of imported beverages. The antiquated, handicraft methods of producing Africa's traditional alcoholic beverages will be unable to support any substantial increase.

* * *

Global

Along with the growth of consumption in the post-war period, there has been a trend towards monopoly in the alcoholic beverages industry and the domination of the industry by powerful trans-national corporations, especially as regards the production and sales of beer and hard liquor. There were 27 such corporations in 1980. The revenues of each topped 1 billion USD, with the overall revenue from their worldwide trade exceeding 170 billion USD (Ashley & Rankin, 1988).

This situation means that almost unlimited opportunities exist for advertising alcoholic beverages. There is a danger that powerful advertising will lead to further growth in the consumption of alcohol. However, strong scientific proof that advertising can have this effect is lacking (Partanen & Montonen, 1991). Science has shown only advertising's effect on the choice of beverages, such as the preference for particular producers. The considerable research in this area suggests that the effect of advertising on the per capita level of consumption has been exaggerated. Unfortunately, the same cannot be said regarding consumers who are children or adolescents (Chapter 2-2).

Chapter 1-3
The alcohol situation in Russia before and after 1945

The attitude of the Soviet government towards its people regarding alcohol consumption was largely prohibitive. A totalitarian state needed a disciplined citizenry. But there was another, very important aspect of the relationship between the Soviet authorities and the populace. Large amounts of money were needed for the rapid execution of the state's often grandiose plans. And infusions of funds from abroad were minimal. There remained one solution – the mobilization of internal economic resources, one of which was the trade in wine and spirits. The contrary tendencies of these two factors badly unbalanced Soviet alcohol policy and largely laid the groundwork for today's alcohol problems. But before proceeding to discuss this, it is important to understand the extent to which the nation's alcohol history determined the present situation. We need, at least briefly, to consider the history of heavy drinking in Russia.

The idea of a long history of heavy drinking that stretches across centuries and which is an inherent characteristic of the Russian people is widespread today. We are usually reminded of the unfortunate saying attributed to Prince Vladimir: "Russians know the joy of drinking and cannot live without it." These words, which may be entirely legendary, are from the Tale of Bygone Years (*Povest' vremennykh let*), a book made up largely of legends. But if the words were indeed spoken, it is noteworthy that they come from a section of the work entitled "Argument over Belief" and are meant as an argument against adopting Islam, whose Prophet stipulated total abstinence from alcohol. It should also be remembered that the transcript of the argument was made more than a century after Russia's adoption of Christianity.

Russia's alcohol history has been affected by an error often made by historians. It is presented mainly through a history of the Russian elite and, although more rarely, through the history of Russia's urban population. In other words, the historians' attention has been focused on the best illuminated and most easily visible areas and not on where the mass of the population in pre-tsarist and tsarist Russia actually lived. Yet it was this mass that determined the basic national patterns of behavior. No one thinks that the heavy drinking of the galas of the Petrine era was an example of the national tradition or the source of a new one.

Vladimir's "Russians know the joy of drinking…" was only the start of the legend of Russian drunkenness that was later and for centuries buttressed by descriptions from foreign travelers. But can these few and localized observations be used to generalize about the entire population, especially when they conflict with the realities of the life of this great people?

The reality was that the ancestors of the Russians lived in an area with mediocre soils and a difficult climate. For centuries, a large part of the population lived in poverty, ate scantily and, for alcohol, consumed only weak beer and mead (a honey-based alcoholic drink). In the course of the 1400s and 1500s, the peasants, who constituted the majority of the population, succumbed to serfdom, a semi-slave condition, and were unable to purchase, let alone attempt to produce strong alcoholic drinks. The alcohol requirements of the urban population in pre-tsarist Rus were met by inns (*korchmy*) that sold food as well as beer and mead.

The start of vodka production in Russia is a matter for dispute during the 1400s and 1500s. But it is well established that taxes began to be applied to alcoholic beverages in 1474. The Russian state henceforth sought to help itself with this added source of revenue. Ivan IV (the Terrible) closed the inns, replacing them in 1553 with royal taverns (*kabaky*) that were allowed to sell only vodka without food; in the 1500s it was believed that a person could drink more without food. Relatives were forbidden to remove their drunken kin from the taverns: "drunkards may not be called out of taverns, nor shall a wife drive out a husband, a father a son, or a son a father" (as cited in Zhirov & Petrova, 1998). The kabaky became dens for alcoholics. They, along with the royal and boyar feasts are the source of almost all of the famous descriptions of Russian drinking in the medieval period – by the Englishman G. Fletcher in 1588, the Saxon A. Oleary in 1634, A. Maierberg in 1661, and the German diplomat Z. Gerbershtein, who visited Russia in 1517 and 1526. The latter recounted that Tsar Vasily Ivanovich created a special establishment for *nalivaiky* (from "nalivai-ka", or "pour already") on Spasonalivaikovsky Lane, between Great Polyanka and Great Yakimanka streets in Moscow. It served mead and beer only to royal servants, while admission was barred to all other citizens of the city.

Later the taverns spread more widely but only in cities, and most often, no more than one per city, and more rarely and briefly, in large villages that belonged to the tsar. Foreigners' descriptions of Russian drunkenness are almost exclusively based on observations of Moscow's taverns and, less often, on those in Novgorod (Velikii Novgorod) and in two or three other large cities to which foreigners were allowed access while traveling. In all, Russia's urban population was only 14.5 percent of the total population as late as 1897. This means that heavy drinking in Russia was, up to that time, a local, predominantly urban phenomenon of the taverns (*kabaky*). Moreover, vodka was expensive: in the 1600s, a cask of vodka (12.3 liters) was 1.5 times more costly than a cow (Kurukin, 1998). It is also worth mentioning that vodka then had a 20 percent ABV. Inns (*korchmy*) continued to function illegally but were remorselessly targeted by the authorities.

Possibly our only source of statistical information comes from the Swedish traveler I. Kilburger, who visited Russia in 1674:

> ... there are not that many taverns, either in Moscow or elsewhere in the country. I encountered on the main land road between Novgorod and Moscow, a distance of more than 500 *versts* [a verst is 1.06 kilometers], no more than 9 or 10. One even finds many large settlements of 40, 50 or even more courtyards where one could not obtain a drop of beer. Almost everyone, and certainly every peasant, has the weak drink known as *kvas*. (as cited by Kurtz, 1937).

So much for drinking Russia! In England, a century before I. Kilburger's trip to Russia, the small, provincial town of Stratford-Upon-Avon had, at the time of the Shakespeare's birth, 20 taverns, "that is, on average, one tavern for every 100 residents" (Anikst, 1964). Every day and especially on holidays, the ale – a strong, thick beer – flowed.

A significant stage in the spread of heavy drinking in Russia took place under Peter I, who made vodka consumption mandatory for the navy and then for the army (up to 600 milliliters of vodka of 10 percent ABV in strength). Another aspect of this new stage took place in 1716, when the tsar, forced by the depletion of his treasury as a result of the cost of various wars, for a short time freed the production of vodka. Thereafter, the number of taverns grew until, in 1885, they numbered approximately 80,000. Alcohol's share in payments to the treasury also rose (Zhirov and Petrova, 1998): from about 30 percent under Catherine II to 38 percent under Alexander II (in 1859). It should be noted that the structure of payments to the treasury was quite different from what it is now.

The next stage is connected with two quite different but temporarily linked historical events: the ending of serfdom (1861) and a significant decline in vodka prices (1863) stemming from a rise in the number of plants producing spirits and a lowering of the price of spirits. Consumption of vodka became possible for the less-well-off layers of the population. By the middle of the 1800s, Russian statistics were quite reliable for their time. For 1863 they record an almost doubling of alcohol consumption (to 6.2 liters per person per year in European Russia, Fig. 1-4). This is the highest level reached in tsarist Russia (Ostroumov, 1914). The following year consumption fell to 4.1 liters, and it continued to drop until the early 1890s (2.6 liters). The decline was, in part, attributable to a deliberate raising of excise taxes by 2.5 times over the course of 30 years. However, the early 1890s witnessed a spurt in alcohol consumption, reflecting the growth of industry, the migration of the rural population to the cities and its transformation into a population of factory workers (3.3 liters in 1913; Fig. 1-4). For purposes of comparison, per capita consumption of alcohol in France at the start of the 1900s exceeded 20 liters; in Italy it was 15 liters, in Spain, Switzerland and Great Britain 10 liters, and

Fig. 1-4: Alcohol Consumption in Russia 1863–2006. 1 – data from official statistics (source: www.naacnt.ru), 2 – weighted average of actual consumption by Treml (1997), State Statistical Committee of the Russian Federation (RussStats), Nemtsov (2000) and chapter-2-4.

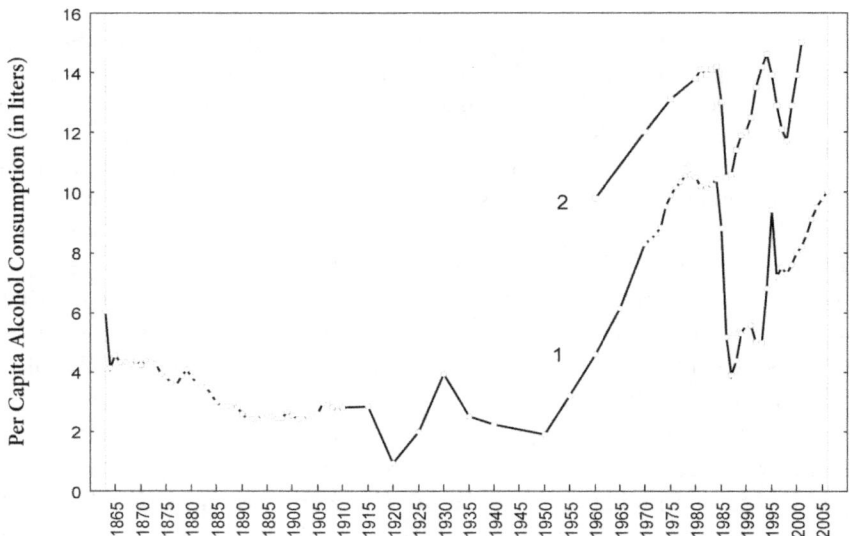

in Germany and the United States 7 liters (Vlassak, 1928; as cited in Afanasyev, 1997, and Fig. 1-2b).

World War I and the "social contract" of 1914, the post-war and post-revolutionary breakdown and hunger, and the "semi-dry" law of 1919 (banning the production and sale of alcoholic beverages with strengths greater than 12 percent ABV) kept consumption of alcohol at a very low level.

However, the 1919 law did not last long. At the June 1923 plenum of the Central Committee of the Russian Communist Party (Bolshevik), the question of a state monopoly on sales of vodka was raised. A heated discussion on the adoption of legislation on the matter took place between Stalin and Trotsky. The latter opposed the idea of a monopoly and called it impermissible "to build the budget on the sale of vodka". The position of Stalin and his adherents prevailed: the 1919 law was annulled as of 1 January 1924, and in August 1925 a resolution was adopted establishing a government monopoly on vodka production. In his report to the 19th Congress of the Communist Party, Stalin said: "If we cannot borrow, if we are impoverished of capital and if… we cannot indenture ourselves to Western European capitalists… then it is necessary to choose between indenture and vodka." In conversations with delegations of foreign workers, Stalin called the introduction of vodka sales a "temporary measure" that "should be eliminated as soon as are found… new sources… of income… for the development of our industry". The "temporary measure" exists to this day, although without a monopoly in fact.

In 1927 state sales of alcohol (3.7 liters per person per year, not counting samogon) reached the pre-World War I level. This is one side of the story; the other involved the adoption, at about the same time, of a law on the struggle against illegal production of alcohol (a second, stricter, version was enacted in 1932). Also in 1927 the government adopted a resolution on the anti-alcohol activity of local organs of power, whose rights in this regard were further widened in 1929 (Zaigraev, 1992). The faith of the Soviet leadership in the power of ideology led it to create and impose branches across the country of an "All-Russia Society of Struggle for Sobriety". An impassioned propaganda campaign against alcohol consumption was set in motion, and there was a countrywide wave of top-down inspired "conferences of drinking" where shoe workers, textile workers and others publicly condemned their lives as drinkers.

By the time of World War II, these measures, and the repressive nature of organization in all spheres of life in the country, had reduced alcohol sales to 2.3 liters per person per year (1940), and home distillation was minimal. In 1950 the consumption of alcohol from government sources fell even further (1.9 liters).

The beginning of the rapid rise in alcohol consumption in the USSR coincided with the beginning of the alcohol boom in Europe. As early as 1958, state production of wine and vodka had doubled in the USSR, and by 1965 had tripled as compared with 1950. Contributing factors included the move to a five-day working week in 1967. The strong rise in sales continued even later (4.5 liters per capita in 1960, 8.2 liters per capita in 1970 and 10.5 liters per capita in 1980; Fig. 1-4). The increase over 30 years amounted to 358 percent.

But these are only the official statistics. The post-war period saw a widespread development of illegal alcohol manufacture, which during the war had been kept under control by the implacably repressive policy of the Soviet leadership. In 1956, in merely three republics of the USSR (Russia, Ukraine and Belorussia), approximately 18,000 persons were convicted of illegal alcohol activities, the number rising to more than 23,000 in 1957. The first resolution on the fight against drunkenness and alcoholism adopted by the Central Committee of the Communist Party of the Soviet Union and the Soviet government appeared in 1958. The militia was ordered to conduct "discovery work". As a result, the population voluntarily turned over or had seized more than 20,000 illegal stills in the first two months of the resolution coming into operation. But these measures did not stop illegal alcohol production, and in 1960, according to Treml (1997), illegal alcohol sales exceeded state sales (5.2 liters per capita as opposed to 4.6 liters per capita). The further growth of illegal production was restrained by the increasing development of the state trade in alcoholic beverages. However, by the late 1970s and early 1980s, illegal production was adding 3 to 4 liters per capita on to the figure for state sales (State Statistical Committeeof the Russian Federation; Treml, 1997; Nemtsov, 1997; Fig. 1-4).

A particularly coarse culture of alcohol consumption formed in Russia in the post-war period, new in quantity and in quality. Heavy drinking in tsarist Russia, if it took the form of what in English is called "binge drinking", was largely limited to holidays. However, it now occurred not only on holidays but also on ordinary working days and in work places, drawing in to it young people and women for whom heavy drinking had until then been viewed as shameful.

Interestingly, worldwide trends of rising alcohol consumption were maintained in the USSR, despite the fact that an "Iron Curtain" had been placed around the country in 1948–1949 and that there were substantial differences in economic conditions between the USSR and the West. Alcohol consumption rose steadily through the period of the "thaw" and in the period of "stagnation". The trend was halted neither by the first (1958) or the second (1972) resolution of the Central Committee of the Communist Party of the Soviet Union and the government on the struggle against drunkenness and alcoholism. This bears witness to the presence in the USSR, along with its particular national reasons for a widening of heavy drinking, of global tendencies in alcohol consumption and the commonality of the changes in the world in the second half of the 1900s. The special national quality of Soviet consumption was its very high level, the predominance of strong spirits and the great share contributed by illegal alcohol to total consumption.

A number of independent researchers have put forward estimates of the actual per capita consumption of alcohol in the USSR at the turn of the 1980s: – 11 liters in 1980 (Zaigraev & Murashov, 1990), – 11.46 liters in 1979 (Treml, 1982), – 12.6 liters in 1980 (Sheregy, 1986), – 12.76 liters in 1975 and 17 liters in 1984 (Segal, 1990; the author has recalculated the non-Russian estimates of per capita consumption for those aged 15 and above). It later transpired that in 1980 the State Statistical Committee of the USSR (and the RSFSR), at the bidding of the government, had compiled secret figures on the volume of illegal alcohol production in the country (5.2 liters of 100 percent alcohol per capita per year). This, together with state sales (8.7 liters) gives an estimate of overall consumption for 1980 of 13.2 liters (and of 13.5 liters for the RSFSR).

With the exception of Segal's figures, the difference among the estimates is not large and comes to 2.2 liters (or 20 percent of the minimum figure). Most likely, Segal overestimated consumption in the USSR. This is likely to have occurred because of his rather free use of ideologically tendentious information found in the Soviet press at the start of the anti-alcohol campaign. The first three estimates, like the figures from the State Statistical Committee of the USSR are quite close and show a very high general level of alcohol consumption in the USSR (on average 12.1 ± 0.5 liters, or 39 percent more than state sales). This is substantially different from the figures reported to the World Health Organization by Soviet researchers (8.7 liters, Urakov & Miroshnichenko, 1991).

By the early 1980s, alcohol consumption in the USSR and Russia, as was the case in many other countries, had stabilized (Table 1) and "a definite 'ceiling' in the dimensions of drunkenness as in incidence of alcoholism had been reached" (Urakov & Miroshnichenko, 1989). In their opinion, "this limit reflected the natural summary result of all the interacting social-economic and psychological factors active at this time". Unfortunately, the authors did not offer proof of this interesting proposition and did not make clear the nature of "the social-economic and psychological factors". However, market reforms showed that the Russians were capable of raising the 'ceiling' higher still.

Among the republics of the USSR, Russia occupied one of the leading, if not first position in terms of alcohol consumption. In any case, state sales of alcoholic beverages in Russia (10.5 liters, 1984) trailed only Estonia and Latvia. However, the estimate of actual consumption in Latvia in 1984 was slightly lower than for Russia (13.4 liters versus 14.2 liters, Nemtsov, 1992c).

State sales, estimates of actual consumption and of unregistered alcohol in Russia from 1970 through to 2001 are presented in Table 1 (the methodology for the calculations of actual consumption is explained in Chapter 2-4). Estimates for succeeding years will be based largely on the average of the estimates from three independent sources for 1980–1994: the State Statistical Committee of the Russian Federation, Treml (1997) and Nemtsov (2000).

One of the most important measures of the alcohol situation before the start of the anti-alcohol campaign was the very high level of state sales of alcohol in Russia (officially, 10.5 liters in 1984), which exceed consumption in other countries such as Great Britain (6.9 liters), the U.S. and Canada (8 liters) and Australia (8.9 liters) (World Drink Trends, 1991).

Another important condition was the very high proportion of unregistered alcohol consumed in Russia in this period (35 percent in 1984; Table 1). For purposes of comparison, the 12 percent consumption of unregistered alcohol in an estimated usage of 6.6 liters in Finland was considered one of the highest indexes in Europe (Österberg, 1987).

State sales of alcohol combined with the consumption of unregistered alcoholic beverages meant that Russia was in the leading position in Europe in terms of its level of overall consumption. France, which had long been the world leader in this regard had seen a steady lowering of consumption through the 1960s (Fig. 1-2b), moved into second place (13.5 liters) behind Russia (14.2 liters) in this same year, while Portugal occupied third place (12.8 liters).

The third special characteristic of Russian consumption was the high share of total consumption attributable to hard liquor. In the early 1980s, without taking illegal production into consideration, this comprised more than half of all consumption (55.9 percent, 1984) and when illegal production was included amounted to about 70 percent. The percentage of hard liquor in Swedish consumption was 43 percent in 1984, while in the Federal Republic of Germany and the U.S. the figure was 31 percent.

For this brief overview of Russian alcohol consumption on the eve of the anti-alcohol campaign, it is essential to note the poor quality of alcoholic beverages in Russia, even though poor-quality fruit and berry wines (the legendary *bormotukha*) made up only a small portion, about 8 percent (1984), of overall consumption and production was falling (5.9 liters in 1980 and 4.8 liters in 1984; statistics from the State Statistical Committee of the RSFSR). But this does not reveal everything about the quality problem. A significant quantity of very poor and cheap port wines were hidden under the label "grape wines". But were these really grape wines? Such wine had been delivered from Algiers, but it was long past its due date for consumption and was sitting in Black Sea ports in tankers cleaned after their earlier use as oil carriers.

Against this background, can it be said that illegally produced alcohol was the chief trouble facing consumers? According to several estimates, small additions of fusel oils (polyatomic spirits – up to 0.5 percent of the volume) increased toxicity by one-quarter (Filatov, 1986). It should be noted, however, that this calculation, like many other estimates of the toxicity of illegal alcohol, was made during the anti-alcohol campaign, which saw an abundance of alcohol "scare stories". It has since been demonstrated that the toxicity of polyatomic spirits (the basic part of fusel oil) has the same toxicity as diatomic (grape or ethyl) alcohol, which constitutes 40 percent of the total volume of grape or ethyl alcohol, with cheap fusel oil providing no more than 1 percent (Nuzhny, 1995).

There was one more widely known but little studied sphere of consumption – the consumption of stolen alcohol. Except for thefts from medical and several others kinds of institution, this was mainly technical alcohol never intended for human consumption whose quality standards did not take possible human consumption into account. Thefts of alcohol in industry were an ordinary, widely occurring phenomenon. Kilometer-long queues formed for stolen *solntsedar* (a cheap and low quality fortified wine), whenever an oil tanker came into port in Odessa with this beverage. Less widely known, but possibly as meaningful in terms of volume, was the theft from rail cars filled with technical alcohol during delivery. This theft was exclusively of the technical alcohol, which contained high levels of iron oxides or, to put it simply, rust. These oxides, or the color they gave to the mixture, are the reason for the last 200 liters of alcohol from these rail cars being called *ryzhik*, or "red-head". At best, it would be filtered through the rolled-up sleeves of an old quilted cotton jacket into which the rail car funnel would be inserted. Again queues of residents from nearby villages would form ready with buckets for this alcohol, or even for the ryzhik, which sold for less.

Although I fear this section is becoming an ode to the "red-head", I must mention that these last 200 liters were, as a rule, to have been destroyed by the plant receiving the delivery. But Russians are not the kind of people who could throw out such a treasure!

Finally, one should note the massive problem of alcohol consumption in places prescribed for it. This is reflected in the sharp increase of the population at sobering-up stations (7.1 million persons in 1980, which was almost six times more than in 1960, during which time state sales of alcohol rose by 2.2 times). One must add to this the increasing consumption of alcohol in industry, often at the work place and during work (Zaigraev, 1992).

All this taken together – the very high level of alcohol consumption, the predominance of hard liquor, the significant quantities of illegal alcohol, the low quality of alcoholic beverages and their consumption in socially unacceptable places – was a product of the post-war Soviet epoch and was new to Russia. It had extremely unwelcome social, economic and medical effects. However, to gauge these consequences, data from the State Statistical Committee, which were declassified in 1988–1989, are of little help (Chapter 2-3). More important in this than the juggling done for political purposes with the final figures was the distortion of the original data at the level of the primary sources of information. For example, in 1984, according to the data of the State Statistical Committee of the Russian Federation, deaths from alcohol-induced cirrhosis of the liver comprised 6.1 percent of all deaths from cirrhosis of the liver. This is 8–12 times less than such figures in the rest of the world (Smart & Mann, 1992).

Another example: according to the data of the State Statistical Committee of the Russian Federation, deaths from alcohol-related accidents, poisonings and physical trauma made up 5.7 percent of all violent deaths; at the same time, the annual reports of provincial Bureaus of Legal-Medical Examiners showed that such causes accounted for approximately 60 percent of the total (1984). This discrepancy stems from the frequent failure of the alcohol-related portions of the diagnosis in the two documents prepared by the Bureau of Legal-Medical Examiners – the death and the autopsy certificates – to correspond with each other. The former document has a legal standing and, in case of an alcohol-related cause of death, can have negative social consequences. The second document remains in the Bureau archive. But it is the death certificate that was the source of information used by the State Statistical Committee (now known as Rosstat) in compiling its summary indexes on mortality.

In exactly the same way, the link between alcohol and other indicators of the social health of the population is partially hidden. High numbers for such measures as absenteeism, workplace injuries and criminal behavior hurt the interests of managers at various levels.

To sum up, the seriousness of the alcohol situation at the start of the 1980s cannot be fully estimated on the basis of official figures. But what was alarming then, even before the lifting of the secrecy surrounding measures of alcoholization: the enormous, 11-year difference in life expectancy in the RSFSR between men (61.7 years) and women (73 years, in 1984). Western researchers working on demographic problems in Russia often pointed to the link between this difference and alcohol. For purposes of comparison, the analogous difference for the European countries is 4–7 years.

Now much more is known of Russia's alcohol problems on the eve of the anti-alcohol campaign, and it is easier to explain the strange phenomenon of the differences in mortality between men and women. In 1984, according to figures from the Bureau of Legal-Medical Examiners, there were 95 deaths from external causes (in particular, violent deaths), per 100,000 of the population of persons found to have been inebriated (Chapter 2-5). The overwhelming majority of these were men. By comparison, in Finland the figure was under 30 per 100,000.

Alcohol-related losses were not tallied in the post-war years, but many other indexes were disturbing to the Soviet leadership. This is evidenced by the anti-alcohol resolutions of 1958 and 1972. The latter was particularly stringent: stepped-up administrative measures, higher prices for vodka, a ban on alcohol sales before 11 a.m. on workdays and a ban on Sunday sales. The early 1960s saw the opening of the first Curative-Labor Dispensaries for the treatment of alcoholics. The dispensaries were given legal standing by a decree of the Presidium of the Supreme Court of the RSFSR (1974) that called for alcoholics found to have disturbed the social order to be sent to the dispensaries by court order (about 150,000 alcoholics were held in the dispensaries in the early 1980s).

In 1976 a special narcological service for the treatment of alcoholics and drug addicts was finally created in the USSR. Before then, such persons had been treated by psychiatric institutions. The year 1976 also saw the organization of an intensive-care service, part of whose mission was to save people suffering from alcohol-related poisoning.

Like all Soviet health services, the narcological service was organized on a territorial-hierarchical principle. Its basic functional unit was the district or inter-district health center, to which patients were assigned to district drug specialists (from 700–800 to 1,500 patients per doctor). Physician-attended and medical-assistant attended narcological stations in outlying areas and at large factories were subordinate to the health centers. In 1984, the health centers of the USSR had on their books 4.3 million alcoholics (2.8 million in the RSFSR); the number of uncounted alcoholics in the country was 2–3 times greater.

The beginning-stage treatment and subsequent periodic observation over the course of five years (after 1988, three years) was obligatory for all patients registered with the health centers. In cases that did not respond, or where there was a deepening of the alcoholism to alcohol psychosis, patients were held at in-patient facilities at the centers in psychiatric hospitals. A great many patients were treated at in-patient facilities created by factories desirous of having a cheap source of labor at hand.

In view of the wide spectrum of alcohol problems in the country, the mission of the narcological service was confined to dealing with the narrow task of treating alcoholism and, to some extent, in preventive efforts. But accomplishment of this limited task was narrowed exclusively to medical means. The more important social and psychological jobs that needed doing were not dealt with, nor were allowances made for their pursuit from the outset. However, the creation of the new service at that time (1976) is testimony to the heroism of its creators as well as to the fact that the Soviet government, under the pressure of real and urgent problems, had begun to give way on some of its harsh ideological positions.

In the course of eight years of work by the health centers, the number of alcoholics on record in the RSFSR doubled (90 per 10,000 of the population in 1976 and 183.9 in 1984; Galkin, 1988), as did the number of alcoholics treated annually in the hospitals (15.1 versus 31.2 per 100,000 over the course of the period). The number of patients registered with alcohol psychosis (54.6 per 100,000 in 1976 versus 35.4 in 1984) and the number of new cases (24.8 per 100,000 versus 20.4) began to decline in 1977.

All this relates to the medical aspects of the problem. But the alcohol situation, overall, changed little: state sales were 10.4 liters per capita in 1977 and 10.5 liters per capita in 1984. In part, this is explained by the fact that, after the creation of the narcological service, local responsibility for almost all alcohol-related problems was given to it, although it was extremely limited in what it could do. The Soviet bureaucracy, aided by the narcological service, shielded itself for several years from the serious and ever increasing alcohol-related problems of the country.

But there was also another barrier to dealing with the alcohol-consumption problem. From the early 1980s, the government found itself caught in an "alcohol vice". On the one hand, it was under pressure from the very high level of alcohol consumption and its serious consequences, which were lowering the country's economic potential. The USSR's direct costs attributable to alcohol have been estimated at 120–150 billion rubles, with indirect costs possibly even greater. On the other hand, alcohol contributed 12–16 percent of budgeted revenues (approximately 50 billion rubles from a total of 300 billion). Some data suggest that these revenues were even higher. Moreover, the USSR had major, long-term commitments to its East European satellites for purchases of their alcoholic products. By 1985, such imports totaled 650 million rubles as compared with 77 million rubles of exports.

All this made the alcohol situation of the country a very difficult problem. How did the new leadership, headed by Gorbachev, deal with it?

Chapter 1-4
The anti-alcohol campaign of 1985

In their official declarations, the leaders of the USSR averred that the anti-alcohol campaign of 1985 was a reaction to the seriousness of the country's alcohol problems. These declarations notwithstanding, the campaign had another, more profound economic and social context and a prehistory of some two decades that throws light on it. The voluntary nature of the campaign's beginning was merely the outward sign of that.

High rates of increase in Gross National Product were characteristic of the post-war period in the USSR, as is often the case with countries with half-ruined economies. That record of growth spurred Nikita Khrushchev's slogan, "To catch up with and pass America". However, the period of reconstruction ended in the mid-1960s, and the rates of GNP growth fell sharply, and the second post-war consumer crisis began (the first occurred immediately after the war). Among the everyday phenomena reflecting the new crisis were the so-called "sausage trains" – people from outlying parts of the country traveling by train to buy food in cities with special allocations of foodstuffs, including, for example, Moscow, Leningrad and Kiev.

The crisis was one of the reasons for the removal of Khrushchev as general secretary and the first "perestroika", which can be called "the Kosygin-perestroika" (Kosygin was chairman of the USSR Council of Ministers from 1964–1980) was an attempt to overcome it. This perestroika was quickly choked as a result of opposition from Communist Party professionals, who would have lost some of their control over the economic leadership of the country as a result of the reforms. The Kosygin perestroika also failed to be realized because the national crisis was overcome in the course of a few years due to the sharp increase in world oil prices after 1973 and the world oil crisis. For the USSR, the oil crisis became a tide of petroleum dollars.

However, in the late 1960s the industrially developed countries of the West and Japan had begun a scientific-technical revolution and transition to a postindustrial society which was brought fully into being in the 1970s. As one aspect of this process, by the start of the 1980s the Western countries had modernized and rebuilt their economies, making them more fuel-efficient and thus overcoming the oil crisis. There were more general preconditions in place for this, specifically, a new organization of the world market on the basis of rules that favored countries developing science-heavy production and unfavorable for countries where natural-resource production predominated.

The highest prices for oil were reached in 1980, after which they fell rapidly and, within two or three years, they were at a level below the actual Soviet cost of production. The influx of petroleum dollars ceased, and again a consumer crisis was in the making.

In conditions of isolation from the world economy, and to prevent a new crisis, the leadership placed its bets on internal resources, on raising the productivity of labor. The brief, 15-month reign of Yury Andropov (November 1982–February 1984) featured a number of steps in this direction. On the one hand, there was an experiment, the so-called *khozraschet*, or relative enterprise independence, in a single narrow sector of the military-industrial complex (material motivation for labor); on the other hand, workers found not at work during working hours were picked up by the police with the idea that fear would "tie" them to their jobs (police methods as motivation for work).

Andropov also tried to use fear to overcome the corruption of the Soviet ruling elite. The most widely publicized of these efforts was the investigative work done by a group under the command of Telman Gdlyan and Nikolaj Ivanov that resulted in most of the leaders of the Uzbek Soviet Social Republic being put in prison. Such police methods, Andropov reasoned, should be the primary methods for imposing iron discipline in the country, from bottom to top, including members of the Politburo of the CPSU. Andropov's agency (the KGB) had long been compiling material on the latter's corruption.

This was one general side of the matter. The other was that the leadership of the country was beginning to acknowledge the dismal condition of the Soviet system and was seeking ways to reform it. To deal with this task, in 1983, on Andropov's initiative, a group of Soviet academics (Abalkin and others) was called together to work under the new, young Central Committee of the CPSU secretaries, Gorbachev and Ryzhkov. For the same purpose, there was a seminar that year of young economists (Gaidar and others). Unfortunately, neither the committee's nor the seminar's "brainstorming" reached the conclusion that it was impossible to reform the unreformable.

Andropov saw a great opportunity to increase the productivity of labor and energize the economy in a sobering up of the nation. Early in 1982 while still KGB chairman Andropov had sent a memorandum to the members of the Politburo of the CPSU on the necessity of adopting a resolution on strengthening the struggle with drunkenness. The Politburo quickly responded by creating a commission under A. Pelshe, who enlisted a number of young and well-versed economists to help prepare a draft resolution.

The draft declared that administrative and punitive measures would not be able to get to the roots of the drunkenness problem. Rather, what was needed was a long-term, systematic effort. As regards the first steps to be taken, it called for an increase in the production of dry wines and beer, a widening of the network of cafes and other enterprises where alcoholic beverages were sold by the glass, and some enterprises of this type quietly began to be opened even before the adoption of the resolution. This liberal draft was soon presented to the Politburo, but it was not destined to be realized: in November 1982 Brezhnev died, as did Pelshe in 1983. Solomentsev subsequently became the head of the commission for anti-alcohol legislation and he also inherited Pelshe's more important post, as chairman of the Central Committee of the CPSU's party control commission. As the new head of the two commissions, with an eye toward the new general secretary Andropov's determination to strengthen discipline in the country, he moved towards a line of harsher measures against drunkenness. At the same time, Andropov sanctioned sales of cheaper vodka, a move very likely taken as a way of making the anti-alcohol measures more acceptable. The new vodka was popularly dubbed "Andropovka" or "*shkolnitsa*" ("schoolgirl"). It went on sale from 1 September. The first draft of Pelshe's anti-alcohol resolution was amended fundamentally to include more stringent anti-alcohol measures. However, the deaths of two leaders in quick succession – Yury Andropov in February 1984 and Konstantin Chernenko in March 1985 – delayed the adoption and realization of the plan.

Less than two months passed between the plenary session of the CPSU Central Committee that elected Gorbachev as general secretary (11 March, 1985) and the adoption of the resolution, "On Measures to Overcome Drunkenness and Alcoholism" by the Central Committee (7 May, 1985). The resolution was the first widely publicized declaration of the new leadership of the country headed by Gorbachev. Why did this leadership begin its work with the anti-alcohol resolution?

It cannot be said that the CPSU Central Committee was of one mind about this decision. Referring to the Georgian practice of making samogon with the left over products from wine production (*chacha*), Shevarnadze spoke against the section of the resolution on samogon. Other participants in the session also sought to soften particular, especially harsh, formulations in the resolution (Politburo member and first vice chairman of the Council of Ministers Aliyev, Politburo member and chairman of the Council of Ministers of the RSFSR Vorotnikov, CPSU Central Committee secretaries Kapitonov and Nikonov). A decided opponent of the resolution in toto was the chairman of the USSR Council of Ministers Ryzhkov, who had just become a member of the Politburo of the CPSU Central Committee. He predicted a sharp rise in illegal alcohol production, breakdowns in sugar supplies, the rationing of sugar and, of greatest importance, a lowering of budgeted revenues. However, all these objections were swept away by the demagogic arguments of Ligachev and Solomentsev, who became the chief and most impassioned defenders of the resolution during the Politburo session. One of their arguments was that the anti-alcohol campaign was needed to halt drunkenness among the leadership layer of the party. In the end, they swayed Gorbachev to join their side.

Ten years after the start of the anti-alcohol campaign and on the occasion of its anniversary, Gorbachev gave an interview to Radio Liberty. The former general secretary explained that the launching of the campaign had been necessary because "they had made the country drunk as a way to solve budget problems" and expressed grief that "consumption of alcohol had reached 10.3 liters per person, including children and old people". But the general secretary might have had access to the secret data of the Soviet State Statistical Committee on the actual consumption of alcohol, including illegal alcohol, showing consumption of 13.8 liters. Gorbachev asserted that the "resolution was moderate" and that "later people, fearful of losing their portfolios and chairs", showed "real bolshevism at the stage of execution".

This "bolshevism" was not only under the control of the general secretary but was ardently supported by him in many of his appearances on television. The rise of Gorbachev's career had been dizzying. It cannot be excluded though that in his first few months as leader of the CPSU Central Committee, Gorbachev felt the weakness of his hold on power, but understood the necessity for change in the country. For that, however, Gorbachev lacked the levers of influence needed in the party apparatus. He sought a soft way of reining in the party's conservative bloc of nomenklatura, or holders of key Soviet posts. He looked to those who had begun to strengthen their positions as early as in the last years of Stalin's rule and who had "brought down" Khrushchev for encroaching on their powers and material privileges. It is possible that Gorbachev's support for the campaign was a "shot at the staffers" (Mao Tse-tung), a message to the Politburo nomenclature that there was more irritation awaiting them after Andropov.

The special political status of the anti-alcohol resolution and the haste and scale of its implementation made clear that the new leadership under Gorbachev had come to power without new ideas and had decided to continue and even further develop Andropov's line, i.e. stepped-up discipline in the country as a basis for hastening the triumph over the Brezhnev stagnation and for creating the economic preconditions for postindustrial development. The anti-alcohol campaign was part of a "speeding up made possible by the human factor" without changes in the political and social sphere. Another part of this political line was a resolution on the struggle with non-labor income, with personal garden plots used as a source of income. Essentially, the Gorbachev-era's "speeding up" was a large-scale and harsh attack on the limited rights of the citizenry, which had been slightly expanded during the Khrushchev "thaw". It is worth recalling how in 1985–1986, volunteer police used crowbars to destroy private forcing frames and greenhouses and how bulldozers cut the houses built on garden plots back down to standard size. There were also campaigns against speculation and prostitution, and dissidents continued to be "sat down", or jailed. All these were signs of a return to the mobilizing the masses style of rule that was characteristic of the Soviet system. The anti-alcohol campaign of 1985 was the noisiest and rowdiest of them all. Unfortunately, it was also the most consistent and in this lies one reason for its "head-spinning success".

In 1987 it became clear that the "speeding up" of the country's development had failed, that the "stagnation" had deeper roots in the political and social spheres. And Gorbachev began to shift course, from "speeding-up" to "perestroika and glasnost" (reconstruction and openness about information). That was the real beginning of a policy aimed at a transition to an information-based, postindustrial society. Democratization and glasnost, freedom of speech, was needed for this. It also meant reducing the power of the party apparatus, strengthening the power of the Soviets and changing the system of elections to the Soviets. On his "pair of steeds", perestroika and glasnost, Gorbachev made his entrance into world politics, throwing the rich West presents from his poor land as a way of improving the image of his country and raising his own prestige. The gifts were accepted with gratitude but without economic benefits for the USSR. Gorbachev snuggled up to Margaret Thatcher and Helmut Kohl and other Western leaders. That was the outer field. On the inner one, there was growing impoverishment, inflation, a looming consumer-goods crisis and a plundering of the country that, as the collapse of the USSR neared, became wider in scale and higher in intensity. The general secretary had to find a balance between various groupings of the Soviet bureaucracy while also "hiding" party funds and property. All of this required enormous effort, and he could no longer tend to the anti-alcohol campaign, which quietly died, although the level of alcohol consumption was fast approaching the level of 1984. But this no longer bothered the general secretary.

Of course, it is necessary to remember that not just the name, but also the activity of Gorbachev is connected with a decisive turn in the history of the Russian state, the positive fruits of which we continue to harvest, although in a seriously reduced form. However, radical changes in the country and Russia's acquisition of a new international status began only after a series of mistaken moves. Chief among them was the neglect of economic reforms in favor of political reforms. This was completed with a change of system and the dissolution of the USSR. But the first mistaken step was the anti-alcohol campaign of 1985, which left a negative impression on the popular consciousness that continued throughout the reign of Gorbachev, who was known to the ordinary citizen as "Lemonade Joe" and the "mineral-water secretary". The anti-alcohol campaign in conjunction with other factors led to the general secretary's loss of the support among most of the citizenry. In part, this was why popular sympathies so easily and quickly shifted from Gorbachev, a truly democratic but naive politician, to another leader, Boris Yeltsin, who was soon to unleash the chaos of "free prices" on the people, deprive them of their savings, become the leader of the Russian "private-seizers" and one of the post-Soviet *turkmenbashi* (a kind of feudal ruler). Indeed, by the time of the August 1991 putsch there were few in the country who felt any sympathy for the "drowning" first and last president of the USSR.

However, it would be wrong to lay the blame for Gorbachev's loss of popular sympathy entirely on one of his personal mistakes – the anti-alcohol campaign. It can be looked at in a wider context, at perestroika as a whole, and to conclude with the words of Gorbachev himself: "The new model was defeated... by the level of culture of the people, by the level of its mind-set. It was rejected by the people. That was the reason for the defeat" (Gorbachev, 1995).

However, let us turn from Gorbachev himself, who gave his name to the anti-alcohol campaign, to the campaign itself and its successful beginning. Only three weeks lay between the resolution of the CPSU Central Committee and the start of the campaign (1 June, 1985), a time devoted to the preparation of the mass, all-Union action, which would have far-reaching consequences. As Yeltsin later declared (1990), such "haste in implementing the resolution, the absence of a scientific workup and the arbitrary character of the decision were witness to the extraordinary personal ambitions of the two initiators of the campaign". I would like to add here that the situation was made much worse by their incompetence. As the saying goes, these people had much ambition but little ammunition. They were the members of the Politburo of the CPSU Central Committee, Ligachev and Solomentsev. It was they who were fiercely active in bringing the campaign to fever pitch, for which they mobilized the bodies of which they were principals, the Secretariat of the CPSU Central Committee (Ligachev) and the Party Control Commission of the CPSU Central Committee (Solomentsev) as well as the entire professional staff of the CPSU. It was these two men who gave the campaign its harsh, sometimes grotesque and at times, sinister form under the slogan "making healthy the moral atmosphere of the country". Under the pressure exerted by Ligachev and Solomentsev, secretaries of district and provincial committees vied with each other to see who could close the largest number of wine-vodka stores, and who could more quickly convert alcohol producers to soda producers. They unearthed even the most "extreme" things imaginable: As a result of its investigations, the Party Control Commission of the CPSU Central Committee revealed deficiencies in the anti-alcohol work of the USSR Ministry of Health, the central agency in the effort to bring the populace to sobriety. Specifically, one of the managers of the USSR Ministry of Health was accused of calling for "sensible moderation" and "a culture of consumption" of alcoholic beverages before the campaign had even started. For this, he was given a severe party reprimand and removed from his position. A new imprecation was then born in the press: "cultural drinker" (*kulturopitejshchik*).

According to the original plan there was to be an 11 percent reduction in the sales of alcoholic beverages each year (this was the number, not anything higher, defended by Aliev), that would have led, in the space of six years, to a 50 percent decrease in government revenues from the alcohol trade. At the same time, it was assumed that the significant losses to the budget would be made up automatically through "the greater healthiness [meaning 'sobriety', author's comment] of workers in industry" as well as in connection with the increased output of consumer goods.

The basic intention of the anti-alcohol campaign in 1985 was a lowering of alcohol consumption through a reduction in the state production of alcohol and state sale of alcoholic beverages. It was also considered important to root out the illegal production of alcoholic beverages (samogon). Somewhat later, in August 1985, prices were raised, including a 25 percent increase in the price of vodka, while in August 1986, there was a further, sharp increase in the cost of alcohol. In parallel with these measures, the network of institutions for treating alcoholism was widened. By a decree of the Presidium of the USSR Supreme Court dated 1 October, 1985, the network of Health Centers (LTP) was widened, as were the criteria for directing patients to these facilities (in October 1990 the Committee for Constitutional Monitoring found this decree to be in violation of human rights and set it aside). In addition to the Health Centers, a wide network of hospitals at large industrial plants was created for those ill with alcoholism. These hospitals were called upon to combine treatment with work at the factories, which thereby gained a source of cheap, if not trained, labor. However, because of the labor provision, these hospitals had minimal health effects; their treatment tasks were subordinate to, and ultimately supplanted by their industrial tasks, specifically, as a result of the night shifts assigned to patients.

The All-Union Sobriety Society had a similar, merely formalistic character. The newly created "alcohol commissions" organized at district soviets and factories were a sham.

In other words, the anti-alcohol campaign was directed at just a few of the more obvious aspects of the alcohol situation (Fig. 1-1): at alcohol consumption, the production of alcoholic beverages and their prices. In no way did the campaign address the fundamental aspects of the situation; the human needs driving it (Chapter 2-1). The attempt to combat the boredom felt in Soviet society through the construction of several hundred sports complexes and movie theaters across the country, many of which were never completed, was insulting. Other such demagoguery was used in large quantities to give ideological support to the campaign, for example, frequent reference was made to Lenin's "dry" decree of 1919. And this took place against a background of yet another noisy campaign in the mass media on "returning to Lenin and unblemished Leninism".

Western Sovietologists were of one mind in regarding the Soviet leadership as having failed to achieve its anti-alcohol aims. Treml, the author of *Alcohol in the USSR* (1982), wrote in 1985 about the recently launched campaign: "Crude pressure and fear of punishment will not be effective ... the nation will begin to produce alcohol underground" (Treml, 1985). Naturally, neither Treml's warning nor the cautious statements voiced by a few Soviet researchers (they did exist) were heeded by the leadership of the country. The campaign was launched and quickly picked up momentum.

The concrete anti-alcohol activities of the Soviet authorities consisted of a partial closing or re-profiling of alcohol-related plants and factories producing containers. Equipment for the construction of eight beer-producing factories, just purchased from Czechoslovakia, ended up almost entirely as scrap metal. Plantations for the cultivation of hops were reduced in number, as was the sowing of a type of special barley used to produce malt for beer. The acreage given over to wine-producing grapes was reduced by one-third, and several types of unique wine grapes developed in the USSR were killed off.

By 1987 in the RSFSR, the network of shops that sold alcohol had been reduced by 80 percent (in Moscow by 90 percent), and the time of sale of alcoholic beverages had been sharply cut (at first, sales were allowed after 2 p.m.). The reduction in the sale of alcoholic beverages also exceeded the plan, and the losses to the treasury amounted to 5.4 billion rubles in 1987, of which 2.4 billion were compensated for by the increased production of consumer goods (Materials of the Commission for the Struggle with Drunkenness of the RSFSR Council of Ministers, 1988). It needs to be noted that all this took place against a background of sharply reduced state revenues because of the low prices for oil in the world market.

Overall, in Russia in 1987, the "consumption of alcohol from government sources" was reduced by 63.5 percent, as compared to 1984 (Table 1), which was substantially more than the planned rate for the reduction in alcohol consumption (11 percent a year or 25 percent in 1987).

Despite such results, no dizziness from the successes ensued: the lines for alcohol at the few remaining specialized stores had sharply increased and now involved hours of waiting, often overnight. Speculative trading in alcoholic beverages also began. To cover the lost but budgeted revenue, the government was forced to increase the sales of expensive beverages – champagne and cognac. In Moscow, for example, sales of these beverages began to be allowed as early as September 1985.

The main problem, however, lay in the sharp increase in the production and consumption of samogon. This can be seen in the calculations presented in Chapters 2-4, as well as in the identical data of the Russian State Statistical Committee and Treml (Table 1). And this occurred despite the fact that, at the outset of the campaign, a significant portion of illegal distilling equipment was confiscated by the militia or voluntarily given up by the citizenry. Indeed, in some areas of Russia, the number of destroyed sets of apparatus was almost equal to the number of homes in the villages (*Izvestiya*, 22 October, 1985). The increase in the production of samogon also occurred despite the fact that the number of persons arrested for illegally producing alcohol had almost doubled every year since 1984, reaching a total of 397,000 persons in 1987 (414,000 in 1988). The total number of violators of anti-alcohol laws and administrative rules exceeded 10 million individuals in 1987.

However, 1987 also marked the turning point in the anti-alcohol campaign. Decisive in this was the budget deficit, which could not be rectified by either the printing of more money or by sales of gold. The government's debt, both internal and external, rose sharply. The country began to encounter difficulties in paying wages, a matter of sacred importance for the Soviet authorities. In addition, 1987 saw a shift in government policy from "speed-up" to "perestroika", means for the realization of which, as for the speed-up, were lacking. This year, too, saw the start of a general increase in alcohol consumption due to a headlong rise in illegal alcohol production, a rise in consumption that was known to the State Statistical Committee of the Russian Federation and, also possibly, to the government.

In 1987, Vorotnikov, chairman of the RSFSR Council of Ministers, sent a memorandum to the Politburo of the CPSU Central Committee on the mistakenness of the methods used to conduct the anti-alcohol campaign. In its discussion of the memorandum, the Politburo decided to give responsibility for deciding the fate of the campaign to the Council of Ministers of the USSR, which at the proposal of its chairman, N. I. Ryzhkov, ordered an increase in the state production and sale of alcohol products beginning on 1 January, 1988. Even earlier, in July 1987, criminal liability for the preparation of surrogate alcoholic beverages without intent to sell was reduced to administrative culpability, and on October 25, 1988, there was a new resolution issued by the CPSU Central Committee "On the Way of Implementing the CPSU Central Committee's Resolution on the Question of Strengthening the Struggle with Drunkenness and Alcoholism", which essentially marked the end of the anti-alcohol campaign, although a few things that it had set in motion continued to resonate for a year or two after.

Some historical recollections may be of some interest at this point. The first resolution (7 May, 1985) contained all the basic articles of the decree of 29 January, 1929, on the struggle with drunkenness and alcoholism; the second (25 October, 1988) used as its model the famous article, "Dizzy with Success" (2 March, 1930; on "Excesses and Perversions in the Struggle with the Kulachestvo" [rich peasants]). Before its fall, the Soviet state was forced to repeat the tactics of its early history.

Chapter 1-5
Consequences of the anti-alcohol campaign

Despite the brevity of the campaign, it was a major shock for the country and affected many aspects of government and ordinary life. The avidity with which party organs, the militia and other power structures took up the anti-alcohol drive had serious moral costs. The prestige of the government had fallen lower than ever since the end of the war. Measures to combat drunkenness were enforced. This became a conflict within the Soviet citizenry. The moral costs were also increased because neither of the warring factions saw the point of the conflict. A militia officer, pouring some confiscated samogon down the drain, like the arrested brewer-culprit, regretted the destruction of so desirable a product. A significant part of the population, possibly a majority, opposed the government's anti-alcohol measures, which ignored a fundamental law of politics, that any reform must find its support in the psychology of people and take into account their basic values and motivations.

The main characteristic of the campaign was the heedless velocity at which government sales of alcoholic beverages were cut back (by 63.5 percent in 2.5 years, that is, by 25 percent a year). At approximately the same time (in 1986), the government of the Netherlands, disturbed at the high level of alcohol consumption in the country (8.9 liters in 1980) and after thorough preparation, introduced a new policy on alcohol (van Ginneken & van Iwaarden, 1989) that also may be termed an anti-alcohol campaign. Its main content was the dissemination of anti-alcohol information to the public through the mass media. There was also a large program of research. The result was a lowering of consumption after three years by 6 percent (that is, 2 percent a year, Engelsman, 1990). This figure was seen as being profoundly positive.

For the USSR as a whole, the result of the sharp drop in state sales of alcoholic beverages was a loss of 49 billion rubles in budgeted state revenue in 1985–1987 (*Pravda*, 24 January, 1989); for the RSFSR in 1987 alone, the budget shortfall came to 5.3 billion rubles, in prices of that time (Materials of the Commission for the Struggle with Drunkenness of the RSFSR Council of Ministers).

A significant part of this money made its way into the pockets of underground producers and sellers of samogon, the consumption of which had almost doubled by 1987 (Table 1). The government was unable to provide consumer goods to attract the money from the lost alcohol revenue. In the USSR 1985–1987, the revenue obtained from consumer goods was 40 billion rubles less than planned and 5.6 billion rubles short in paid services. This unspent money by the public began to exert pressure on the consumer goods market, which was the anti-alcohol campaign's contribution to the depreciation of the ruble and the exacerbation of inflation.

By 1985 the technical base of the wine and vodka industry was outdated. As a result of the campaign, the rates at which it was being updated – already the lowest in the food industry – fell by more than half. The anti-alcohol campaign reoriented the nation's viticulture to growing table grapes at the expense of the technical grapes that go into the making of wine. Acreage for these types of grapes fell by 29 percent, and government purchases of them fell by 31 percent. The sharp decrease in the production of alcoholic beverages was accompanied by a reduction in the production of the bottles needed for wine and vodka products (by about two-thirds) and for beer (by one-third). Many glass factories were re-assigned to produce bottles for other purposes.

Samogon distilling was not only "not liquidated", as the initiators of the campaign presumed, but significantly widened. In 1990 alone, as calculated by the State Statistical Committee of the USSR, such alcohol production diverted approximately one million tons of sugar (3.6 kilograms per capita) from other food uses. Home-based alcohol-beverage production seamlessly grew into an underground vodka industry. As a result of the campaign, speculative trading in alcoholic beverages and their illegal production rose to such a level that it enabled the first all-Union school of market relationships to form and to lay the basis for the contemporary alcohol-related criminal structures and the powerful capital accumulations of the "vodka kings". Indeed, by the time the market reforms started, as a result of the anti-alcohol campaign, an infrastructure of illegal production of alcohol and a market in alcohol products had formed which covered the whole of the Soviet Union. As a result this infrastructure stood poised to take advantage of the new market relationships perhaps more so than any other actor.

The Narcological Service, which had been created in 1976, was more alive to the needs created by the introduction of the alcohol campaign than other government agencies. The campaign breathed new life into this branch of medicine: the number of narcological health centers in the USSR increased by 3.5 times in the course of four years and by 4.3 times in the RSFSR. More than 75,000 beds for those suffering from alcoholism were made available in new narcological institutions, attached to industrial and agricultural enterprises. This obviously excessive number of beds was filled, often by force, by patients who then became common laborers in these enterprises. Forty percent of the patients' earnings went towards their treatment. Work schedules though, which included night shifts, were often not compatible with treatment schedules meaning in many cases treatment was not received.

The ranks of the narcological service had been quickly filled by physicians, most of whom had no special narcological training. Up to the start of the campaign, their retraining had been slow. Thanks to the anti-alcohol campaign, the qualifications of physicians and other medical personnel sharply improved; narcological knowledge spread through the entire medical system. As a result of the campaign, the qualifications of practicing narcologists, overall, rose.

This cannot be said about scientific narcology. Unlike the practical service, the science of alcohology at the start of the campaign was in a dire state due to its ideological direction and political limitations. Soviet scientific narcology amounted to two or three dozen specialists, mostly clinicians, scattered in small groups in three or four institutions in Moscow and a few of the other large cities of the Soviet Union. The closed V. P. Serbsky Institute of Forensic Psychiatry had a department of narcology which largely concerned itself with the biological problems of alcoholism. The social and other aspects of heavy drinking and alcoholism remained virtually closed to research. The rare narcological publications of this kind were, for the most part, stamped "for service use" or were treated as top secret.

At the beginning of the campaign, in 1985, the only existing department of narcology was reconstituted as the Center for Narcology for the entire Soviet Union. However, organizational disarray and a mistaken direction with regard to its aims hindered the start of systematic work at the center for several more years. In addition to the Center for Narcology, several laboratories and small departments were created in the country.

Thus, somewhat strengthened, Soviet alcohology continued to follow in its general footsteps – the study of the problems of alcoholism, which hardly exhausted all the problems connected with alcohol. Thus, by the early 1970s, at the behest of the World Health Organization, world alcohology had taken a considerable turn away from the problems of alcoholism to "the problems connected with consumption of alcohol" (Room, 1984). One could mention here that the National Institute of Alcohol Abuse and Alcoholism was created in the United States in 1970. By 1985 it had become a major, world-class research center.

Despite the creation of a "single goal-directed complex program", almost nothing was done in terms of studying and quantifying the alcohol situation in the country or forecasting the immediate future. Thus, the campaign left no noticeable trace in the scientific sphere, despite the forced enlistment into the campaign of a large number of general research institutions and an increase in the number of publications in the field of alcohology (Chapter 2-3). On the whole, the great possibilities offered by the sort of "experiment" that the anti-alcohol campaign represented, were missed.

In contrast, the anti-alcohol campaign did bring about significant demographic changes. As early as in June 1985, the campaign's first month (Andreev, 2002), a substantial lowering of the mortality of men was noted and consequently an increase in male life expectancy, which by 1987 had increased by 3.2 years for men (by 5.2 percent) and 1.3 years for women (by 1.8 percent), reaching 64.9 years and 74.3 years, respectively (Chapter 2-5). The anti-alcohol campaign in Russia saved the lives of more than 1 million individuals (Chapter 2-5). This was the main positive outcome of the campaign.

As a result of the anti-alcohol measures, not only mortality but also morbidity, in particular that related to alcohol consumption, decreased. For example, in 1987 the incidence of alcohol psychoses in the RSFSR fell by three quarters compared to 1984. This fact shreds the widely held and firmly entrenched myth that, during the campaign and despite the significant lowering of average consumption, "alcoholics drank as they always drink". But that was not so. Alcohol psychosis only affects alcoholics, and if the number of psychosis cases fell, there had to have been a drop in alcohol consumption by alcoholics. This was mostly the case with those who were ill and relatively protected – both clinically and socially (Vorobyev & Khudyakov, 1988).

The mass anti-alcohol propaganda campaign, on which much was spent, had little influence on the attitude of Russians toward alcohol, whether among those sick with alcoholism or among half of all healthy men, whose critical attitude towards the abuse of alcohol remained "laughably low" (Morozov, 1988).

One might have thought that, having for the first time in 20 years raised life expectancies and reduced mortality, the campaign would again have demonstrated the dangers of heavy drinking. There was less vandalism and criminal drunkenness. But the lesson fell on deaf ears. For the public, the compulsory nature of the campaign, and the violent methods used in carrying it out, had a far greater impact. This significantly narrowed the psychological and social support for the idea of the campaign, which was that excess consumption of alcoholic beverages is as great an evil for the individual as it is for society. The failure of the campaign's struggle with illegal alcohol production also worked to reduce the number of people with anti-alcohol views. Above all, what the authorities failed to learn from the campaign was that alcoholic beverages and their consumption in the company of others is a part of the culture not only of Russian society but, more broadly, of contemporary society, which has a need for alcohol (Chapter 2-1). And needs cannot be changed by declarations, and certainly not in short order. This is why the anti-alcohol campaign did not liberate Russian life from its alcohol problems.

In discussing the consequences of the anti-alcohol campaign, it seems appropriate to consider the popular view that the campaign brought on Russia's epidemic of drug abuse, drug addiction and the drug trade, or narco-business. However, the increase in drug addicts in Russia began several years before 1985 and took place as a result of the influence of other factors, both domestic and international.

These factors were largely linked to the saturation of the American market with drugs in the 1970s. As a result, the international narco-business began to infiltrate the Western European market and develop new routes for supplying it from Central Asia. An additional stimulus in this direction was a temporary closing down of two of the world's three "golden triangles", or principal regions, of drug production and the narco-business: the Colombian (Colombia, Peru and Bolivia) and the Thai triangle. As a result, the third "triangle" of Pakistan, Iran and Afghanistan stepped up its activities. The USSR was chosen as a transit territory for moving its drugs. The poor technical equipment possessed by the Soviet customs service and its unpreparedness to find freight of this kind were among the reasons for choosing this path. Thus, drugs camouflaged as innocent cargo easily passed through Russian borders. However, the soil on which all forms of narco-business, including the transportation of drugs, feeds is the drug addict or abuser.

The war in Afghanistan had great significance for the rise of drug addiction in Russia (it began in December 1979). That was followed then in time by the openness of the Afghan-Tadzhik border, the narco-business pursued by the Tadzhik opposition and, mainly, the factory production of narcotics that was perfected in Afghanistan by the Taliban, who dealt harshly with private narco-business. Afghanistan became one of the main sources of opiates for the markets in Russia. At virtually the same time, Iran began imposing a very tough policy on drugs. This had the effect of eliminating it as a member of the third "golden triangle" and cutting it off as one of the main routes for transporting drugs to the West. All this led to the formation of a new, powerful "triangle" (Pakistan, Afghanistan and Tadzhikistan-Gorny Badakhshan). The new route for transporting drugs across the countries of the Commonwealth of Independent States (CIS) was widened and consolidated. There were also other, internal, factors for the rise in drug abuse in the USSR in the period before the start of the anti-alcohol campaign.

The anti-alcohol campaign triggered a rise in drug addiction in Russia but almost exclusively in the form of the abuse of medicines, which began to decline with the increase in the consumption of alcohol (Luzhnikov et al., 1989; Fig. 1-5). However, drug-related problems widened steadily, continuing the tendencies that had arisen before the start of the campaign. Since the early 1990s, drug addiction has itself become a major problem in Russia.

That said, it is necessary to keep in mind that, overall, the problems associated with drugs are in no way comparable in scope with those associated with alcohol. Some examples may be offered as illustrations. First, deaths from external causes, including violence, during alcoholic versus drug intoxication comprise 52.3 percent compared to 0.1 percent, respectively. Second, deaths from alcohol poisoning versus deaths from drug overdoses: more than 40,000 compared to 3,500 (2004). Finally, the number of persons registered as having alcohol problems far exceeds the number registered as having drug-related problems (Fig. 1-6). Even if we allow for the greater secrecy surrounding drug addiction, these numbers indirectly reflect the seriousness of problems related to alcohol consumption and of illicit drug use in Russia.

Fig. 1-5: Number of registered drug addicts in Russia (1985–2000). 1 – the total number of registered, 2 – new registered (source: State Statistical Committee of the Russian Federation).

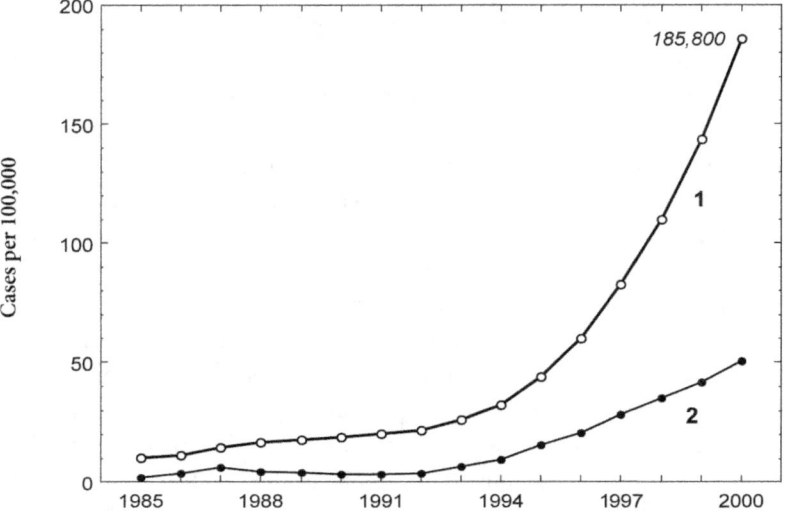

Fig. 1-6: Number registered with chronic alcoholism + alcohol psychosis + alcohol abuse (A), drug addiction + toxicomania + consumers of narcotic and psychoactive substances (D); (1991–1999) (source: Koshkina et al., 2000).

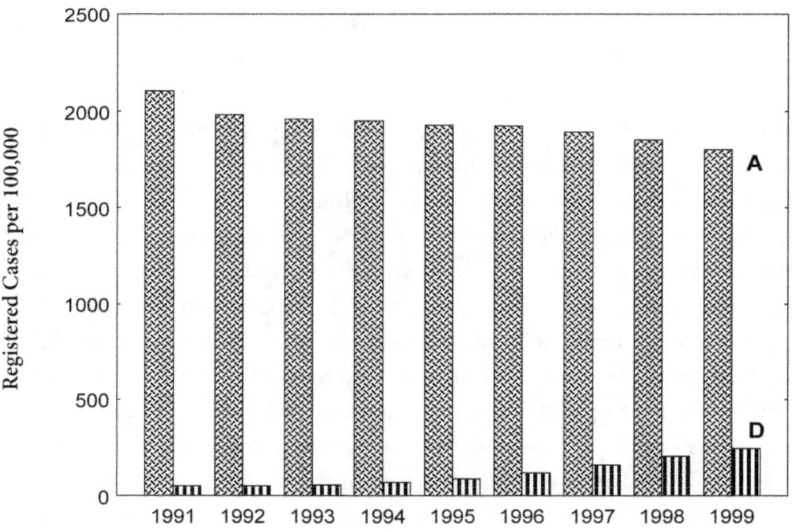

There can be no doubt that drug dependency entails more serious problems for the individual than alcohol and affects relatively younger people. Moreover, a tendency to drug addiction at younger ages is in process (Fig. 1-7). This is why the widening of the narco-business and of the drug culture in Russia constitutes a grave danger. However, overall, the country's alcohol problems so far dominate over drug problems that a careful reconsideration of Russia's priorities has long been in order. A predominating interest in the problems of drug addiction has long been evident in the press, in some administrative agencies and some scientific groups. For these sources, the way the West looks at the matter is what is important. And there alcohol problems have been declining since the 1980s, while drug problems remain acute. But even in the industrially advanced countries, where alcohol consumption is 30–50 percent lower than in Russia and where the drug addicts are more common than in Russia, alcohol remains the most widely used narcotic and causes enormous economic losses. Thus, for the U.S., material losses attributable to alcohol abuse amounted to 54.7 billion USD in 1986, with those attributable to drugs coming to 26 billion USD (Reisch, 1987). Without doubt, the (analogous relative) difference in Russia is even larger because of the large difference in alcohol consumption between Russia and the U.S..

Fig. 1-7: Age distribution of persons with drug addiction and toxicomania in 1985 and 1995 (Moscow, hospitalized patients; Shamota et al., 1998).

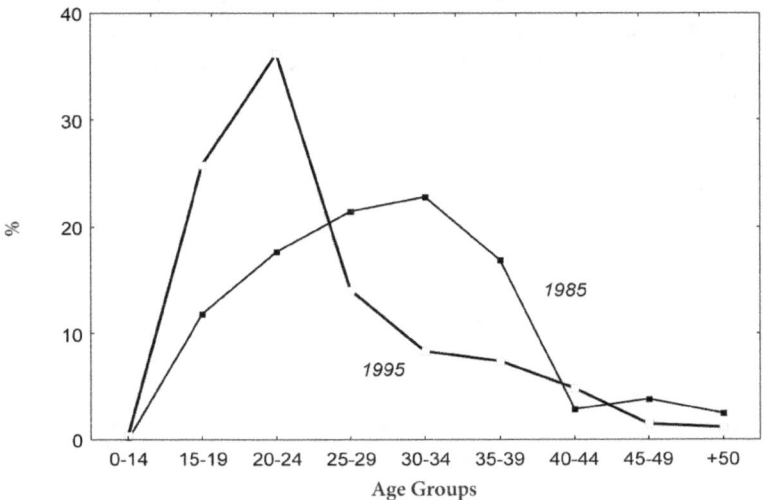

However, the heavy-drinking traditions of Russian life which took shape in the post-war period, the fact that society has grown used to Russian drunkenness and, consequently, the apparent naturalness of the material and human costs associated with alcohol – have all acted to push the problems of alcohol into the background. Further abetting this was the failure of the anti-alcohol campaign and a powerful alcohol lobby. Moreover, the abundance of new, non-alcohol-related problems for Russia – the poverty of a large portion of the population and the breakdown of social and moral norms (Emile Durkheim's "anomie") – have concealed the dramatic nature of the alcohol situation in Russia but have not reduced its scope.

In the context of this discussion of the consequences of the anti-alcohol campaign, it is necessary to point to one very important circumstance: the campaign took place during the years of the remaking (perestroika) of the economic and social life of the country, the break-up of the state apparatus and a change of leaders. Essentially, this was a point of deep fracture in the history of Russia. In this historic time, the efforts of Gorbachev and the state apparatus were diverted to the tasks of implementing the anti-alcohol resolutions, while the attention of the public was narrowly focused on resisting these measures. Many people's major concern was where they might obtain a bottle, and the authorities' concern was with how to prevent that happening or taking the offending bottle away. This was a part of why neither the authorities nor the public had time to think about where perestroika was heading. Had it moved even halfway along a path strictly towards the democratization of society, then either in parallel or in turn, it would have been necessary to carry out economic reforms, legally divide the three branches of government, make a clear division between the government and private property, conduct an assessment of the value of government properties (land, minerals, forests, etc.) and lay the foundations for meeting the social needs of the bulk of the population. No activities of this kind were carried out. Part of the reason for this was the enormous waste of resources which went into conducting the anti-alcohol campaign.

Chapter 1-6
The alcohol situation 1987–1991

It was not just the anti-alcohol campaign that reached a turning point in 1987. By this time, Gorbachev had finally felt his way to his own political line – perestroika in tandem with glasnost was launched in 1987. That year saw the appearance of the Law on Cooperatives and on Individual Labor (private businesses). The introduction of full cost-accounting for enterprises was underway. The Law on Enterprises was adopted. In late 1988 cooperatives were permitted to borrow money.

All of these new initiatives had serious consequences for the economic and social life of the country. A shifting of assets from the government to private hands began, with the creation, at first, of Komsomol and later nomenklatura property. Meanwhile, the wholesale and retail market was breaking down, and the public found itself facing a growing shortage in the supply of food and other goods. Empty shelves in stores became the particular symbol of this period, especially in 1990–1991. This was the surface manifestation of things. Below, the administrative system or, to put it more generally, the system of state power was collapsing.

Obviously, in this chaos and under the pressure of significant shortfalls in budgeted revenues, it was easy to curtail the anti-alcohol campaign, beginning in 1987–1988. There was a substantial decline in the number of legal actions taken in connection with samogon; for example, in Moscow there was a decline from 1,445 cases in 1986 to 23 cases in 1989 (there had been 114 in 1984). Beginning in 1989, the number of narcological hospitals and health centers began to fall (from 339 to 260 in 1993), as did the number of physician-narcological specialists (a drop of 1,345 in five years). In 1990 the period of active or, more accurately, compulsory observation for alcoholics was cut from five years to three years. And all this occurred against a backdrop of a rise in cases of alcoholic psychosis that began in 1989 (up 37 percent for the year). The growing budget deficit forced the government to increase the hours of trade for the sale of alcoholic beverages and change the time when they could be purchased from 2 p.m., as called for in the Resolution of 1985, to 8 a.m. (February 1990).

The wrapping up of the anti-alcohol campaign was helped by alarming information about the increase in the consumption of samogon, non-beverage alcohol-containing substances and other intoxicants. Sales of BF glue (a medical adhesive used to strengthen alcoholic beverages) rose by 26 percent between 1985 and 1987, glass-cleaning liquid by 13 percent and diclofos (a household insecticide), by 15 percent (USSR Ministry of Trade figures). The volume of sales of perfumery-cosmetic goods grew by 29 percent. According to the figures of the Ministry of Internal Affairs, 11,000 deaths occurred from such substances in 1987. For balance, it should be noted that there were 28,000 deaths from alcohol poisoning in 1984 and 11,500 in 1987 (State Statistical Committee of the Russian Federation).

The return to an increase in alcohol consumption, which began in 1987, was slower than the decrease of 1985–1987 (Table 1). For 1987–1989, the average was 3.8 percent a year, and for 1990–1991 it was 2.1 percent. The biggest incremental increase occurred in 1989 (5.3 percent), and the smallest in 1991 (1.7 percent). In other words, after 1989 the rate of increase in consumption began to slow, and in 1991 it reached 12.3 liters per capita per year, which was 2 liters less than consumption had been on the eve of the campaign. The rise in alcohol consumption occurred primarily because of the production of underground samogon, which increased with the weakening of state controls and the production know-how that had accumulated over many years. Data from the RSFSR State Statistical Committee and the estimates of specialists show that the consumption of unregistered alcohol began to prevail over state-produced alcohol even in 1987 (Table 1). The succeeding years would witness a further rise in the share of consumption attributable to unregistered alcohol.

A way of characterizing underground production is through sugar sales, the chief ingredient of samogon. Those sales stood at 7.9 million tons in 1985; in 1986 at 8.6 million, and by 1987 the figure had reached 9.3 million tons. It has been possible to follow this process in more detail for Moscow (Chapter 2-4). A decline in purchases of sugar was evident as early as June 1985, which means that it coincided with the start of the campaign, and continued until September. However, in the period October-December of that year, sales of sugar exceeded the level of the year before. Purchases stepped up in 1986 and 1987, especially in the second half of these years. In 1988 the increase led to interruptions in the supply of sugar and, as a result, to a "sugar panic", when the public began to buy and store sugar at home in fear that it was going to disappear. In May–June 1988, sales of sugar were double the level of the year before, which had already exceeded the previously highest 1984 level. Beginning on 1 June, 1989, sugar was rationed.

Samogon production increased in step with the rise in sugar sales, as did the number of persons brought to trial for illegal alcohol production: almost 400,000 individuals in 1987 and 414,000 in 1988.

The emergence of new cooperatives in the country brought with it new ways of producing illegal alcoholic beverages, for example, by the use of technical alcohol ostensibly purchased for technical use but illegally transformed into surrogate, or counterfeit, alcoholic drinks. This and other methods of underground surrogate production now supplemented the amounts of samogon produced.

The increase in consumption had its response in changes in phenomena dependent on alcohol use: as early as 1987, the decreases registered in most of the alcohol indexes had ceased (Fig. 2-11), and several kinds of violent death involving drunkenness (from road traffic accidents, homicides and suicides) began to climb (Chapter 2-5). The same year saw the beginning of a rise in admissions to medically staffed sobering-up stations (Gukovsky & Kolomin, 1989).

In the following year, 1988, an increase in the overall number of violent deaths was noted, and in 1989 increases in deaths from cirrhosis of the liver, pancreatitis, alcohol poisoning and alcohol psychoses, that is, increases in the indexes most sharply linked to alcohol consumption. The lag in these increases in relation to the rise in actual alcohol consumption is attributable to the time required for abuse of alcohol to fully form the ailments, including alcohol poisoning, which would become the cause of death of some alcoholics (this is discussed in more detail in Chapter 2-5).

The period 1989–1991 saw a stabilizing trend in the data for alcohol-related road traffic accidents and crime. Violent deaths, fatal alcohol poisonings and homicides continued to rise, but the share of drunks among the dead remained at close to half of all violent deaths, a proportion typical for the earlier years of Russian statistics-keeping. There was also stabilization in the number of suicides, but at a very high level.

As a result of untimely deaths, 2.23 million man-years of labor were lost in 1991, of which 1.02 million were the result of accidents, poisonings and injuries (Ermakov et al., 1998). According to the figures of the Bureau of Forensic-Medical Reviews, 52.4 percent of these deaths were among persons who were inebriated at the time of their death. Taking this into account and also the fact that the consumption of ethanol raises the risk of death by an order of 10 (Nemtsov & Nechaev, 1991), direct losses of labor potential from alcohol came to 0.48 million man-years for the year. To this must be added the loss of labor potential from deaths from heart and artery disease, stomach and intestinal diseases and other illnesses for which drunkenness and alcoholism are complicating factors, as well as the deaths of sober persons caused by intoxicated persons (approximately, 150,000 man-years). Thus, in 1991, more than a quarter of Russia's labor potential was lost due to deaths for which the direct or indirect cause was alcohol.

By the start of the 1990s, in the view researchers in Siberia (Bokhan et al., 1991), the alcohol situation had "accumulated the powerful negative energy of medico-social complications", evidenced in particular by changes in the forms of alcoholization and the public's growing acceptance of surrogate alcoholic beverages, which, as mentioned, were now predominant in consumption.

There was a flourishing business not only in underground sales of samogon but also in a black market in alcohol produced in state factories. The chaos in the country was so great that truckloads of alcohol could easily "disappear" without consequences, on the way from the factory to the store, and find their way into the hands of underground merchants. Stores routinely sold alcoholic beverages under the counter to middlemen who resold them at very high prices. Thus, as early as December 1991, the state price for a half-liter bottle of vodka was 10 rubles, but the black-market price was as much as 50 rubles. For all practical purposes, the state's alcohol monopoly had been replaced by a monopoly of a caste of middlemen, which by this time had produced its own "vodka kings", whose underground work already covered the entire Soviet Union and thus made them the actual rulers of the country's alcohol market and quite able to hold their own against state production of alcoholic beverages.

According to figures compiled by the State Statistical Committee, samogon and black-market trading in alcohol engendered revenues of 23 billion rubles in 1989 (*Argumenty i Fakty*, No. 43, 1989) and 35 billion in 1990 (*Vechernyaya Moskva*, 10 July, 1991), which was the main part of the income of the "shadow economy" (40 percent and 42 percent, respectively). For purposes of comparison, illegal income from drug sales, prostitution and smuggling made up less than 2 percent of the income of the shadow economy in 1989 (*Argumenty i Fakty*, No. 43, 1989). The high profitability of the underground alcohol business attracted criminal organizations, often armed. Increasingly immersed in this business were groups of veterans of the war in Afghanistan, including those left handicapped by the war, who by this time already had acquired considerable trading privileges, which were steeply bolstered after the putsch of August 1991, when the "Afghans" joined the side of Yeltsin against the Committee for the State of Emergency.

In summing up the results of this five-year period (1987–1991), it should be mentioned that the level of alcohol consumption rebounded strongly during this time (12.3 liters per capita per year). This level of use and the broad dimensions of speculative activity in vodka and samogon ought to have alerted both society at large and the government, and again given life to an anti-alcohol policy. However, once again there were neither individuals nor organizations in the country which understood the alcohol situation, could see where it was heading or had the authority to put any conclusions before the country's leadership. Indeed, was there a leadership of the country at all in 1991? What was more, a leadership supported by the nation? Gorbachev's perestroika was defeated – the country had rejected the rapid and profound modernization of its life and, with it, the leaders carrying it out.

The political reforms of the late 1980s had undermined the power of the Communist Party, which itself was so tightly grafted onto the state that the blow to it was a blow to the state. This hastened the degeneration of the Union and the rise of separatism. The high point of these processes came in August 1991 with the putsch. A sweeping disintegration of the USSR was underway, climaxing in

December 1991 with Yeltsin's abrupt change of direction (the Belovezhsky accords – 8 December 1991, on the breaking-up of the Soviet Union.).

In 1991 the budget deficit came to 22 percent of gross national product. The increasing political and economic tension was accompanied by social tensions, at the base of which was the collapse of the consumer market, the almost complete emptiness of store shelves and alarming communications concerning the exhaustion of bread supplies in one city after another. Consumer prices began to rise in the early spring of 1991, before the introduction of market reforms. People began to grab empty bits of land along railroad tracks, for instance, or near high-tension wires and plant potatoes on them.

That spring saw the start of a wave of miners' protests in Vorkut, climaxing in a mass strike that had the support of many miners in other areas. For several months, these events were widely discussed in the mass media. All this contributed to the growing mood of panic felt by the public. It is possible that 1990–1991 was the culmination of the social tension in the post-war period.

At the same time, it should be noted that, despite the sharp increase in tensions in the country, this was the very time that the increase in alcohol consumption began to slow down, not having reached the level of 1984. Moreover, this was happening at a time when the public had accumulated considerable disposable income with which there was almost nothing to buy and when alcohol was more easily available, that is, by this time the harassment of the anti-alcohol campaign had ended.

The author does not have an unambiguous explanation of the disjunction between the level of alcohol consumption and of social tension in the country. One can only offer possible suppositions. One is that the alcohol market, together with the market for food and other commodities, had broken down to such an extent as a result of the economic chaos in the country that it could not fully meet the public's demand for alcohol. The large difference in price between state and black-market alcoholic beverages offers support for this view. The shortage of alcoholic beverages arose, in part, from a shortage of containers and is reflected in the fact that, up to the end of 1990, there was a rationed sale of alcoholic beverages in many cities; tokens for alcohol purchase were issued through trade unions (1 liter of vodka per worker per month). An additional argument for the view that the alcohol market was unable to meet demand at this time may be found in the fact that, in the succeeding two or three years, when new market relations came into being and state control of the alcohol market disappeared, consumption rose sharply.

But that is the simplest explanation. It should also be kept in mind that 1990–1991 was also a time of social tension caused by acute shortages of food products, especially in the cities. The deficit was almost at its limit. Daily and hourly, the vital task of finding food might have supplanted the desire for alcohol in much of the population, as happens during war or natural disasters.

The market reforms that followed resulted in a market filled with food and other products and, in consequence, there was a lessening of psychological stress in the country. There arose new, entirely different concerns about adapting to the sudden emergence of market relations. Now, indeed, there was demand for extra portions of such an "adaptive gene" as vodka. A swift rise in alcohol consumption began. There were other reasons as well for this "leap" and we will come to them in the next chapter.

Chapter 1-7
The alcohol situation 1992–1994

The five or six years preceding 1992 were essentially preparation for a new, fateful shift in Russian history. The main contours of the new stage were well laid out in those earlier years.

By 1987–1988 it was clear that the efforts to mobilize the population under the banner of "speeding-up" (*uskorenie*) had not worked and that the new leadership was in no condition to lead the country to capitalism while maintaining state (that is, party) control over the economy. Instead of a democratization of political life, there was a collapse of government structures and a consequent conversion of power into capital, the so-called "nomenklatura privatization": "He who runs things comes to own things." The economic infrastructure, the system of management, distribution and finance, was now in private hands, the ministries were businesses, the State Committee for Material-Technical Supply (Gossnab) a series of markets. The three specialized state banks, with their many sections, became commercial banks and in turn the seed of what would become the banking system of the Russian Federation, operating with abundant infusions of assets from the Communist Party of the Soviet Union and mafia money.

1987–1988 were also the years that saw the start of large-scale transfers of Communist Party and government funds outside the country, a process made possible with the help of the KGB (the central figure was Kruchina, manager of affairs for the CPSU Central Committee, who, after the putsch of 1991, "fell" out of the window of his own apartment, the fate of two of his predecessors as well). In the early 1990s, too, even before the economic reforms, prices on a third of all commodities sold in the country were already free. Many of the then extraordinarily flourishing cooperatives were used in the transfer and laundering, not only of mafia money, but also of party and state funds. That was why the government granted the cooperatives the right to convert assets into currency.

Even before the onset of market reforms, a significant portion of criminal activity had become organized. This was the basis for the start in 1987–1988 of a fundamental redivision of criminal property and spheres of influence. This so-called first criminal war had an all-Union character, although the media mistakenly linked it exclusively with the Kazan (Tartarstan) group. "Shadow owners" (*teneviki*) controlled about 40 percent of the country's economy and, in some spheres, dominated, as was the case in the alcoholic-beverages industry. The fact was that the government had lost its monopoly on the production and sale of spirits even before 1992, when the demonopolization was made law or, more accurately, when lawlessness was given legal sanction. "Black money" or dirty money, had already become a substantial portion of Russia's capital flow and, specifically, of the alcohol market.

All this and much else besides gave rise in 1991 to an extremely acute shortage of goods throughout Russia, money's loss of value, and the collapse of the country's financial system. Industrial production and wages fell sharply. By the end of 1991, these phenomena had acquired a critical mass and were ready to burst through the dam. This pressure was converted into the market reforms. Of course, they were late. The crisis had arrived in the middle of the 1980s, a crisis of government and of society, a society that not only lacked ideas that might be fruitful but also, the readiness to act on them. There were no far-sighted and strong leaders with national priorities.

The new, "market-oriented" government of Gaidar, unlike its predecessor Soviet governments and their redistribution of material resources, moved on to the redistribution of state property and funds. These "pieces of the pie", were sold dirt cheap, that is, at a loss to the government, and went to a narrow circle of rich people who had made their riches through semi-legal and illegal activities. Oligarchic capitalism and its uncivilized market were thus born.

All this took place under the flag of liberalizing the economy, a liberalization that was to make the market the sole regulator of the economic life of the country. The market helped with the shortage of goods. But, in Russian soil, it grew into a liberal extremism that led the country to economic degradation and, in the sphere of the alcohol economy, to catastrophe. Liberalization here took the form of a revocation of the government's monopoly on the production and sale of spirits and thus eliminated the last barrier to total recklessness in the alcohol market with its calamitous consequences for the health and lives of the country's population.

Under the cover of liberal phraseology and the guise of democracy, the country's new leadership created for itself a bulwark in the form of a financial-economic oligarchy, thus strengthening the gap, historically typical, between government and society in Russia. The first government of this new Russia did not allow the nation as a whole to participate in the redistribution of property and finances, nor its middle class, which might have created a civil society and thus protected itself and the country from runaway corruption and theft. Russia's market reforms exclusively served the interests of the uppermost, oligarchical slice of the population, "our people". But this became obvious to all only later, as a result of the voucher system of privatization that turned into, or was planned to become, a masked comedy for the transfer of government property, for virtually nothing, to a narrow circle of the "chosen".

It is naive to think that the haste with which the new course was pursued and the many mistakes that ensued can be justified by the need for a root-and-branch destruction of the former party-bureaucratic system. It is obvious today that all that was destroyed was the party-state element of the system and even that not entirely. The state bureaucracy was strengthened. Karl Marx's formula, "the government is the bureaucracy's property", was realized in Russia. The price of this version of chess castling was enormous: among the many negative consequences of the market reforms was an extraordinary increase in mortality in 1992–1994 (Chapter 2-5), largely as a result of a debauch of drunkenness. The long-awaited restocking of the food and general commodities market quickly exhausted the buying power accumulated as reserves in the preceding period.

The chief milestone of the new stage was the sweeping liberalization of trade and the freeing of prices as of 2 January, 1992. Prices began to skyrocket (President Yeltsin had earlier promised "to lie down on the rails if prices go up"). The liberalization of prices in China, it ought to be mentioned, was stretched out over 15 years (1978–1993).

Prices of alcohol products, like those for bread, remained regulated, for political reasons, until April 1992, after which they were freed – the alcohol lobby winning out over political considerations. But even earlier, state prices on alcohol products had risen by 200 percent-300 percent and were comparable with black-market prices (120–150 rubles for a half-liter of vodka). Private sellers of alcohol though charged much higher prices than the government for additional services: covering the deficit in state trade in terms of volume, time and place of sale. This "coverage" was provided by taxi drivers whose baggage compartments were "bars", by *toptuny* (loiterers) in shops and metro stations with bags full of bottles, by underground vodka shops in apartments and by after-hours shops by way of the "back door". This merely scratches the surface.

The changes profoundly affected the alcohol situation in the country. The Russian market in alcoholic beverages was flooded with imports. Previously unseen beverages such as tequila, grappa, Bacardi, prepared cocktails appeared. The variety and qualitative differences of imported beer and, later, Russian beer and its presentation in cans quickly and radically changed the tastes and preferences of a large portion of Russian consumers, who had been denied this kind of taste variety during the Soviet period. Now there was a wide range of choices, but only a relatively small number of people could avail themselves of it. As was the case before the market reforms, cheap vodka, whether legal or surrogate, remained the predominant drink after the introduction of market reforms.

In May 1992, President Yeltsin signed into law the government resolution that essentially ended the state alcohol monopoly. The resolution principally affected the production of spirits and strong beverages, including cognacs. Production of beer and wine was permitted by enterprises of any kind as long as they were licensed. Control over the manufacturing and sale of alcoholic beverages was vested in the local authorities, who were to issue licenses and supplement their budgets with income from the trade in alcoholic beverages. Alas, just over 100 persons applied for licenses countrywide! Nonetheless, the alcohol market widened very rapidly, and it was run by the same old "vodka kings", "samogoners" and countless middlemen, who set their own prices.

This particular decision was part of the general debauch of liberalism, the cornerstone of which was minimalization of the role of the government in the economy and a fond hope that "the market will correct itself". But liberalization turned into a kind of anything-goes situation, especially in the alcohol market. The leadership of the country once again forgot that most important given – that alcohol is a special commodity, loaded with more social functions, many of them negative, than other commodities. The public became the victim of a generally heedless and, in the case of alcohol, criminally reckless economic liberalism. The alcohol market was part of the general race to raise prices while avoiding excise taxes, thanks to "black cash".

The prices of spirits had a special feature, and it is important to understand it in order to understand the alcohol situation in the entire succeeding period: their increase lagged behind both the general rise in monthly wages and the general consumer price index. For example, in 1990 the average monthly wage was equivalent to the price of 16 liters of vodka, in December 1992 it was equal to 29 liters of vodka, while in December 1993 it was 33 liters of vodka (*Izvestiya*, 24 February, 1994). As a result of hyperinflation, the combined index of consumer prices for food products rose 2,263 times between December 1990 and December 1994, but only by 654 times for alcoholic beverages (Russian State Statistical Committee; Fig. 1-8). For the four-year period, thus, the actual price of alcoholic beverages fell by over 70 percent.

It should be noted that Fig. 1-8 primarily reflects the increase of prices of legal alcohol products. If illegal vodka and surrogates are included, the difference is even greater. According to figures compiled by the Accounting Chamber (2003), illegal vodka made up 65 percent of total alcoholic beverages sold!

An especially rapid fall in the relative price of alcoholic drinks occurred in 1994. Thus, in June 1994, it rose by only 5 percent compared to May, while inflation rose by 8.1 percent for the same period (*Argumenty i Fakty*, Life and Pocketbook supplement, No. 2, 1994).

The question arises, how could prices of alcohol-related products have lagged behind the prices of food and other goods so strongly? Calculations show that, assuming there was an average level of consumption of 14 liters of alcohol per year while using 1993 government prices, the Russian people should have spent 12.5 trillion rubles on alcoholic beverages that year. Half this total should have gone to the government in the form of excise taxes. In fact, such payments to the budget amounted to 1.1 trillion rubles (figures from the Budget Department of the Russian Finance Ministry), that is, to less than 20 percent of what should have

Fig. 1-8: Consolidated price indexes for alcoholic beverages and food products (1990–2005). Indexes for 1990 accepted as unit growth measured in multiples of unit (figures from RussStat). Relation of Prices of Alcoholic Beverages and Food Products in 1990 onwards (1990 considered 100 percent).

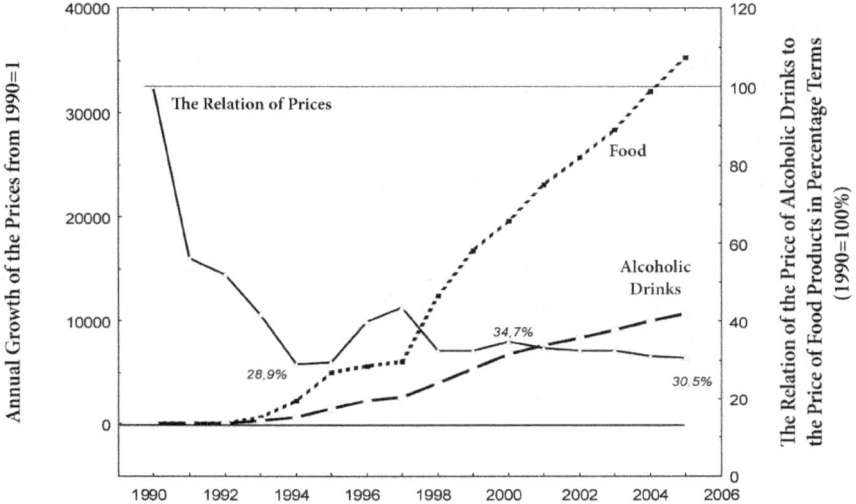

been received. According to officials, "the state budget had never, in all its history, received so small a portion of the sales of trade in alcohol" (*Vechernyaya Moskva*, 9 February, 1992). As an excise tax, its full collection would have led to a growth in the price of alcoholic beverages and to the evening out of their prices with the prices on other commodities. At the same time, this would have resulted in a decline in consumption, if illegal production were eliminated.

As calculated by the Ministry of Economics of Russia and including wholesale purchase prices, transportation costs, excise and customs payments and retail mark-ups, a liter of imported vodka should have cost 16,000 rubles in Moscow in the summer of 1994. In fact, the cost was 6,000 rubles. This large discrepancy can only be explained by the absence in the actual price of a significant portion of the excise duties. The use of actual currency ("black cash") in the wholesale market for alcohol facilitated the avoidance of taxes.

Another source of the lower prices for alcoholic beverages was the place in the market of counterfeits made from technical alcohol and spirits made from non-edible substances. The base cost of this alcohol was much less than the price of spirits made from edible substances and in addition excise taxes did not apply to them. In the period 1992–1994, a decrease in demand from the main users of technical alcohol continued: use by the paint and lacquer industry fell by 57 percent and production of synthetic rubber by 61 percent. There was also a drop in demand for technical alcohol from the defense industry. Nonetheless, the reduction in the output of technical alcohol amounted to only 14 percent. It is easy enough to imagine where the technical alcohol that industry did not need went.

It should be noted that, since 2000, the difference in the rate of price increases between alcoholic beverages and food products has been minimal because the difference had to have a limit (even underground vodka has to cost something). However, the huge difference created in the 1990s continues to be in place to this day and makes alcoholic beverages accessible to the very poorest strata of the population.

An informational-analytic memorandum of the Research Institute of the Russian Interior Ministry (dated 19 January, 1995) states:

> The activity of organized criminal groups involved in the production of illegal vodka and cognacs has significantly increased. The distinctive features of these groups are: carefully coordinated criminal activity, a significant number of participants (10 or more), the presence as a rule of interregional ties, and most important, a readiness to actively resist the organs of the militia – with weapons in hand, it may be assumed.

Another contribution to the Russian bacchanalia came in the form of fraudulent Chechen bank orders. For example, in the spring of 1992 a single small criminal group used these means to swindle more than 30 million USD from banks in the Moscow region, money that was used for the production of the relatively low-priced Kremlyovskaya Vodka that, at one time, flooded Russia. These funds were also used to create the powerful Moscow-region-based Topaz company (based in the city of Pushkino), whose vodka advertisements were seen all over the Moscow metro and highways for a long time. There is speculation that some of the earnings from the sales of this vodka returned to Chechnya and were controlled by Dzhokhar Dudaev (President of the Chechen Republic of Ichkeriya 1991–96). And in this story, like many others of its kind, there was a victim – Topaz's first director, who was shot dead.

The National Foundation of Sport inflicted great harm on the country when it obtained an exemption from tariff payments for all goods imported in connection with the conduct of international competitions (Presidential Decree No. 1973 dated 22 November, 1993) and later for all goods purchased by the Foundation (government order dated 13 May, 1994). In the course of several months, the Foundation concluded approximately 140 contracts that for 1994 alone required the delivery into Russia of foreign excisable goods, mostly vodka, worth 500 million USD. These goods were chosen primarily because they would be the most profitable, even though they were sold at minimal prices, well below the average prices for the country. Thus, the Foundation used its privileges extremely irrationally, adding only a little to the price that it had paid for the imported goods. The loss to the budget (4 trillion rubles in 1994) caused by the granting of these privileges far exceeded the gains to the foundation brought by the tariff exemption. But something else is more important: the domestic alcohol industry was entirely denied tariff protection and made uncompetitive in the domestic market. As a result of this, for example, the Kristall factory in Moscow was forced to reorient most of its production for export.

Such a situation could not last long. As early as 29 August, 1993, on the initiative of the Finance Ministry, a decree (No. 1787) was signed annulling all privileges as of 1 September, 1994. However, this was the start of a sixteen-month tug-of-war to protect the tariff exemptions. Nineteen days after issuance of Decree 1787, a decree was published extending the exemptions until 31 December, 1994, and on 29 December, 1994, there was a new decree (No. 2221), keeping the exemptions in place until all already concluded contracts were fulfilled. A few days later, there was another decree which gave 1 March 1995 as the end date for all exemptions. However, the Foundation won another two-and-a-half month extension. Still, this was not the end of the matter because there remained a large number of unfulfilled contracts. And yet this was only one of the foundations granted exemptions. In addition, there were NFS-Neva, the Hockey Federation of Russia, the Russian Foundation for Invalids of the War in Afghanistan (RFIWA) and others. The exemption bandwagon was joined by the Moscow Patriarchate in the form of its Department of External Relations, which energetically brought excise-exempt cigarettes and vodka into Russia. It fell to the government to pay out 37 trillion rubles (9 billion USD) to cover the contract forfeitures of all the privileged groups (based on a communication from Boldyrev, vice chairman of the Accounting Chamber).

However, the trouble went even beyond this. After payment of the external debts, there remained very large internal debts. Moreover, the foundations, and other organizations granted exemptions had now accumulated large amounts of capital, amounting to hundreds of thousands or even millions of dollars (USD). All this led in 1996–1997 to a very harsh settling of accounts, with physical attacks, contract killings and bombings. Likhodei, the chairman of the RFIWA, was killed and, a year later, 14 other people, including the new chairman of the RFIWA, Trakhirov, died in a bombing at the Kotlyakovsky Cemetery, where they were attending a memorial service on the anniversary of the death of Likhodei. In all, 34 persons were killed and 62 wounded in this settling of accounts, merely with respect to the RFIWA. In addition, V. Sych (president of the Hockey Federation of Russia) was shot dead, and there were attempts on the life of S. Fyodorov (first vice president of the NFS – The Russian National Hockey Federation). This is a very partial list of the bloody results of the history of the privileges.

The relative fall in prices for alcohol products is explained by a Russian paradox – a rise in alcohol consumption occurred against a background of economic crisis and hyperinflation, although the world experience in recent decades has clearly demonstrated a different relationship: economic collapse or even mild recession lead to a decline in the consumption of alcoholic beverages, especially of hard liquor (Österberg, 1995).

The lawlessness of the alcohol market and the shortfall of budgeted state receipts forced President Yeltsin to issue a decree on 11 June, 1993, "On the Restoration of a State Monopoly on Production, Storage, and the Wholesale and Retail Sale of Alcohol Products" (Decree No. 918). The decree was designed to halt the bacchanalia in the production and sale of alcoholic beverages by establishing control over the country's market in alcohol using a system of licensing and quotas. Control was also to be established over the quality of beverages by a system of certification. To implement the decree, a binding government resolution was prepared, entitled "On Confirming the Method of Retail Sales of Alcoholic Beverages and Beer on the Territory of the Russian Federation". However, thanks to the efforts of the alcohol lobby and a series of underhand maneuvers, the signing into law of this government resolution was delayed for more than a year (26 September, 1994, No. 1088). One can say that almost the only result of the resolution was the change in the name of the "State Inspection for the Control..." into the "State Inspection to Ensure...", which was later disbanded without having dealt with its tasks. A state monopoly on the production and sale of alcoholic products has not been revived to this day, and approximately half of all vodka production remains illegal (2007).

There is no doubt that the relative cheapness of alcohol products in respect to the wages and earnings of the population, and in respect to the price of food and other goods, acted as an important stimulus to consumption. It is, thus, not surprising that the market reforms were accompanied by a sharp rise in alcohol consumption in 1992 (by 13.8 percent as compared to 1.6 percent in 1991; Table 1). For the same period, state sales of alcoholic beverages fell by 10.7 percent, but sales of unregistered alcoholic beverages rose (by 34.3 percent). There was also a change in the makeup of the alcoholic beverages and the channels used in bringing them to the market.

Before 1992, the principal portion of unregistered alcohol in Russia was made up of samogon. However, beginning in 1992, increases in the price of sugar and other food products used in the process made samogon production unprofitable. Moreover, by then new, cheaper sources of alcohol for the production of illegal vodka had become available in Russia and elsewhere.

In 1993–1994 the Russian Interior Ministry uncovered numerous instances of pure alcohol, some of it technical alcohol, being delivered to individuals and commercial enterprises producing alcohol products without a license. During the course of 1993, for example, a single biochemical firm, Krasnoyarskgidrolizprom (a typically long abbreviation), increased the percentage (from 20 percent to 69 percent) of its sales of raw material that went to commercial structures that, largely, turned out to be suppliers of technical alcohol for the production of illegal alcoholic beverages.

Using false documents, the Vikom Company in the Krasnodarsk region stole more than 3 million liters of pure alcohol for the underground production and sale of illegal vodka during 1993–1994. This was possible because the manufacture and distribution of technical ethyl alcohol in the country was neither regulated nor subject to control by quotas as food-based alcohol was.

Another source of unregistered alcohol was the importation or smuggling of significant amounts of non-standard and, thus, cheap alcohol products, principally, vodka. Most often, this consisted of deliveries of low-quality goods from countries of the CIS (Azerbaijan, Moldova, Armenia, Georgia) and from the further afield (China, Poland, Germany [Royal spirits], Belgium [Rasputin vodka], Holland [Smirnovskaya vodka], Italy [Terminator vodka], France [Rossiya and Golitsin vodkas]). In Hungary counterfeit Absolut vodka, a Swedish brand, was produced and reached the Russian market via Ukraine. The Swedish embassy made frequent but unavailing protests against this falsification.

According to figures from the State Commercial Inspection Service, approximately two-thirds of all imported cognacs and liqueurs were rejected, as were half of all champagne imports. Vodka imported from China, for example, showed the presence of aldehydes at a level 4.7 times greater than acceptable and of fusel oils, a byproduct of refining ethyl alcohol, at a level 13.4 times greater than acceptable. A significant portion of such shipments arrived after avoiding customs stations, without any inspection or control and without payment of customs duties.

It is difficult to estimate the quantity of illegal alcoholic beverages on the domestic market. According to figures from the State Trade Inspectorate, in 1991 in the course of selective checks its organizations rejected 5.6 percent of all alcoholic products in the territories of Russia, 12.4 percent in 1992, 25.6 percent in 1993 and 31 percent for the first half of 1994 (*Argumenty i Fakty*, Life and Pocketbook supplement, No. 10, 1994). By the year's end that figure was 37 percent. The figure for wine taken out of circulation in 1994 was 33.4 percent and for cognac 46.9 percent. But imported vodkas were of particularly poor quality – 68.3 percent of vodkas tested were scrapped. Selective inspections by the Interior Ministry revealed an even higher percentage of illegal alcohol – from 40 percent to 70 percent.

There was still another concern in Russia's alcohol market – the monopoly situation arising in connection with the official control of quotas on ethyl alcohol made from food products. It has already been said that, in the wake of the market reforms, the government gave up state distribution of material resources. However, a small group of industrial products continued to be distributed by the state as before, including food-based ethyl alcohol. And this was done while technical alcohol, widely used in the production of illegal alcoholic beverages, was not controlled or regulated.

An overwhelming share of the food-based alcohol (70 percent in 1994, or 672 million liters) was, as in the former Soviet era, intended for the Ministry of Agricultural Products (figures from the State Statistical Committee of the Russian Federation). Despite the fact that all the enterprises of this ministry that produced alcoholic beverages had been privatized, the Agricultural Products Ministry fought hard to increase its quota of alcohol and the right to distribute it as it saw fit. Such a product in the hands of a monopoly in a country given to drinking offered great criminal possibilities. This and the make-up of the staff of the Ministry of Agricultural Products help explain why about one-third of the alcohol allotted to the ministry for supplying the entire country ended up in North Ossetia (the future Alania). This took place even before the start of the anti-alcohol campaign and the market reforms and was the reason for the rapid emergence in the small republic of approximately 20 major enterprises (the largest was Terek) and approximately 200 small plants and workshops that together employed one-third (!) of the adult population of the republic. During the anti-alcohol campaign, these factories stopped working but were not destroyed (as was the case in the rest of the country) and were protected. Within a year or two, they resumed operations. The increasing production of alcohol products demands ever more raw material, and the republic began to buy cheap spirits in Ukraine, where excise charges were 75 percent (as compared to 85 percent in Russia). Ukrainian alcohol entered the republic under false documents in which Russia was listed as a transit country, with Georgia listed as the country of destination. By customs rules, alcohol in transit is not subject to Russian taxes. The alcohol was unloaded from railroad cistern cars in Vladikavkaz, from where it was transported to factories in North Ossetia. According to the documents however, the alcohol was transferred to trucks and sent to Georgia.

North Ossetia produced about 40 percent of the vodka consumed in Russia. Almost all of it was illegal. This became the chief, if not the sole, source of the republic's prosperity (recall the sporting glory of the Alania football team). This history will have its dramatic continuation – the retribution for having an alcohol mono-economy (Chapter 1-8).

Every illegal product is a sharp knife plunged into legal producers. This is true, too, of vodka. To impose order on the alcohol market and counteract vodka from Ossetia, Russian producers formed an association, Rusalko, which "forced" through the Duma, a new form of extracting customs duties on alcohol in transit. This halted the flow of Ukrainian alcohol into North Ossetia. But new sources of cheap alcohol were quickly found (see Chapter 1-8).

The precipitous leap in alcohol consumption led to an increase in almost all of the indexes dependent on alcohol (more detail is provided in Chapter 2-5). Thus, for example, violent deaths increased in 1992 by 22.3 percent (the figure was 6.3 percent in 1991) and amounted to 173 deaths per 100,000 of the population, which was two to three times higher than Western European indexes (France: 88.3 deaths per 100,000; 1989). In 1993 the increase was even larger – 31.7 percent. What is most important for our topic is that, with the start of market reforms, the tempo of the increase in deaths of intoxicated persons from external causes, including violent deaths, exceeded the tempo of the increase of such deaths for the sober by two times (Chapter 2-5).

The same tendency is evident in the figure for total crimes committed, with the share by drunken persons rising at an increased rate (Chapter 2-5, Fig. 1-9). It is important to bear in mind that it is easier to determine that a perpetrator of a crime was drunk rather than sober. Nonetheless, it is unlikely that the relation between these figures would change substantially over the three years beginning in 1991, and in 1994, 77 percent of murderers were found to have committed their crime while drunk. In other words, the increase in criminality at the start of the reforms was largely the result of crimes committed by persons while drunk. These figures, like the mortality indexes for death from external causes, show that, in Russia, alcohol is a powerful stimulus for crime or, to put it more broadly, a perverse factor that sharply worsens the country's unfortunate social situation.

Fig. 1-9: Number of persons found to have committed crimes whilst sober (1) or drunk (3). Overall number of homicides committed whilst Sober (2) or drunk (4). All percentages relate to 1991, accepted as 100 percent.

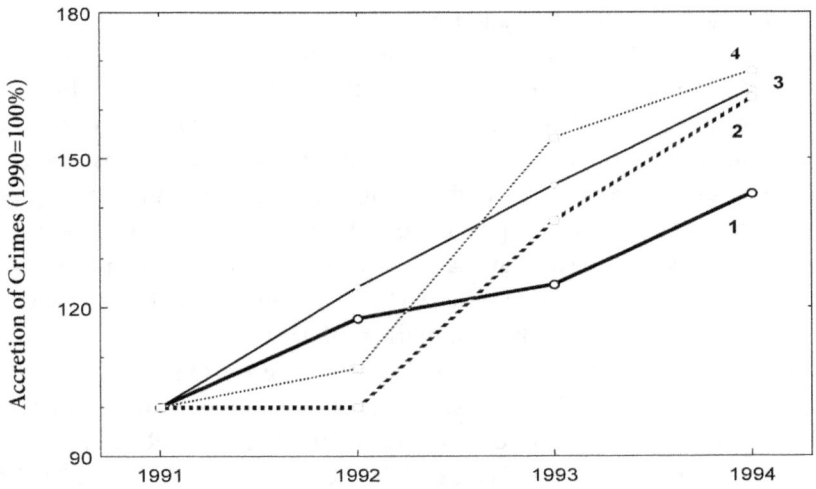

1992–1994 saw increases in all the negative medical and demographic phenomena associated with alcohol consumption, but especially significant was the rise in alcohol psychoses (an increase of 249.2 percent as compared to 1991) and deaths from alcohol poisoning (up 237.5 percent), which stood at 167,900 and 55,500, respectively, in 1994. 1993 was particularly dramatic for Russia. The number of cases of alcohol psychoses rose by 141.4 percent and the mortality from alcohol poisoning by 75.6 percent in a single year, although the preceding five years had seen average yearly increases of 2.5 percent. Moreover, alcohol consumption in 1993 increased by only 5.1 percent. A detailed explanation of this paradox will be given in Chapter 2-5. Here it is worth noting that the headlong rise in deaths from alcohol poisoning in 1992–1993 was a function of the lag time coming to an end (Chapter 2-5) but, even more, reflected the growth in a cohort of alcoholics whose lives had been saved by the anti-alcohol campaign. It is also linked with the appearance in the alcohol market of a larger quantity of illegal alcoholic beverages with excessive toxicity. Thus, according to figures compiled by the Moscow's Health Inspection Services (SES, 1993), approximately 40 percent of alcohol products did not meet government's normative requirements. Some batches of the widely known Royal Vodka were found to contain significant amounts of foreign admixtures: acetone, aldehydes and sulfur compounds, evidence that non-edible spirits were used in making the beverage.

Unfortunately, not all of Russia's Forensic-Medical Review Bureaus had the technology to determine the particular toxic additives at work in the event of deaths from alcohol poisoning. However, typically, in cases of alcohol poisoning, people die with lower concentrations of alcohol in their blood. Thus, in a single year (1992) in the Republic of Karelia, deaths from alcohol poisoning tripled, but the average lethal concentration of alcohol in the blood among the victims dropped by 1.4 times (observations by the author), most likely because of the presence of indeterminable toxic additives.

It is thus not surprising that such a universal and integral index as life expectancy should have fallen especially sharply at the start of the reforms. In 1992–1994, this index declined 6.0 years for men and 3.3 years for women, to 57.5 years and 71.0 years, respectively. In 1992, life expectancy for a man in Russia was 11 years less than male life expectancy in the countries of the European Community.

In 1994 deaths from alcohol poisoning were probably at their highest ever level in Russia – 55,500 deaths or 2.4 percent of all fatalities (for purposes of comparison, the rate was 1 percent in 1964 and 1.7 percent in 1984). That was the price paid for the starting phase of market reforms. One may say that history's gift of freedom was partly paid for with death at the vodka stall.

It is worth comparing the loss caused by alcohol with other Russian losses in 1994. In that year 48,200 persons died as a result of homicide in Russia, of which 60–70 percent were intoxicated. The first Chechen war cost Russia 35,700 civilian and military deaths (Mukomel, 2005). Calculations of the "alcohol loss", in comparison with the number of killed, gives an approximate idea of the dimensions of Russia's alcohol problems in relation to other problems.

It can be objected that the 48,200 homicides were not the whole picture of Russian criminality. Neither, however, do the 55,500 deaths from alcohol poisoning in any sense exhaust the whole of the losses to alcohol, which were almost 10 times greater if other causes of death are considered (Chapter 2-5). Moreover, the loss to alcohol includes losses to industry, family problems and divorces, drunken vandalism and thefts, problematic children, an army of actual and future alcoholics and much else besides. A survey conducted by the Russian Public

Opinion Research Center (VTsIOM) in the summer of 1993 found that 43 percent of those surveyed considered drunkenness the most serious problem of family life (*Izvestiya*, 14 August, 1993). This figure can be interpreted as meaning that 43 percent of Russian families contain, at least, one alcoholic in the family or close to it. More generally, this can be seen as indicating how closely linked to alcohol the social, psychological and health problems of current and future citizens of Russia are.

To this must be added the huge budget shortfalls caused by the failure to collect excise taxes. It was assumed that the measures listed in Presidential Decree 918, dated 11 June, 1993, on the return to a state monopoly in alcohol, would bring in much of the money to the budget that had been shielded from payment as excise tax. Insofar, however, as nothing of this kind occurred, a new presidential decree (No. 2270), issued on 22 December, 1993, raised the tax on hard liquor by 5 percent (effective from 1 January, 1994). In other words, the new decree resolved only one problem, a problem not openly expressed in the preceding decree, namely, the budget problem or, more precisely, the search for means to meet the government's obligations, above all to pay wages.

The story of the second decree is further notable in that it made clear the presence in Russia of a powerful alcohol and spirits lobby, which conducted a brief, but very intense propaganda campaign in the mass media. The authors of countless articles threatened that, were the excise tax increased, "unemployment would soar", "the widespread collapse of a whole sector of the Russian economy would ensue" and that "the treasury would lose more than 1 trillion rubles". They even raised the frightening possibility of a "Russian uprising" (all quotations from various publications).

The speed with which the campaign came into being and its breadth attested to the considerable means at the disposal of the alcohol lobby. The propaganda campaign climaxed with an "extraordinary convocation" of the directors of all the alcohol and spirits factories in Russia (3 February, 1994). Its aim was to "work out anti-crisis measures for the sector"; in fact, the aim was to pressure the government to rescind the new excise tax.

Also impressive were the speed and completeness of the government's capitulation – within days the former 85 percent excise tax was reinstated. As asserted by the journal *Russkaya Vodka* (p 55, No. 6, 2003), "the cost of the decrease was 800,000 USD", which "certain well-known persons in the Russian parliamentary building" received; the directors of alcohol producing plants simply "chipped in together".

With all due respect to the organizational abilities and financial possibilities of the alcohol lobby, one must also speak of the government of that time, busily patching up holes in the budget. The fact is that a mere 5 percent increase in an excise tax would have approximately caused a 1.5 times increase in prices because of the increase in value-added tax, transportation costs and retail markups. Once again the rulers of the country ignored the special character of a commodity like alcohol, which demands that, in addition to economic aspects, its psychological, social and cultural aspects be taken into account, which the alcohol lobby did for its own benefit.

After its defeat, the government returned to more civilized methods of managing the alcohol market. On 22 April, 1994, Prime Minister Viktor Chernomyrdin, in further developing the first presidential decree (No. 918), signed Resolution No. 358, "On Measures for the Re-establishment of the Government Monopoly on the Production, Storage, and Wholesale and Retail Sale of Alcohol Products". The Ministry of Economics began work on a "federal program specifically on the production and sale of alcohol products", where the task was to determine the quantity of alcohol needed in the country and its price. Beginning from 1 January, 1995, it was intended that all imported alcoholic beverages would be marked. However, this deadline was subsequently put off a number of times, which was typical of how the government conducted itself in the alcohol market.

Meanwhile vodka continued to fall in price, sometimes in absolute terms, as, for example, in April 1994, when its cost fell by 1.6 percent, but more often, in terms relative to the increase in wages and the prices of other goods (Fig. 1-8) or to inflation, and this, undoubtedly, spurred the rise in alcohol consumption.

Unfortunately, this was the very time when the destruction of the narcological service, a process that began in 1989 (Chapter 1-6) and continued into the early 1990s went even further. The Law on the Militia, adopted in 1991, among other things freed the militia from "functions not natural to it" and, thus, from the Medical-Labor Clinics (LTPs), which housed up to 150,000 of the most abusive alcoholics as a way of preventing their socially harmful behavior. The law called for the closing of all LTPs by 30 June, 1994. The result was that approximately 150,000 of the most abusive alcoholics were out on the streets again and swelled the cohort of the chief consumers of alcohol. This took place just when alcohol mortality was reaching its highest level ever in Russian history (Chapter 2-5).

As part of the freedom granted entrepreneurial efforts in the country, there arose a large sector devoted to narcological help. It worked on a principle of anonymity and, for the most part, had a single contact with sick alcoholics. The positive side of this sector was that it offered an alternative to and provided competition for state narcology, which found itself forced to supplement its own service with subunits that adopted similar principles. But there was a negative side, too: the private sector was to a significant extent staffed by non-specialist doctors or simply by self-elected individuals, who discredited narcological methods of treatment. Moreover, one-time medical contact with a patient is a poor basis for lasting remission. It can be justified only in the sense that a single contact with a sick person (if the contact is by a narcological specialist) is better than no contact at all.

In summing up the results of this brief but highly dramatic period in the alcohol history of Russia, one must state that there was a sharp increase in alcohol consumption to 14.6 liters in 1992–1994, which exceeded the level (14.2 liters) on the eve of the anti-alcohol campaign. This took place

- because of a sharp rise in the production and consumption of unregistered (by the state) alcohol, with such alcohol becoming the main source of all alcohol consumption;
- because of a relative fall in the price of alcohol products that reflected the non-payment of most excise taxes and customs duties as well as the production and smuggling into Russia of a large quantity of illegal alcoholic beverages.

In addition

- in terms of alcohol consumption, Russia now ranked first in the world (France was second, at 13 liters; for purposes of comparison, U.S. consumption was 7.5 liters in 1992);
- the state had entirely lost control of the largest part of the alcohol market in the country, while the state budget failed to receive a significant portion of budgeted tax receipts from the alcohol industry;
- alcohol abuse was seriously worsening the socioeconomic crisis in Russia;
- the negative consequences of alcohol consumption reached levels that threatened the physical, psychological and social health of the Russian population.

Chapter 1-8
The alcohol situation
1995–1998

In previous periods, the sharp changes in the alcohol situation were the result of sharp changes in socio-political conditions in the country in 1985 and 1992. Unlike those times, the new stage that began in 1995 was not accompanied by any such substantial changes in political life or the economy. The factors that determined it had built up in the preceding period. The well-being of the bulk of the population began a sharp decline as a result of an enormous rise in inflation. Prices increased by 1,000 percent and output was down by a third. The climax was the default of 1998, which "wiped out" the public's savings.

The principal indicators of the onset of this new stage in Russia's alcohol history were those phenomena that are strictly linked to the level of alcohol consumption: deaths from alcohol poisoning, alcohol psychoses among other things – its negative consequences. There were no reliable indexes of the actual level of consumption of alcohol in Russia at this time, as there were none for the other periods. The figures compiled by the State Statistical Committee of the Russian Federation on the "quantity of sales" cannot be accepted as tallies of actual consumption. They were much lower than the official figures on alcohol consumption before the start of the anti-alcohol campaign (Table 1), although the alcohol losses to the country in 1994–1995 were fully on par with those in the early 1980s (Chapter 2-5). Unfortunately, Treml (1997) took his estimates of Russian consumption only up to 1993, but the present author, using a methodology worked out earlier, has brought the estimate up to 1994 and, with the help of a supplemented methodology, to 2001 (Chapter 2-4).

There are, in addition, a host of estimates made by foreign writers or with their participation, which are based on survey data from samples of the population (this is dealt with in greater detail in Chapter 2-3). But none of the estimates work as estimates of actual consumption, including the largest of them, which surveyed more than 10,000 respondents over 10 years (Zohoori et al., 1997a and 1997b, http://www.cpc.unc.edu/rims). Chapter 2-3 will present proof that this estimate, like most of those by other researchers, is very low because of the way in which it was calculated.

There are many estimates of the production figures for alcoholic beverages in this period made by specialists from Russia's alcohol industry. Thus, for example, the Declaration of the 1st Congress of Russian Producers of Alcohol Products gives a production total of 137 million decaliters of pure alcohol for 1996, which yields an average per capita alcohol use of 9.3 liters. As it happens, this is the highest estimate of the many estimates of this kind that exist. The absence of a description of the method used while calculating the figure makes it difficult to judge its usefulness for estimates of the actual level of alcohol consumption in Russia after 1994.

Using the new methodology, one sees that a decline in alcohol consumption was underway from 1995 to 1998. This corresponds well with such indirect measures as deaths from alcohol poisoning, pancreatitis and cirrhosis of the liver, the incidence of alcohol psychoses and violent deaths. All these measures began to decline in 1995–1996, as did the figures for overall mortality.

Most likely, the sharp and synchronous diminution in these measures was a function of the action of a single factor, and the linkage of these measures with alcohol attests that the factor was the decline in the level of alcohol consumption. This is similarly attested to by the increase in the tempo of decline of the number of crimes committed by inebriated persons in comparison to crimes by sober individuals after 1995 (Fig. 1-9) and official figures on the decline in the production of vodka and other alcoholic goods from 124.8 million decaliters in 1994 to 86.4 million dal in 1998.

The question then naturally arises: What reasons lay behind the decline in alcohol consumption that began in 1995? To answer this, one can compare alcohol consumption with other phenomena, alcohol-related and non-alcohol-related, that occurred in the country not long before or after 1994. In this connection, it is useful to recall the multi-component character of the diagram of the alcohol situation presented at the start of this book (Fig. 1-1) A small number of key elements were the basis for changes in earlier periods, but in 1985 there was only one or almost only a single one, the anti-alcohol campaign, which sharply limited the accessibility of alcoholic beverages and in this way lowered alcohol consumption. Most likely, the same factor – reduced accessibility – lay at the base of the new decline in consumption in 1995–1998. But in 1985 this factor had a very elementary composition, the reduction in state production and state sales of alcoholic beverages, then the major sources of the alcohol consumed in the USSR and Russia. By 1995 there were many channels through which alcohol products reached the market, and the state had, to a significant degree, lost control over the production, importation and sale of alcohol in the country. However, the government still had several ways to affect the alcohol situation, one of which turned out to be a factor, though not a substantial one, in the lowering of consumption that began in 1995.

The preceding chapter took up the long, painful and sometimes tragic history of the rescinding of customs and excise-tax privileges for a number of organizations. This relates above all to the National Sports Foundation and the Russian

Foundation of Invalids of the War in Afghanistan. The struggle to remove these privileges, which had begun in 1994, continued in 1995 and 1996. Even as late as 1997, there is documentation of the arrival of some shipments of privileged alcohol products stemming from earlier contracts, but these were already arriving under the guise of humanitarian aid. However, 1995 was the turning point: imports of alcoholic beverages fell sharply, by almost three-quarters (figures from the State Customs Committee of the Russian Federation), with a consequent increase in prices and fall in demand. Such were the dimensions of the importation of privileged alcohol that the sharp reduction in 1995 substantially affected prices across the alcohol market. The relationship between prices of food products and alcoholic beverages changed (Fig. 1-8).

At the same time as the channels of the privileged were being closed off with considerable difficulty, a new way for cheap vodka to reach Russia appeared – the so-called "Belo-Russian corridor". In November 1995, President Alexander Lukashenko of Belarus exempted the state trading-exporting company, Torgekspo, from payment of customs duties and excise and value-added taxes on purchases made in Britain of consumer goods. This was done as a new year's gift to the nation and was worth half a billion USD. Belarus did not then have funds enough to cover gifts to the public and allowed "third parties", which happened to be Russian companies, to make contributions.

As a result, a significant portion of the "gifts" to the people of Belarus came in the form of vodka transited through Belarus en route to Russia, where it crossed the border unhindered in light of the customs union between the two countries. In such fashion, Russian firms working with Torgekspo avoided paying taxes and excise duty and were able to sell vodka at reduced prices. There was only one positive thing about the deal – its brevity. It ended in mid-1996, when the final and decisive government resolution (No. 816, dated 18 July, 1996), ending all privileges and thus the flow of vodka not subject to excise taxes, was published. According to figures of the State Customs Committee of the Russian Federation, for the first nine months of 1996, as compared with the same period in 1995, imports of alcohol from countries outside the former Soviet Union fell by an additional 75 percent, as had been the case in 1995. Accordingly, there was a reduction in sales at dumping prices, which had to be reflected in retail prices, which began to "catch up" with prices of food products and other goods (1995–1997; Fig. 1-8). The rise in prices of alcoholic beverages is precisely one of the factors limiting the accessibility of alcohol (Österberg, 1995).

Another way in which the government can affect the alcohol market is through a struggle against underground production of illegal vodka and other alcoholic beverages that had also brought down market prices for these products. This struggle has intensified in the mid-1990s. Thus, in 1994, agencies of the Ministry of Internal Affairs eliminated more than 1,500 underground workshops making illegal alcoholic beverages; in 1995 the figure was more than 2,300 and in 1998 it was 3,400. So great was the volume of confiscated spirits and illegal beverages (10.9 million liters of alcohol products in 1995, and 33.3 million in 1998) that a serious problem arose concerning what to do with these materials. Most often, they were reprocessed into chemical items of everyday use, which is what was done, for example, by the Khimkinsky and other factories in Moscow, which made brake or glass-cleaning fluids from the sequestered materials. But there were also instances where confiscated materials of this kind moved on to another underground workshop from which, after a change of label, they finally made their way to the retail market.

A major problem for the Russian alcohol market involved the production in North Ossetia (Alania) of good quality vodka that, through machinations with excise taxes, sold much more cheaply than locally produced vodka. This aggrieved legitimate Russian producers. It was noted in the preceding chapter that the personnel makeup of the Ministry of Agricultural Products had led to the bulk of food-based spirits, allotted by quota to the ministry, being concentrated in North Ossetia. Using these spirits and spirits purchased in Ukraine, a network of several very large and a great many small plants formed. This network produced vodka which was distributed throughout the country and that amounted to approximately 40 percent of all vodka consumed in Russia.

The market reforms deprived North Ossetia of the quotas assigned to the Ministry of Agricultural Products, but new sources of cheaper spirits were found, at first in Ukraine but later raw material supplies for vodka production also reached North Ossetia by truck from Georgia. The port of Poti became expert in handling tankers arriving with cheap spirits from Turkey, Ukraine, the United States and Canada. Georgia earned considerable income from the receipt and trucking of spirits across its own territory. The official cost of merely transporting one liter of spirits was eight cents. Georgian truck drivers earned a lot, but even more went to the Tbilisi authorities, who took part in this profitable arrangement. Although at the head of the organization of the receipt and transportation of spirits stood the Georgian mafia.

The spirit was transported by rail from the city of Poti to Gori, where it was reloaded into trucks. For the most part, these were large-capacity spirit-tanker-trucks that traveled by the Trans-Caucasian and Georgian Military Road to the Roki Tunnel in the Darial Gorge, upon exiting from which they crossed the border into Russia. A smaller flow of contraband spirit went by the Ossetia-Military Road and the Alagir Gorge. On the transit documents, all the spirit was listed as "wine materials" or "cognac spirit", which was not subject to taxes on crossing the Georgian-Russian border. The Georgian and Ossetia mafia spent a good deal of money to make sure that Russian customs personnel would fail to "notice" the discrepancy between the actual contents of the trucks with what was described on their accompanying documents.

In July 1997, the director of the Federal Border Service, General Nikolaev, acting with the support of the president of Russia, ordered the Russian border to be closed to Georgian alcohol trucks and, on his own initiative, had the border posts moved 1.5 kilometers into the neutral zone to the exit from the Roki Tunnel. Customs officers were transferred there, and they now began demanding payment of duties on the alcohol being moved. These were large amounts of money that no one wanted to pay. In the course of several months, 2,300 alcohol trucks, carrying about 30,000 tons of spirit, were stopped, while tankers with new shipments of alcohol continued to arrive at Poti and other Georgian ports. The losses to Ossetia's vodka makers as well as to the Ossetia and Georgian mafia and the Tbilisi authorities cooperating with them were so high that, in addition to the protests by "students" at the Roki Tunnel and the attempted breakthrough by five trucks that cost one driver's life, both Georgia's Ministry of Foreign Affairs and the president of Georgia joined in the protests to demand a return to the old border control. The president of Russia ordered Nikolaev to capitulate, and, as a result, in December 1997, the general tendered his resignation, which the president accepted. The flow of alcohol across the Russian-Georgian border resumed, though at a somewhat reduced level. While the vodka war ended with the defeat of the Russian side, the quantities of raw material reaching Ossetia's vodka industry were cut, as were its earnings. From time to time until even as late as 2006, large shipments of illegal vodka from Vladikavkaz were still stopped on Russian territory, while other shipments probably still passed by unnoticed. But the overall quantity is not what it was before the events at the Roki Tunnel.

Although the underground production of alcohol products was reduced, a new approach was born – non-excise alcohol, that is, illegal alcohol production at legal plants: two shifts produced legal vodka, while a third shift produced the very same vodka, but on this vodka no excise taxes were paid. Production of "third-shift vodka" could not have existed without corruption.

What is most striking in the official reports is the very low percentage of their capacity that Russian alcohol plants were then using (from 3 percent to 15 percent). According to figures from the Ministry of Economics, when used capacity falls to under one-third, plants become unprofitable. Despite their apparent unprofitability, there was a steady increase in the number of alcohol plants (from 373 in 1995 to 830 in 1998). The situation continued into the new stage. According to figures from the State Statistical Committee of the Russian Federation, in the year 2000, with capacity to produce 400.7 million decaliters of vodka, Russia's vodka and other alcohol plants produced a total of 122 million decaliters, or 30.4 percent of capacity. This means that the actual production of strong alcoholic beverages by legal plants significantly exceeded the reported amounts. Naturally, taxes were not paid on such unaccounted production and brought extremely high profits to the shadow economy. Naturally, too, in order to produce this unaccounted vodka, one must have unaccounted spirit.

The main source of raw material for the illegal production of alcohol products in 1995–1998 was spirit smuggled across almost the entire length of the Russian border. The Darial Gorge and the Roki Tunnel were merely one road to the border and one point on it, but they were, for the time being, the most important for the flow of spirit.

Government activity in the field of alcohol legislation intensified after 1994. It had, in fact, begun in 1993 with the issuance of the presidential decree, "On Restoration of the Government Monopoly on the Production, Storage, and Wholesale and Retail Trade in Alcohol Products" (11 July, 1993, No. 918). That year, too, the Duma passed the "Bases of the Legislation of the Russian Federation for Protecting the Health of Citizens", which prohibited the advertising of alcoholic beverages in the mass media. The latter measure had virtually no effect, which necessitated, less than two years later, issuance of the presidential decree, "On Guarantees of the Right of Citizens for Health Protection in the Dissemination of Advertisements…", in which, unlike in the "Bases of the Legislation", some degree of responsibility for violations was stipulated. This does not mean, however, that violations did not occur after the decree. On every occasion, for example, when Moscow found itself short of money, the city was beautified with advertisements for alcohol products.

Presidential Decree No. 918 and the subsequent government resolution (26 September, 1994, No. 1088) that made it legally binding had no effect on the alcohol market. That is why the government was forced as early as in February 1995 to adopt a new resolution on measures to stabilize the Russian market in alcohol products; its principal aim was to increase payments to the state budget. It assumed that this effort would enlist the services of the Customs Committee of the Russian Federation, the Ministry of Internal Affairs and the State Security Service – the FSK. In the very same year, the Duma (22 July, 1995) and Federation Council (15 November, 1995) revoked a presidential veto and adopted a law, "On State Regulation of the Production and Sale of Ethyl Spirit and Alcohol Products", which was signed by the president on 22 November, 1995. The law again established a state monopoly on the production and sale of alcohol products and sharply limited imports of such products in to Russia (no more than 20 percent of all alcohol sales, with no less than 80 percent of imports being wine). The law prohibited the creation of organizations with foreign investments for the importation, or sale of drink and other sales of alcohol products containing more than 12 percent ethyl spirit. The latter stipulation was the main reason for the presidential veto, which was dictated by the country's obligations to the European Community. The law stipulated the licensing and declaration by producers and sellers of alcohol products of the quantities of production and sales. There were, of course, to be punishments for violations.

It was assumed that the law "On State Regulation of the Production and Sale of Ethyl Spirit and Alcohol Products" would act as the basic regulator of the alcohol market. However, this does not seem to have occurred, judging by the continuing efforts (2007) by the country's authorities in this direction.

In parallel with the difficult creation and passage of the law "On Government Regulation...", the government also convened an interagency commission under the leadership of Yakov Moiseevich Urinson, the first deputy of the minister of economics of the Russian Federation. It included high-ranking representatives of all the immediately concerned ministries and departments, including the so-called *siloviki*. The commission's task was to find the ways and means to increase receipts in the budget from the production and sale of alcohol products. This was necessary because the share of tax receipts from sales of alcohol products had fallen to 2 percent! For purposes of comparison, the share, even during the heyday of the anti-alcohol campaign, had never fallen below 10 percent. The commission planned to raise the share of domestically produced alcohol products, which at that point constituted barely half of all the alcohol consumed.

Urinson's commission created a whole package of "vodka" documents, many of which soon became presidential decrees or government resolutions: an increase in the fines for violations of the law from 100 times the daily level of social benefit to 5,000 times, privileges for domestic producers, the establishment of a minimum price for drinks with a strength higher than 28 percent ABV, that had been in practice earlier but which was now given the force of law.

1996 was especially rich in legislation. Changes in the law "On Excise Taxes" (14 February, 1996), three presidential decrees (Nos. 161, 165 and 1213) and more than 10 government resolutions were aimed at increasing receipts coming in to the budget and at making the alcohol situation in the country healthier. One of the resolutions introduced, as of 1 January, 1997, a system for marking all alcohol products with excise stamps denoting the payment of the excise tax. On 10 January, 1997, this measure was made legal by an amendment to the law "On Government Regulation...." But as early as on 1 September, 1997, because of numerous instances of counterfeit stamps, principally in Ukraine and Belarus, the original offset-printed stamp had to be replaced by a new, metallographic one. The introduction of the new excise stamps increased the cost of the final product, for both hard liquors and weaker beverages. This is why the Duma, under pressure from the "beer-lobby", as early as December 1996 had decided that beer would not be considered an alcoholic beverage.

A new presidential decree prohibited, as of 1 July, 1997, the sale of alcohol products of more than approximately 12 percent ABV strength by smaller retailers (e.g. stalls, kiosks, booths etc.) without their own separate sales room. Undoubtedly, such an innovation did help bring order to the trade in alcoholic beverages. But one cannot dismiss the possibility that the decree also had a quite different subtext: the competitive struggle between the large alcohol businesses and small entrepreneurs, who had the advantage of greater commercial dynamism and, were thus, "interfering" with big business.

In all this activity of the leadership of the country, one important characteristic of contemporary alcohol policy in Russia was clear: its priorities lay in the economic sphere and principally sought to increase budget receipts. The problem of preserving the health and lives of citizens was taken up only in passing and only insofar as greater orderliness in the sales of alcoholic beverages led to decreases in consumption and the improved quality of alcoholic beverages.

It is difficult to estimate the effectiveness of all these fiscal and legislative actions by the leadership of the country. On the basis of accessible materials, it is hard to say to what extent the decline in consumption in 1995–1998 was attributable to the government's actions during these two or three years. After all, the first group of government resolutions (Nos. 127–132), which were developed in accord with the federal law "On Government Regulation of Production and Sale of Alcohol Products", were adopted on 8 February, 1996, and the next (Nos. 915, 938, 943 and 948) in July 1996, while the decrease in consumption began in 1995. Thus, one must conclude that by far the most effective government measure was the struggle against privileges, which began in 1994.

In moving away from the topic of excise tax exemptions, the author cannot refrain from commenting on those who opened the doors to privileged vodka and thus, under the banner of Russian sports, aid for war invalids or support for the Russian Orthodox Church, paved the way for the deaths of hundreds of thousands of Russian citizens and deprived the Russian budget of trillions of rubles! It is just as well, indeed, that the matter of the privileges appears to be over, at least in its former amplitude.

An important factor that might have helped to lower alcohol consumption beginning in 1995 was the increasing pauperization of the population, which reduced its purchasing power. One of the reasons for this impoverishment was the rise in wage and salary arrears, which stood at 0.9 percent of the wage fund in 1992, 4.8 percent in 1994 and 11.7 in 1996 (Gordon, 1997). The income of the population was cut. Thus, in 1992 income exceeded expenditure by 13.6 percent, stood at -4.5 percent in 1994 and then at 1.4 percent in 1996 (figures from the State Statistical Committee of the Russian Federation). In line with this, spending on alcoholic beverages declined. It equated to 4 percent of consumer outlay in 1992, 2.9 percent in 1994 and 2.5 percent in 1996 (data from the State Statistical Committee of the Russian Federation). This was occurring while wage increases were lagging behind the increases in prices for consumer goods overall and for alcoholic beverages. A sharp decline took place in the quality of life of the population. This can be seen in the indexes for the consumption of food products, and also in the decrease in the overall caloric value of food consumed and in its protein content which started in 1994 (Fig. 1-10).

Fig. 1-10: Life expectancy for men and women and calorie and protein content of food consumed by Russian population (1992–1996) (RussStat).

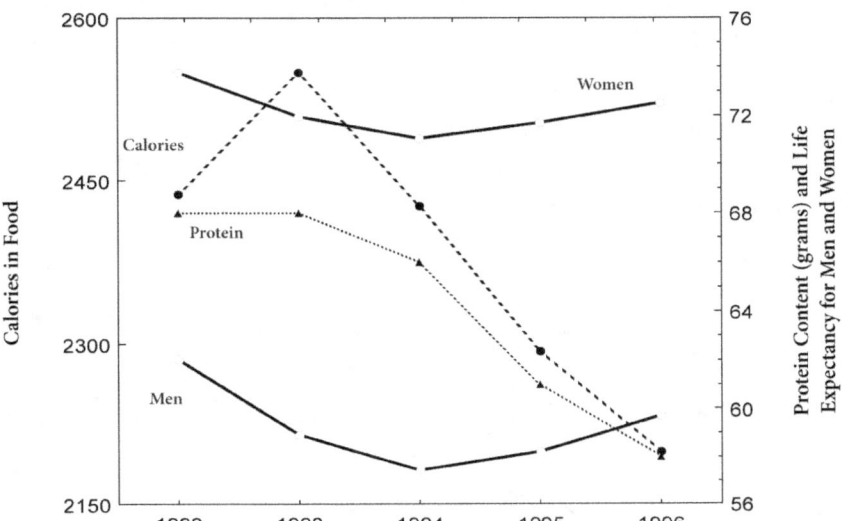

It is necessary to note that, despite all the negative social phenomena just listed and many others, an increase in life expectancy occurred for men as well as women (Fig. 1-10). This is important because 1995 saw the start of the decrease in alcohol consumption and because the gain in life expectancy happened despite a sharp deterioration in the quality of life of the population. This again shows the significance of alcohol consumption for the mortality of the population of Russia and, accordingly, for its life expectancy.

An important factor in the overall decrease in alcohol consumption that began in 1995 may have been the increase in deaths in the country that began in 1992 which resulted from the increase in alcohol abuse (Fig. 1-11). Those who died were mostly in the age range 20–69 years, the group with the highest alcohol consumption rate. And this cohort included the many alcoholics whose lives were saved during the years of the anti-alcohol campaign, but who still faced the risk of an alcohol related death in the form of illnesses contracted during their earlier periods of alcohol abuse.

The coincidence of the rise in general mortality and mortality caused by alcohol poisoning (Figs. 1-11, 1-12) makes reasonable the supposition that among those who died in this period there were many alcoholics, that is, persons who were prime consumers of alcohol. The decrease of such a large cohort of heavy alcohol consumers could substantially lower overall consumption.

The disjunction between the age distribution of general mortality and mortality from alcohol poisoning among 15 to 34 year-olds (Fig. 1-11) is a function of the fact that alcohol poisoning usually occurs among alcoholics and that, in order to become one or the other, a relatively protracted and massive alcoholization is required (six or more years, Nemtsov & Pokrovskaya, 1997). It is not difficult to suppose that the increase in mortality in 1992–1994 among persons aged 15–34 years was linked with alcoholization (for example, due to road traffic injuries, drowning etc.).

Fig. 1-11: Age distribution of men's deaths in 1985–1986 in relation to 1984, and in 1992–1994 in relation to 1991. The thick lines and squares refer to overall mortality and the thin lines and points to deaths from alcohol poisoning.

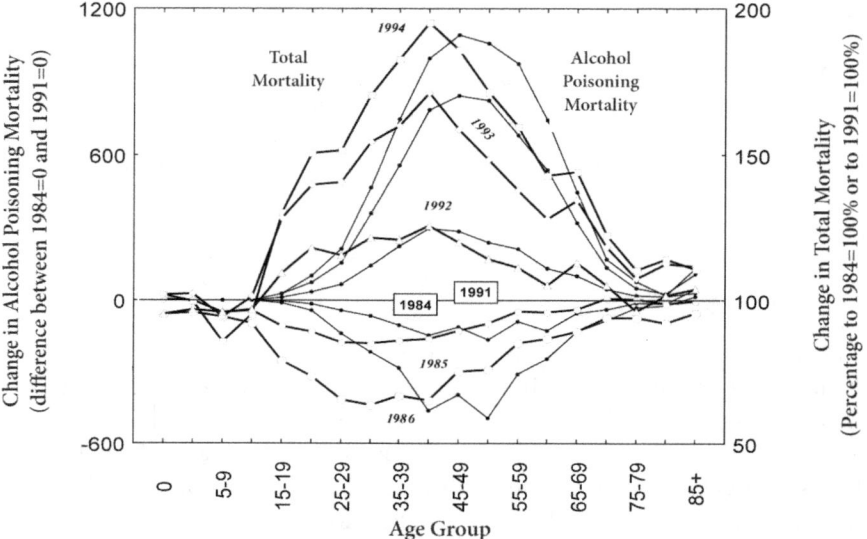

As a result of the processes listed above, the year 1995 witnessed a slowing down of the rate of increase in the price difference between food products and alcohol products (Fig. 1-8), and in 1996–1997 prices of alcoholic beverages began to catch up with food prices, although prices on both kinds of goods increased both before and after this period. In 1996 the combined price index for food products rose by 8 percent but by 48 percent for alcohol products. The speeding up of the increase in prices for alcohol products is an important indicator of the normalization of the alcohol market. A lowered level of alcohol consumption moved hand-in-hand with it.

It is also worth mentioning another important factor that may have influenced the general decline in the level of alcohol consumption in 1995–1998. In recent years, many alcohol consumers, especially young people, have begun to develop a preference for weak alcoholic beverages, principally beer. According to figures compiled by the State Statistical Committee (Fig. 1-13) as well as in estimates offered by Business Analytica Europe Ltd., a firm that specializes in consumer market research (*Itogi*, 12 December, 1998), beer is the only drink in

Russia whose consumption has risen sharply, in quantitative terms reaching the level of consumption of vodka in 1998 and continuing to rise in succeeding years (Fig. 1-13).

Fig. 1-12: Overall mortality and mortalities from alcohol poisoning (1965–2005). Dotted line is regression for 1965–1979.

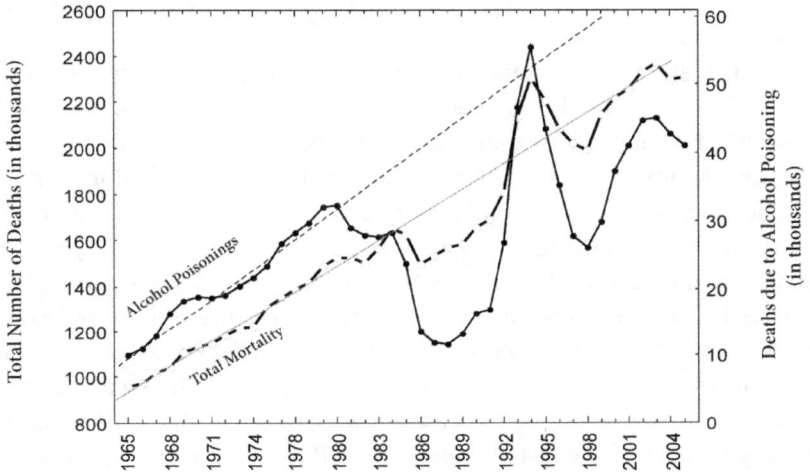

Fig. 1-13: The production and sales of vodka and beer (1990–2000) (in millions of decaliters). The shaded area represents the difference in the official figures for sales and production of vodka.

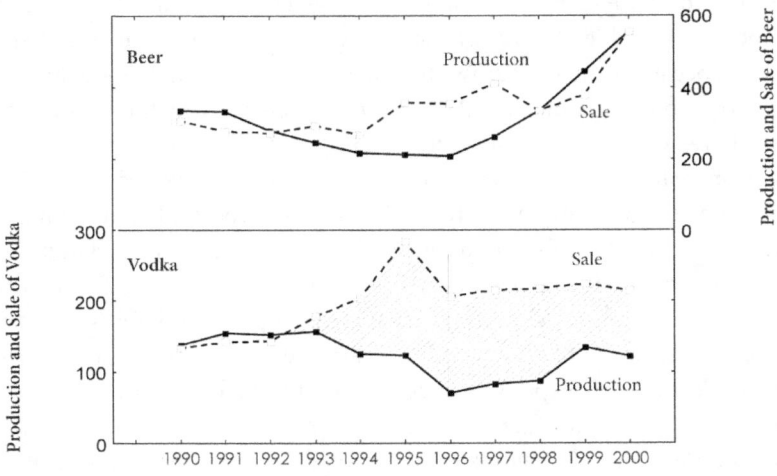

Business Analytica Europe Ltd.'s estimates cannot be dismissed as empty words. Their estimates of average per capita consumption of alcohol (for 1998) attribute

10.8 liters of alcohol to vodka and 1 liter to beer. The total alcohol from these two sources is close to the figure for overall consumption for the same period (Chapter 2-4). Also characteristic is that demand for imported alcoholic beverages, principally hard liquor, fell by almost 75 percent in tandem with the increase in their prices in the second half of the 1990s. After the default of August 1998, the structure of alcohol consumption swung in the direction of greater consumption of beer (Fig. 1-13). Although beer prices rose, they rose less than prices on stronger beverages and even less when compared with other food products and consumer goods.

But the crux of the matter concerns not only a change in the quantity of beer consumed (Fig. 1-13) but also the new character assumed by beer consumption, a quite significant change in the attitude toward beer, which for a large segment of young people now became an element of their lifestyles. This, along with the relative cheapness of beer, was probably one of the reasons for the increase in beer consumption nationwide.

In addition, until the start of the 1990s, beer often played a "supporting" role and was used as a basic component of *yersh* (i.e. a mixture of beer and vodka) where it was an "intensifier" of the action of vodka ("vodka without beer is money thrown to the wind") or, in hot weather, as a cooling drink. The variety of imported beverages arriving in the country as a result of the market reforms significantly broadened the taste preferences of Russian consumers, theretofore very limited. The cohort of beer lovers significantly increased, who not long before had had to satisfy themselves with choosing between the Zhigulevsky and Moskovsky brands. There was even a "Party of Beer Lovers" registered.

The Russian brewing industry quickly responded to the widened circle of beer consumers and their preferences and was encouraged by regional authorities, who looked to beer as an added source of income for local budgets. Large and small beer breweries began to emerge across Russia, mostly producing low-quality beer. But there were also beer giants, like Baltika (St Petersburg), which began producing in 1990. Three years later, a controlling interest in the brewery was acquired by a Scandinavian concern, Baltic Beverages Holding, which invested 105 million USD to upgrade the operation. As early as 1998, Baltika produced 45 million decaliters of beer per year (of 9 different kinds), and owned, in addition to Baltika in St Petersburg, three plants in other cities (Rostov-on-Don, Yaroslavl, Tula), which were earmarked for upgrade using credit from the European Bank for Reconstruction and Development. Baltika intended to distribute its beer throughout Russia. In all likelihood, the firm's expansionist activity cost the life of its financial director, Ilya Vaisman who was murdered 10 January, 2000.

Another marketing tack was taken by Baltika's (Baltic Beverages Holding) principal rival, the international company Sun Brewing Ltd. The quantity of its beer output lagged only slightly behind its rival's and by 1998 it owned a controlling interest in breweries in Ivanovo, Saransk, Kursk, Volzhsk, Ekaterinburg,

Perm and in St Petersburg (the Bavaria plant). The company followed a principle that dictated that beer should be made where it is consumed.

According to expert estimates, 20–30 percent of the beer produced in Russia in this period was already controlled by foreign companies, which invested funds even in smaller breweries on the assumption that the market for beer in Russia would broaden, especially in the cities. And there was a basis for such thinking: beer consumption in large cities is approximately twice the average of consumption nationwide. Small cities and rural areas were and remain "indifferent" to beer, that is, its price was at the level or slightly lower than a bottle of samogon or illegal vodka. Moreover, even the pricing of legal vodka and beer was not to the advantage of beer: 1 gram of alcohol in the beer was 2.5 times more costly than the same gram in vodka (Andrienko & Nemtsov, 2005).

The broadening of the brewing industry in Russia was also encouraged by the default of August 1998, one result of which was to make imported beer uncompetitive, to reduce deliveries of it and to allow Russian-made beer to come to dominate the market (Fig. 1-13). Foreign beer companies/importers and their Russian dealers began to experience huge losses. In connection with this, millions (USD) were spent on lobbying efforts to have beers included in the list of alcoholic beverages. This would have led to higher excise taxes and, thus, higher prices for domestic beers and their greater price equivalency with imported beers.

As early as September 1998, the Duma adopted an amendment to the law "On Government Regulation of Production and Sale of Ethyl Spirit and Alcohol Products" which stated that beer was an alcoholic product. In the mass media this provoked a storm, "stirred up" further by the largest domestic producers of beer, who for the time put aside the fierce competitive struggle between themselves. As a result of this, and possibly with good reason, the Federation Council did not approve the amendment, thus maintaining the price discrepancy between domestic and imported beer. According to figures from the State Statistical Committee of the Russian Federation, imports of beer fell by 64.8 percent in January-November 1999 as compared with the same period in 1998. It was likely then that there would also be further declines in beer imports and that the consumption of domestic beer would continue to climb, aiding the slight shift of interest away from vodka to beer and lead on to the new drink fads that would flare up in the next few years (Chapter 1-9).

The events just described in and around the alcohol market were an inspiration for several of the country's leaders. First Deputy Prime Minister Boris Nemtsov declared proudly in October 1997 that, in a single year, receipts of excise taxes from vodka had soared so much that "today the government truly controls 50–60 percent of the Russian market in alcoholic products". It may be noted in passing that this is very questionable grounds for pride. According to Nemtsov, the gain had been achieved after "we destroyed all the vodka factories in North Ossetia, stopped the uncontrolled importation of alcohol via Belarus and Ukraine and established use of excise stamps for enterprises in Russia". It is remarkable that, at the very time that Nemtsov was making his declaration, 20 carloads of illegal alcohol from North Ossetia were discovered, and their occupants arrested, in Moscow.

In January 1998, the chairman of the Russian State Committee for Ensuring the Monopoly on Alcohol Production, V. Berestovoi, reported that in 1997 excise collections were up 1.8 times as compared with the year before and that the legal share of the market had risen to above 50 percent. The director of the Federal Tax Police Service, S. N. Almazov, used the same figure for the sales of legal alcohol products at the end of 1997. He gave a figure of 30 percent for the beginning of the year.

In summing up the results of 1998, Finance Minister Zadornov reported that taxes on spirits at the beginning of the year made up 5 percent of the budget's income and that in December, as compared with September, growth had been 50 percent; the sales of excise stamps had also gone up, which, in the minister's view, signified an increase in the production of legal alcohol products.

Meanwhile, and despite such questionable optimism, the leadership of the country had in no way gained control of the alcohol market. Moreover, the leadership had a poor understanding of the actual dimensions of this market and its structure. Evidence of this is to be found in the preamble to a draft federal law, signed by the prime minister, "On Introducing Changes and Supplements into the Federal Law 'On Government Regulation of Production and Sales of Ethyl Spirit and Alcohol Products'". It stated that the "legal manufacture of vodka and liqueurs in 1999, overall, came to approximately 120–125 million decaliters of an estimated production of more than 240 million decaliters. Thus, about 50 percent of vodka and liqueurs products in 1999 were in illegal commerce". Consider, too, that 120–125 million decaliters of vodka comes to 3.3 liters of pure alcohol per capita per year, while 240 million gives a figure of 6.5 liters. Later (Chapter 2-4) it will be shown that in 1999 average per capita consumption of alcohol stood at 14.3 liters a year (Table 1). Hence it follows that the government, while thinking that it controlled half of the alcohol market, actually controlled only one-quarter of it. It must be assumed that the leadership of the government, for one reason or another, was misinformed about the actual dimensions of the country's alcohol problems. And this was of little use in making the alcohol situation in the country healthier or in bringing about a welcome shift in the country's alcohol history.

Chapter 1-9
The alcohol situation after 1998

It has already been noted that the division into stages of the latest alcohol history of Russia has been done on the basis of striking changes in the level of alcohol consumption. With this approach, a new stage began in 1999, when consumption increased, as demonstrated by both figures compiled by the State Statistical Committee and estimates made by this author (Table 1). Also moving upward were measures of all the phenomena that are dependent on alcohol, such as total mortality and mortality from alcohol poisoning (Fig. 1-12).

The preceding chapter described a quite high level of government activity in the sphere of alcohol policy. It continued for five or six years and sought to bring order to the alcohol market. In 1999–2000, new measures along these lines were introduced. Thus, on 3 December, 1999, the Duma approved the third reading of the law "On Excises" which raised the excise tax on alcohol products. The government of the Russian Federation adopted a resolution (12 June, 1999, No. 623) on creating "An Interagency Commission to Conduct a Single Government Policy for the Prevention and Stoppage of Illegal Production and Sale of Ethyl Spirit and Alcohol Products". The Federation Assembly of the Russian Federation also created a Consultative-Expert Council on questions concerning the production and sale of ethyl spirit, alcohol- and spirit-containing products. In addition, a working group on the alcohol industry was created in the presidential administration's economics division.

Despite these political decisions and the many actions of the preceding period, alcohol consumption began to grow again in 1999. Among other things, this shows that, in Russia, politics has little influence either on the alcohol market or on the principal measure of the alcohol situation – the level of consumption of alcoholic beverages. This is why changes in consumption little coincide with political activity, unless the latter bears an extreme character, as was the case in 1985 and 1992.

Preceding the rise in alcohol consumption in 1999 was a distinct lagging of price increases for alcoholic beverages behind the rise in prices of food products (Fig. 1-8) and other goods. At this time, the market in alcoholic beverages was significantly less dependent on imports than the market for food products and other consumer goods, the prices of which rose rapidly because of the default

(Fig. 1-8). A new, major spike in the difference between the price of food products and other consumer goods as compared with the price of alcoholic beverages took place – again there was a new relative cheapening in the price of alcoholic beverages and thus an increase in their accessibility, a factor in the rise of consumption.

The default of August 1998 provoked a sharp drop in the exchange value of the ruble, as a result of which prices increased on foreign hard liquors and as a result imports of them fell, by 43.6 percent for January to November 1999 as compared with the same period of 1998 (figures from the State Statistical Committee of the Russian Federation). After the default, such products constituted a fraction of a percentage point of total consumption. Especially unprofitable were imports of cheap German and Belgian vodka. These factors, together with the ending of the privileges for imports of alcoholic beverages, resulted in the fact that, in 1999, for the first time in several years, legal production of strong beverages began to increase (Fig. 1-13). In 1998, 864 million liters of vodka and liqueurs were produced, but in 1999 the figure was 1,346 million liters, or a rise of 56 percent, or 3.3 liters of pure alcohol per capita for the year. This kind of speed in increasing industrial output is suspect. Most likely, it is due to the legalization of a portion of production that was previously illegal. And this is linked with the fact that the default had its effect on the underground production of alcoholic beverages, that is, many of them were made from imported spirit illegally brought across the border, in particular, across the border with Georgia. This spirit was purchased with dollars, but the "illegal" products were sold in rubles. As a result of the fall in the exchange rate of the ruble, the profitability of the underground production of vodka from imported alcohol dropped sharply and the illegal production of vodka was severely curtailed. However, legal production was able to compensate for these losses.

Moreover, also helping the growth in total consumption in 1999 was the appearance of new forms of illegal vodka production. This was now taking place in completely legal enterprises, which (not without the help of regional authorities) "stepped aside" from the payment of taxes. There were various ways to "step aside", the main one being tax preferences (commercial "privileges") granted by local authorities who, independently, lowered excise rates or gave exemptions from payments of value-added taxes. North Ossetia (Alania), Kabardino-Balkaria, Karachayevo-Cherkessia, Tatarstan and Bashkortostan, all of whose governments were becoming more independent of the center, were particularly active along these lines. As a result of preferences, the price of vodka from these and several other regions arrived on the market at a cost of 15–16 rubles for a half-liter bottle as opposed to 22 rubles for vodka on which all taxes were paid (in 1999). "Normal" vodka was now uncompetitive. It was more profitable for retailers to work with these cheaper and thus more rapidly turned over goods.

Another way to avoid taxes was use of non-standard containers with volumes of more than 0.25 liters and less than 0.5 liters (excise taxes and thus the excise stamps applied only to these sizes). For example, on a bottle containing 0.475 liters, a stamp for a volume of 0.25 liters would be placed, thus substantially reducing the excise payment.

There were other ways to avoid paying taxes, in part or altogether, for example, by the sale in the producer's territory of fictitious exports of alcohol, exports not being subject to value-added and excise taxes. There was also "third-shift" vodka, use of cash payments, barter arrangements and imaginative bookkeeping. The result was that a significant share of illegal vodka was produced in legal plants in 1999. This was the "creative contribution" of the default to alcohol production. Clearly, the "contribution" was a factor in the new rise in consumption.

Another factor contributing to consumption growth might have been the replenishment of the cohort of heavy consumers of alcohol, that had dwindled at the start of the market reforms (1992–1994; Chapter 1-7) but revived its consumption potential six or seven years later. It is possible to think that the process of revival began together with the start of the rise in consumption in 1992–1994 and in parallel with the soaring death rate for heavy consumers. A feature of the revival and growth in new users was that it advanced more slowly than the loss of the old because alcoholism and heavy drinking take years to come into being. The death of individuals, meanwhile, with a high risk of dying an alcohol related death takes less time, or may happen in an instant. It is also possible that the difference in the "speed" of losses to, and the restoration of the cohort of alcoholics, in part explain the fluctuating character of Russian mortality over the past 20 years.

The period after 1998 is notable for two political "battles" in the alcohol market. The first flared up in the passions aroused by the excise stamps. 1 July, 1999, was set as the final date for implementing government Resolution No. 601, "On the Marking of Goods and Products on the Territory of the Russian Federation with Stamps of Conformity Protected from Counterfeits". The resolution had been adopted on 17 May, 1997, and had missed several "final" deadlines for implementation, a pattern that has been typical for Russian alcohol policy. The new marking system applied to computer, audio and video equipment as well as to alcohol products. The stamp was to offer assurance of legal conformity and provide an indication of the region of origin, which would make it easy to determine the producer.

As already stated, the new deadline was 1 July, but at a meeting attended by the Minister for Agriculture and Food Shcherbak, on 11 June, a decision was taken to "put the brakes on" the implementation of Resolution No. 601 for vodka until 1 October. A long struggle had preceded the meeting: inquiries by deputies addressed to the government, press briefings, memoranda from government functionaries about the already existing excise stamps and calculations showing the supposed loss to the government from the introduction of the new marking system and consequent higher prices for alcohol products and lowered demand for them. The decision, of 11 June, 1999, to once again keep vodka out of the marking system, even if only temporarily, may be understood to mean that the government had again suffered defeat at the hands of the "vodka kings" and the regional authorities backing them.

Moreover, by this time more than 30 regions of Russia had established their own marking systems for alcoholic beverages designed to keep alcohol products from other regions out. This was an attempt by regional authorities to increase the receipts to their own budgets. At the same time, it reduced payments to the federal budget and acted as a brake on normal competition. The government tried to eliminate the right of the local authorities to impose their own identification systems, sought to transfer all such questions to the federal level and to make uniform the rules for sales of alcoholic products throughout the country. This would have increased receipts to the federal budget and would have made possible a struggle with the many, virtually official forms of "sidestepping" taxes.

As it transpired, it was not necessary to wait until 1 October, 1999 (the deadline ordered by Shcherbak). Within a month on 12 July, 1999 the government of the Russian Federation issued a new resolution, No. 797, "On the Obligatory Marking with Special Marks of Alcoholic Products Made on the Territory of the Russian Federation".

In addition a new attack continued on the alcohol market with the aim of bringing in funds to the budget. On 3 December, 1999, in the Russian Federation, the Duma, adopted on third reading, an amendment to the law "On Excises" (M2-F3) which called for an increase of 40 percent in the excise duty on vodka and other alcoholic beverages (with the exception of natural wines and beer). The Federation Council approved the amendment, with minor changes, on 22 December. In accord with these actions, on 3 February, 2000, the Ministry of Economic Affairs accepted a new minimum price for vodka of 62 rubles per liter for retail sale which was to come into effect on 25 February, 2000.

However, before the implementation of this decision by the Duma and the Economics Ministry, the presidential election took place. On 15 February, 2000, acting President Vladimir Putin declared that the "price [of vodka – author's comment], as it stands, is at a level at which, approximately, it will remain", which was a signal to work out a series of measures designed to restrain any rise in the price of "40-proof". Despite such repeated assurances from the head of the government, the people of Russia continued to make mass purchases of cheap varieties of vodka. And this time the people were proved right in their distrust of the declarations of the authorities. On 25 February the minimum price of vodka was raised in accordance with the decision of the Economics Ministry.

But on 7 May, 2000, by decree of President Putin a state holding company, Gosspirtprom, was created. The new holding company was intended to bring together under its roof all of the enterprises in the alcohol industry in which the government owned controlling shares. Moreover, the plan was that in the future this holding company would buy up the controlling shares in large private enterprises and, in this fashion, achieve a monopoly position in the industry. This was a reflection of the new policy of a bolstered role for the state in the country's economy. Looking ahead, it should be noted that the monopolization of the alcohol industry by means of Gosspirtprom failed as a consequence of the illegal machinations of the holding company's leaders. In 2002 the functions of Gosspirtprom were substantially cut back, specifically its control of the distribution of quotas on spirit, which had been transferred to it from the Agriculture Ministry, and its managers were dismissed and then subsequently had criminal charges brought against them.

At the very end of 2000, immediately after the passions over the "marking system", the "beer" turmoil flared up. On 15 December, 2000, a resolution from the first deputy minister for health and chief public health physician of the Russian Federation, Onishchenko, was published, "On Strengthening the State Health Sanitary-Epidemiological Inspection of Beer Production" (No. 16; December 15, 2000). The document expressed uneasiness over the rise in beer consumption in the country and the attraction of young people to beer drinking and proposed a prohibition on beer advertising.

Besides this entirely sensible demand, the letter contained several unproved assertions, for example, on the increase in the country of alcoholism based on beer consumption, for which there was no statistical evidence provided, nor had any scientific work on the topic been undertaken. But the main surprise was that the new action on alcohol, the first since the campaign of 1985, touched only on the problem of beer consumption. According to official figures, the beer consumed in 2000 made up only 17.4 percent of the alcohol consumed in Russia (Fig. 1-14). Moreover, the Onishchenko resolution in no way touched on questions concerning the quantity and quality of strong beverages, principally vodka, which made up the lion's share of consumed alcohol (in 2000, the share was 73.1 percent, according to official figures; Fig. 1-8). Vodka did incomparably more harm to the health and lives of the Russian population than beer and these official figures do not take into account illegal alcohol, by far the greater part of which went into vodka surrogates. And this means that their real share of per capita consumption was substantially higher (possibly 80–90 percent).

A result of the resolution was the "crusade" of local sanitary inspectors against breweries and the harsh fines imposed on them. One might have had the impression that the sanitarian services under Onishchenko had until then not concerned themselves with the sanitation of beer production. Several plants were instantly closed for failure to observe sanitary norms.

All these actions bore witness to the fact that an active anti-beer campaign had started. The initiative of the chief public health physician was strongly supported in the mass media, the statements of which were often uninformed and irresponsible.

Fig. 1-14: Official figures and estimates of actual alcohol consmption in Russia (1990–2000). The shaded area represents the difference in pure alcohol content in vodka and beer according to official figures.

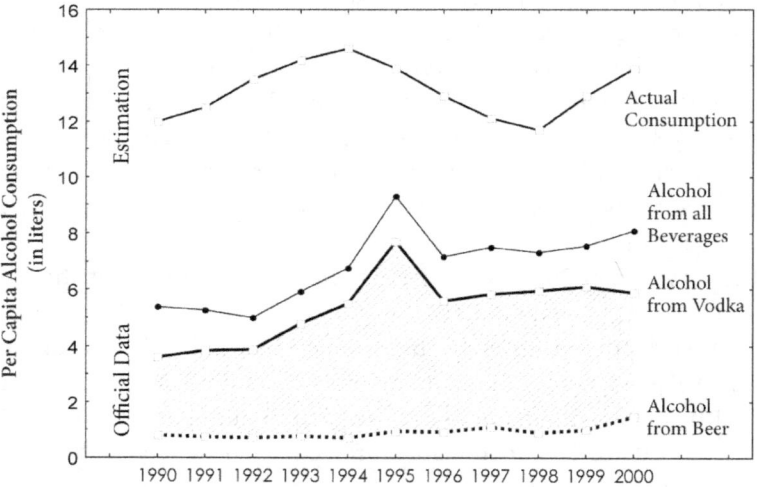

"Doctors attest that ... the consequences of beer alcoholism are terrible: brain cells die, the heart is weakened, the metabolism breaks down ... [A]mong young men under the influence of beer more female hormones are produced, which leads to a widening of the pelvic area, breast growth ... [A]mong young women there is an increased risk of breast cancer" (http://www.regnum.ru). Much was said and written, with passion, about the increase in beer alcoholism in general and, with special emotionality, about beer alcoholism among adolescents and the fact that beer producers, in their headlong quest for profits, were "forcing our young people to drink".

In the tide of accusations, no one, literally no one at all, seemed to realize that the problem lay less in adolescents appearing on the streets with bottles of beer in hand, than in the fact that some adults had sold them the bottles of beer. And this is the cardinal fact about adolescent beer consumption. There should have been a legislative initiative four or five years earlier when the consumption of beer began to increase in the country. That was when the Ministry of Health could and should have analyzed the situation and sounded the alarm. And when it belatedly did so, it should have been done properly.

Personal observations of young people and adolescents drinking beer on the streets and on public transportation are very worrying. Nonetheless, these are just impressions, and government policy needs proof. But Russia still did not have it even though the rise in beer consumption had by then been underway for seven years. Why did the chief public health physician and later first deputy health minister, that is, the state official and member of the government with full authority to act, not initiate scientific research on the matter? Moreover, while there was a declared increase in beer alcoholism among adolescents, the fashion in that group had already shifted to 9 percent ABV alcohol cocktails and gin and tonic.

The first scientific publication on the character of consumption of alcoholic beverages by adolescents with alcohol dependence did not appear until 2002 (Egorov). However, unlike the many stories carried in the media, there was not a single use in this scientific article of the phrase "beer alcoholism" (more details in Chapters 2-2 and 2-3). Moreover, Koshkina and her coauthors (2004) showed that in 2003 as compared with 1999 consumption of beer by 16-year-olds had fallen substantially, especially among males. For example, 39 percent of those surveyed said they had drunk beer three or more times in the preceding month as compared with 47 percent in 1999. At the same time, wine consumption was up, both among boys (16 percent versus 9 percent) and girls (19 percent versus 11 percent), although, clearly, beer remained the principal alcoholic beverage among adolescents, most likely because of its availability (Koshkina et al., 2004) and relative cheapness.

The level of alcohol consumption in Russia is terrifying (Chapter 2-4). In line with this, alcoholism among adults and "early-onset alcoholism" (Egorov, 2002) is a widespread Russian phenomenon. Its pernicious effect demands that the problem be looked at comprehensively and that priorities be established for an alcohol policy. This is an absolute necessity. In the context of "beer alcoholism", the following questions must be asked. Has there in fact been a rise in alcoholism in tandem with the rise in beer consumption? What are its dimensions? If so what portion does it constitute of the major losses caused to the country by alcohol? Which beverage is most responsible for these losses? Which beverage is next in terms of the harm it has caused, and so on? At the moment we do not know the answers to any of these questions and so can only speculate (Chapter 2-3).

However, the problem is not merely a matter of beverage types. The alcoholization of certain groups in the population has a special social role. This applies first of all to adolescents and young people. Aside from the generally acknowledged humanitarian side of the matter, in this case there is an economic side: the irrecoverable losses in the event of early social degradation or death. And these risks can and should be measured in terms of age and in terms of the predominant beverages involved. Unfortunately, it must be concluded that we do not have in Russia a proven answer to any of these questions and specifically not to those concerning beer consumption by adolescents.

In the detailed research by Koshkina et al. (2004), as in the foreign scientific literature of the past decade, there has not been a single publication on the topic of "adolescent beer alcoholism". However, there is to be found alarming information on the wider problem – beer and adolescents. These data show that the early use of beer by adolescents can lead to a higher level of consumption in the future, and that beer advertising has the effect of increasing the consumption of alcoholic beverages by adolescents (Chapter 2-2).

Let us return, however, to the rash action of Onishchenko, which on a personal level was ill-conceived due to an absence of factual information. But it had its social consequences – the anti-beer campaign stirred up bitter protests from brewers. Accusations of incompetence rained down on the chief public health physician and on his idea of "ruining the New Year's holiday for the brewers".

The Union of Brewers demanded that the prime minister force Onishchenko to resign. Although no such thing happened, the brewers were victorious, and the order issued by the chief public health physician was overturned by an order from the Ministry of Health. This is one example, among many others already described, of the absence in Russia of a clearly directed and systematic policy on alcohol. It appears that the leadership of the country is badly coordinated and that one hand doesn't know what the other is doing. However, the question remains: Is it only a lack of coordination that makes Russia's alcohol policy so unbalanced?

The climax of the "beer turmoil" came when the Duma joined in the anti-beer campaign. In April 2002 it passed a law limiting beer advertising on television and in March 2005, after protracted attempts to fashion an agreement with the Federation Council and President Putin, a law "On Limitations on the Retail Sale and Consumption (Drinking) of Beer and Beverages Made from It" (who knows what they had in mind with "beverages made from it" or why they had to decode the word "consumption"). The law forbids the sale and consumption of beer in children's, educational and medical organizations, on all forms of public transportation, in cultural organizations and in health and fitness and sports buildings. It is especially important that the law forbids the sale of beer to minors and its consumption by minors "in any public place". One might have hoped, though it was hardly believable, that as of 14 April, 2005 (when the law went into effect), we would no longer see adolescents on the streets with bottles of beer. At the time of writing, in 2007, such adolescents are still encountered on the streets of Moscow.

The preceding chapter (1-8) mentioned the quite rapid growth in the production and consumption of beer and in the variety of beers that began in the mid-1990s. Along with this went a change in the structure of the production and consumption of other alcoholic beverages, both in terms of overall quantity and in per capita consumption. However, judgments about this have only the very approximate figures of the State Statistical Committee to go on (Figs. 1-13, 1-14). For example, the figures pertaining to vodka for 1993–1994 are paradoxical. According to the Committee's data its sales were 1.5–2 times greater than its production (Fig. 1-13). The paradox is easily resolved if we take into account that only 23–27 percent (1995–2000) of the productive capacity of the vodka and liquor industry was being used, according to official reports. Dependence on such a small share of capacity would have made plants unprofitable. However, the industry continued to exist and, moreover, with no signs of impoverishment. It is easy enough to assume that this was the case because of the production of illegal products, as the sales figures significantly exceeded official production figures. As a result, of this, in 1998 the budget received only 14.8 billion rubles in excise charges instead of a planned 25.8 billion.

The excess sales of beer over beer produced in 1995–1997 (Fig. 1-13) had different reasons behind them, principally beer imports, which were sharply curtailed after the 1998 default. One might mention here the unprofitability of illegally produced beer because of its relatively low price; it is easier to earn "extra" money by producing legal beer of lower quality.

It is important to underline that, along with the continuing rise in the production of beer (446 million decaliters in 1999 and 525 million decaliters in 2000), production of vodka and other liquor products decreased (134 million decaliters in 1999 and 122 million decaliters in 2000; figures from the State Statistical Committee). Vodka producers link the decline in sales of their product with the increase in beer consumption. They found this disturbing, especially in view of the plans of the brewers to increase their output, although the rate of increase subsequently declined (33 percent in 1999, 23 percent in 2000, 15 percent in 2001, 10 percent in 2002 and 8 percent in 2003. These are the percentage increases in the volume of production; figures from the Union of Russian Producers of Beer and Non-Alcoholic Products).

The unease of the vodka producers was evident as early as in the summer of 2000 and was expressed in statements in the media about a law on the state regulation of the beer sector expected in the fall of 2000. Articles declaring that Russia would "be drowned in beer" proliferated. The world-famous sculptor, Ernst Neizvestny, agreed to create a memorial to "Russian vodka" in the city of Uglich (he and the city were eventually unable to agree on the terms of the memorial's production), and in St Petersburg, a vodka museum was organized. While difficult to prove, all these measures appear to be links in a single chain that stretched back to vodka producers disturbed by the fall in their output.

At the same time, the decline in the consumption of strong alcoholic beverages and the increase in the consumption of weaker beverages, mainly wine and beer, was part of a worldwide pattern of recent decades. Thus, in the 22 nations of the Organization for Economic Cooperation and Development, the general consumption trend for 1970-1990 had led to the following distribution: 50 percent beer, 35 percent wine and 15 percent strong beverages (Griffith et al., 1994). This has resulted in the lower per capita consumption of ethyl spirit – the chief culprit of all the ills associated with alcoholic beverages. The rise in beer consumption in Russia was very constrained (38 liters per capita0020per year in 2000 and 51 liters in 2003). Russia, together with countries like Iceland, Italy and Poland, has a low rate of beer consumption. For purposes of comparison, the populations of the Czech Republic, Germany, Britain and the United States consume on average from 100 to 150 liters of beer per capita per year while their overall average consumption of alcohol is lower or much lower than Russia's.

One might merely have welcomed the fact that Russia had joined in the trend toward increased beer consumption. However, unlike most other countries, where replacement of hard liquor by weaker beverages was accompanied by a lowering of overall alcohol consumption, in Russia only the first stage of this process (1995–1998) was accompanied by a lowering of per capita alcohol consumption (Fig. 1-14). Moreover, beer's role in the decline was minimal or nil. The further increase in beer consumption took place against a background of increasing alcohol consumption. The world's laws are not written for Russia; we go "our own way".

The official figures do not offer an answer to the question of how, in the face of declining vodka consumption and an approximately equal (in terms of quantity of alcohol) rise in beer consumption, there could have been an increase in overall alcohol consumption (Fig. 1-14). This probably occurred as a result of the illegal production of vodka and surrogates. The drop in the production of legal vodka may have reflected the fact that legal producers were increasingly producing shadow vodka ("third-shift vodka"). This is suggested by the official reports of a significant underuse of vodka-making capacity and sales of legal vodka exceeding the production of legal vodka.

No one can give the exact dimensions of the illegal production and sales of vodka and other liquors, but figures from the State Statistical Committee of the Russian Federation (30 November, 2001) showed that the alcohol in hard drinks accounted for 73.1 percent of overall alcohol consumption. These are the official figures. But there is a memorandum from the Committee, entitled "Analysis of the Alcohol Market in the Russian Federation in 2000". After an abundance of numerical calculations, the information sheet ends with these words: "It is possible that in 2000 almost every second bottle of vodka sold was *on the left* [illegal] [emphasis added Nemtsov], and it is almost certain that this was true of one out of three."

There are yet more dire conclusions from the Accounting Chamber of the Russian Federation. As regards the consumption of vodka and other liquor products in 2002, the share held by illegal alcohol production was 56 percent, and, if the production of samogon and alcohol surrogates is included, its share in overall consumption stands at 65 percent. Unfortunately, this estimate can be believed. Using the official statistics for 2002, which give the volume of sales of vodka and other liquor as 138.3 million decaliters and assuming that this constitutes 35 percent of overall consumption, the actual per capita figure for consumption of hard liquor comes to 11 liters. Approximately 2 liters of alcohol are attributable to beer (1.86 liters, or 17 percent of overall alcohol consumption) and half again as much from wine. This gives a total of 13.8 liters, which is very close to our independent estimate for 2002 – an annual rate of 15.1 liters of pure alcohol per capita. Thus, the main burden of alcohol consumption in Russia lies in the realm of hard beverages – vodka and its surrogates, which together make up the lion's share of Russian alcohol consumption.

The "beer war" was still not over as a new one was ripening in the depths of the vodka market – the struggle over vodka brands, at the source of which stood the future vodka magnate Yury Shefler and ZAO Soyuzplodimport. Starting quietly in 1997, the struggle over brands has become even more acute and dramatic in the more recent period that this book does not extend to, underlining the unbroken continuity of negative trends in the Russian alcohol sector.

To conclude, it is important to dispense with the "alcohol" myth that is unconsciously or deliberately used to manipulate public consciousness and sometimes serves as the basis for government decisions. This is the matter of the so-called "toxic" additives contained in vodka and its surrogates. These toxic substances have been the frequent subject of research (Gadalina et al., 1986; Nuzhny, 1995; Rumyantseva et al., 1999; Nuzhny et al., 2002a,b; Vyazmina & Savchuk, 2002). As a result of studies of the acute and chronic toxicity of various spirits, vodkas and surrogates, it has been established that food-based, synthetic and hydrolyzed spirits with a high degree of purity do not differ in their toxic effects and that alcohol-containing liquids with denatured or medical additives, such as samogon, cannot be a substantial reason for the high level of fatal alcohol poisonings. And from this it follows that the presence of substandard vodka in the legal or shadow economy is not the cause of the high alcohol morbidity and mortality. What then, kills people? It is ethyl or grape-based spirit, the main component of strong alcoholic beverages, consumed in enormous quantities. This means that the nub of the alcohol problem in Russia lies not in the quality of alcoholic beverages but in their quantity.

Part 2

The alcohol history of Russia in the light of epidemiology

The anti-alcohol campaign of 1985 and the related market reforms of 1992 can hardly be described as a successful alcohol policy. It can be said, however, that these mistaken and in many ways perverse political decisions gave the country's alcohol problems a rare dynamism. For 15 years, starting out from a base of very high alcohol consumption, there has been a succession of periods of sudden cuts in alcohol consumption followed by periods of sudden increase. The results of such policies, conducted with the rigor of laboratory experiments, have provided a vast amount of material for scientific study, especially on a large-scale population level. Never before has such a large mass of people been subject to such rapid changes in alcohol consumption. In this way, the contemporary alcohol history of Russia has provided unique conditions for the development of the science of alcohology.

The term "alcohology" was first used in 1903, and in 1927 it was applied to the branch of social medicine associated with alcohol consumption. Its definition came only in 1987: "alcohology is the discipline dedicated to the problems of the relationship of human beings with ethanol, including its production, storage, distribution, consumption, and the individual and social consequences of consumption" (Gadard, 1990). In this sense, the term "alcohology" (also English "alcology", "alcoologie" in French) is used in official World Health Organization documents.

The term, still not accepted in Russia, is useful in that it allows us to single out and specifically name alcohol problems within the very broad concept "narcology" and deal with them separately from the problems associated with narcotics. This is particularly helpful in that alcoholism in Russia is not considered a drug addiction. Another advantage of the term lies in the fact that it allows us to take into consideration not only the problems of alcohol pathology (including alcoholism), but a wide range of phenomena that lie outside the boundaries of medicine and whose social impact exceeds that of alcoholism and other alcohol-related pathologies.

Alcohology was born as a science, although not yet defined, in the 1920s and 1930s in connection with the explosive development of cities. In 1800, 3 percent of earth's population was urban, but by the 1920s and 1930s this figure was approaching one-quarter of the total. This required regulation of the relations of large masses of people living in small spaces. Predominant among the urban residents of that time were migrants who were used to consuming much more hard liquor than their longer settled neighbors. This, together with the pressure of city life, to which the migrants were not accustomed, gave rise to serious alcohol problems.

Prohibition in the United States (1919–1933) was an unsuccessful response to these problems. Active enforcement of the law was accompanied by an increase in mortality in the U.S. and a startling increase in crime: in 1926 alone, fines for illegal sales of alcohol came to more than 500 million USD, and 20,000 ships and 60,000 trucks carrying alcohol and alcohol products were taken into custody. Yet it is believed that the confiscated alcohol was no more than a tenth of the total. In economic terms, prohibition had a catastrophic effect on U.S. grape production, the U.S. wine industry and the workers in the industry. The resounding failure of the United States' "dry law" had a worldwide effect, including acting as a stimulus for the formation of a new science – alcohology.

At that time, the relation toward alcoholism and drunkenness in the social consciousness began to shift away from the purely moral and social towards social conceptualizations in the fields of psychology and medicine. This helped change the status of alcohol problems, helped move thinking away from condemnation toward the necessity of treating alcoholics. There arose interest in scientifically understanding the problem.

The diagram of the alcohol situation presented earlier (Fig. 1-1) is essentially also a description of the totality of alcohology's objects of study. Even so generalized and, thus, incomplete the diagram shows that alcohology is an interdisciplinary science. Its separate character arises from the specificity of the principal, central subject – the drinking person and the special features of his daily behavior and biography, which can be catastrophic. Alcohology is also interested in those who eschew alcohol. What explains their sobriety, and what alterations in the alcohol situation can bring them into the ranks of the drinking cohort?

The consumption of alcoholic beverages is a mass phenomenon. The problems associated with it affect every nation in the world (Chapter 1-2), all strata of the population and almost all individuals, including non-drinkers in view of their voluntary or involuntary contact with persons who drink. Alcohol is the most widely used psychotropic substance in the world. This characteristic of its consumption, as well as the increase in drinking in the post-war world, has stimulated the use of population and epidemiological methods that have long since moved beyond the boundaries of describing infectious diseases. They are the basis for one of the most important branches of alcohology – "the epidemiology of alcohol consumption and its abuse" (Plant, 1991).

This branch of knowledge in its contemporary form took shape and developed primarily in industrially advanced countries. Many of the patterns discerned by alcohology and described by epidemiology have a universal character and can be applied in countries other than the one in which the observations originated. However, there are also characteristics relating to the consumption of alcoholic beverages that have a national aspect and thus require national means for dealing with them in social and political terms. This is why a specialized epidemiological knowledge applicable to particular countries and to the regions of those countries is needed.

Unfortunately, population alcohology was a subject long barred from study in the USSR. It is not surprising, then, that this branch of knowledge did not exist in the USSR, nor does it exist in contemporary Russia. Only a small amount of work that might be considered epidemiological has been done in Russia, and that which has been done, in terms of its methodology has often been far removed from international standards. This makes it difficult to accept these results or to compare them to Western findings. Moreover, many epidemiological studies of alcohol problems in Russia have uncritically used official statistical data that give a far from complete picture of the alcohol reality of the country, and thus distort it.

The situation in Russia as regards the epidemiology of alcoholism is somewhat better. The restrictions on this narrow sector of alcohology in the USSR were not so severe, and the official record of at least one-third of the country's alcoholics may be considered satisfactory because of the extensive network of narcological health centers.

At the present time, obstacles to the development of epidemiological alcohology in Russia include, first, inadequate material resources and, second, the underestimation of the seriousness of the country's alcohol problems by both the leadership and by the population at large. The backwardness of Russian epidemiological alcohology is not only to be explained by the "pause" in its history in the Soviet era, but also by the weak background of Russian specialists in contemporary epidemiological methods and statistics. Another problem is the scanty acquaintance with Western alcohology and, sometimes, an attitude of contempt towards it. All this is slowing the formation and development of epidemiological alcohology in Russia.

Yet Russia remains the biggest alcohol-consuming country in the world and faces serious consequences due to alcohol abuse. Everyone knows this, but mostly in terms of everyday life, strictly in the sphere of alcohol itself, they know it intuitively but not intellectually. The development of epidemiological alcohology would significantly encourage recognition of the seriousness of the Russian alcohol situation and the dimensions of the losses caused by it.

But before moving on to epidemiology, with its quantitative calculations, laws and patterns, it is necessary to clarify "the problem of the human relationship with ethanol" on the level of psychology, on the level of want. In other words, we must first know why the masses consume alcoholic beverages. Only then can we move on to the characteristics of consumption, to the factors that modulate it and to what follows from this.

Chapter 2-1
Alcohol consumption as a human need

Alcohology has largely avoided the topic referred to in this chapter title. The mass nature of the degrading behavior stemming from alcohol abuse and the heavy burden felt by society make it difficult to deal with the fact that alcohol has positive effects. Few studies have looked into them (Chapter 2-2). Yet they are the point of origin for the entire spectrum of alcohol problems. Alcohol has been a fixture of life for four millennia. But we will not venture so far back. The anti-alcohol campaign of 1985 clearly showed that the desire for alcohol cannot be eradicated.

Most Soviet people subjected to the campaign were born and raised in a totalitarian system that for decades had repressed non-conformist thinking, demanding obedience and loyalty. The post-war period, before the campaign, had seen instances of active resistance to the authorities, but by individuals, perhaps groups of as many as 10 or 100 and even, once, several thousand people (Novocherkassk, 1–2 June 1962).

The situation was quite different during the anti-alcohol campaign. In the second half of 1985 alone, 507,000 individuals were detained "for drinking alcoholic beverages at work or being in an un-sober condition at work". The number of persons brought before the courts for producing samogon almost doubled, reaching 397,000 in 1987. The following year the figure was 414,000 (USSR State Statistical Committee, 1991). The overall number of known violators of the Soviet anti-alcohol laws topped 10 million per year, while uncounted violators bloated this figure even more. Essentially, this amounted to an illegal protest against the barriers to consuming alcohol put in place by the country's leadership.

Legal resistance was expressed in the kilometer-long or half-day waits in queues for alcohol. Thousands of people across the country spent their nights waiting, sometimes in freezing weather, to buy their liter of vodka the following day. These lines of hundreds of people queuing for alcohol were not exclusively made up of alcoholics. Most of the "standers" were "ordinary" Soviet people. Such extreme willingness to sacrifice in order to obtain alcohol leads to the question: What exactly is the attraction of alcoholic beverages? What drove millions of people to resist the harsh anti-alcohol policy of the government in 1985–1988? And, why did the resistance succeed?

Of course, the Soviet system on the eve of its dissolution was weak both politically and economically. It could not exile, imprison or execute people for this kind of mass disobedience. Soviet power had never been total, but now it had finally and fully lost its foothold. The main thrust of the victory of the population, however, was the unconquerable desire to drink.

It would be simplest to link the reckless Russian drunkenness of the second half of the 1900s with customs and traditions, but massive heavy drinking in Russia has its roots in the post-war period (Chapter 1-3). So, firstly, the traditions of serious Russian drinking are in their infancy. Secondly, given that heavy drinking increased, and that there was a very rapid growth in alcohol consumption beginning in the mid-1950s, new factors must have been at work beside traditions, and running contrary to past habits of consuming alcohol in comparatively small quantities, as prevailed in the pre-war and pre-revolutionary periods (Chapter 1-3).

It was demonstrated in Chapter 1-2 that growth in alcohol consumption in the second half of the 1900s was a virtually worldwide phenomenon with consequences that had a global impact, despite the substantial differences in the economic and social conditions in various countries and regions of the world. This suggests the presence of general causes for this phenomenon, although various countries and social groups might have their own specific stimuli for the rise in consumption. What then are these causes and why are they linked specifically with alcohol? It is important to know the preconditions of drunkenness so as not to repeat the mistakes in alcohol policy that were made in 1985 and 1992.

It is worth beginning with the most simple of matters, the psychoactive features of alcohol, its ability to alter the user's psychological condition. In this regard, alcohol's effect is multi-faceted, but mood elevation, the surfacing of positive emotions (the euphoric effect), is the leading one. This capacity of alcohol is closely linked with its capacity to end bad moods (the anti-depressive effect). Another important quality of ethanol relates to its ability to eliminate emotional stress (the tranquillizing effect). Thanks to these effects, alcohol in moderate doses makes it easier to relax and mobilize.

The potential effects of alcohol are often learned by exposure to them in one's peer group. This learning is important as it presents standard ideas with regards to intoxication to the individual. But for our purposes it is not as important to know exactly how an individual comes to experience the euphoric, anti-depressive and tranquilizing effects of alcoholic beverages. What is important is the fact that for most Europeans these effects of alcohol are the main reasons for becoming intoxicated.

Other psychotropic characteristics of alcohol are derivatives of these three: a heightened sense of self-worth, a psychological reduction in the complexity of real problems, a false sense of need satisfaction. Alcohol helps overcome barriers to socializing and eases contacts between people ("communicative doping"), thanks to euphoria and the repression of individuality, through the alienation of the individual from himself.

Contemporary civilization finds it necessary to resort to so-called "symbolic consumption" (e.g., pornography as a sign of and substitute for sex) when people's needs grow more quickly than the possibilities of gratification. In this context, alcohol helps symbolic consumption, possession and gratification.

Intoxication helps to create a friendlier and more attractive self-image. It liberates the individual from personal responsibility and allows him to put his conscience on hold for a time. Finally, alcohol is an aid in myth creation, which has always been an important element of human existence.

These and many other qualities of alcohol make it possible to distort one's perception of reality so as to create the illusion of agreement between wish and actuality. In other words, alcohol is capable of giving rise to an illusion of happiness. The positive emotions felt during the experience often leave deep traces in the form of vague but pleasant memories, often referred to with the trivial remark, "We sat well" (*khorosho posideli*).

In this manner, alcohol acts as a remarkable psychotropic substance, combining in itself the power to elevate mood, end boredom, relieve weariness and do away with psychological stress. These capabilities of alcohol, in combination with its low cost, might well make it the ideal psychotropic substance for wide use were it not for the sinister ability of ethanol to lower social and physical control and, when used regularly, to raise the individual's necessary dosage to reach inebriation and, in this way, increasing alcohol's toxic effects, that take the form of a number of somatic illnesses. Alcohol abuse can cause alcohol dependency (alcoholism) with its resultant degradation of the alcoholic's personality. Finally, all this pathology substantially reduces the life expectancy of drinkers (Chapter 2-5). Put simply, the price alcoholics pay for this escapism is an early departure from this mortal coil!

This has probably been the case over the course of the entire four-millennia-long history of alcohol consumption. In the long distant past, however, abuse of alcoholic beverages created basically individual problems. Only in the past 100–150 years have the troubles associated with alcohol begun to acquire a national dimension (Germany, France), and only in the past 50–60 years has the immoderate consumption of alcohol become a global problem.

But the human race does not use alcohol for its negative consequences. And why do a great many people now often feel a need to experience the positive psychotropic effects of alcohol?

One must search for the answer to this question in the sharp change in the conditions of life that occurred in the middle of the 1800s. A series of phenomena occurred with exponential speed bringing with them global impacts that had their beginnings then or somewhat earlier in time. They are described as explosions (in demography, urbanization, in terms of information), revolutions (scientific-technical, technological, computerized) or booms (communication). All of them have been accompanied by an increase in the weight of burdens felt by a significant part of the population.

In the 1960s people everywhere began to talk about the environmental pollution brought on by the sharp increase in industrial production. However, the social milieu as well as the physical milieu was being polluted. What weight should be attached to the threat of atomic war as a factor in human psychological stress? The youth revolts of the 1960s and the increase in drug addiction were marks of this social pollution. The reverse side of Western individualism was revealed in an epidemic of loneliness ("alone in the crowd"). One of the reactions to all these changes was a rise in alcohol consumption.

The exponential growth in the population of the planet and in the size of its urban population, the increase in the economic potential of Western society, the formation of the "golden billion" and the poverty faced by the remaining billions, the rapid rise in mobility and migration that led to radical changes in social structures were all defining factors in this and many other phenomena.

Over the millennium just past, Earth's population grew by 172 percent in 900 years, or about 19 percent per 100 years on average, and by 294 percent in the past century. In 1800 the population of cities made up 3 percent of the population of Earth; by 1950 the proportion had topped one-quarter, and it is now approaching one-half. In pre-war Russia city dwellers made up one-third of the population (34 percent in 1940) while in the year 2000, the total was a little less than three-quarters (73 percent).

The assimilation of new regions and their industrialization have been accompanied by intensive migrations and, as a result, a rise in alcohol consumption and alcoholism (Artemyev & Minevich, 1989). In Siberia and the regions in the north of Russia, these factors are supplemented by extreme natural conditions, which also raise alcohol consumption (Korolenko & Botchkareva, 1990). In addition, there have been voluntary and involuntary flows of millions of refugees into Russia and other regions of the world in recent years.

All this bears witness to the fact that a great mass of people living in the modern world need some way of adjusting to conditions altogether new to them. To put this in more general terms, for millennia the population of the planet was primarily rural, but during the past 100 years half has become urban. Accordingly, there has been a sharp rise in human crowding and a related increase in emotional tensions among city dwellers. This is why, almost everywhere, rural people consume less alcohol than city dwellers.

Among the changes that took place in the 1900s, the sharp increase in economic potential played a special role. For all the unevenness of its distribution, the material welfare of a significant portion of the population improved and, accordingly, its purchasing power, which in itself might increase consumption of alcoholic beverages. What is important for the topic of alcohol, as a felt need, is that working conditions grew more comfortable, time at work sharply decreased and as a consequence, free time increased. For much of the population, this free time was consumed by the difficult problem of dealing with spiritual emptiness and a meaningless existence, or more simply put, of boredom, for the overcoming of which many have turned to alcohol.

Post-Soviet society had its specific reasons for needing alcohol: the collapse of the USSR, perestroika and the market reforms destroyed the world-view to which people were accustomed and robbed a large number of them of the last of their social illusions. At the same time, the rapidity of the changes hampered the formation of a new world-view. Moreover, the changeability of the socioeconomic conditions, general instability and the galling enrichment of a few, while many millions were experiencing unaccustomed poverty, only made matters worse.

The automation of industrial processes clearly depersonalizes labor as it reduces the importance of the "human factor". Where the "human factor" cannot be realized and where there is a state of boredom in one's free time the potential for social pathologies that seek new sensations is created. This can clearly be seen in the sexual revolution, the many marginal youth movements that have sprung up and in the epidemic of drug use. Much "credit" for the spread of drunkenness belongs to boredom.

Urbanization and the scientific-technical revolution sharply altered the conditions of existence of contemporary people as compared with their distant and not-so-distant forebears. While the quantity of human contacts increased enormously, they became to a significant degree formal, superficial and technically mediated. Mass communications, especially the visual, do not give the individual opportunity to regulate the speed of their transmission and receipt (unlike printed communications or oral conversation) and make it difficult to deal with them thoughtfully. The visual principle has triumphed over the verbal, and somewhere on the heights of the victory stands the video clip, which may well be the leading art form of the coming decades. While this may be a welcome change for one portion of humanity, another part will strongly feel the absence of the verbal, of actual human contact, the virtually sole means of human communications for millennia at whose center stood dialogue. The new conditions of existence leave little room for dialogue, and the telephone and internet deprive dialogue of its natural quality, its facial expressions and gestures, while calling for quite different and new psychological capacities. In essence, the old form of dialogue is dead. Yet it was this form of communication that from time immemorial served to unite people on the basis of emotional interactions, the absence of which drives many people to alcohol as a kind of "communications doping". How many people are there who would be prepared to "share a drink" for the sake of conversation?

Today, as compared with the not-too-distant past, material independence keeps people, even close neighbors, apart. No longer is it necessary jointly to oppose external forces and the dangers of everyday life that for centuries was the basis for mutual relations and mutual assistance. New possibilities of borrowing money have even shunted aside the old way of borrowing among acquaintances.

Contacts between people grow increasingly more impersonal. All this leads to a kind of loosening of the ties between individuals and groups and nourishes a feeling of loneliness. Alcohol is capable of artificially compensating for the absence of the genuine, that is, for emotional interaction, and creates its mirage (note the typical drunken query, "Do you respect me?").

The weakening of ties between individuals and the increase in loneliness has been accompanied by the structuralization of daily life. This may take the form of monotonous work or a severely demanding schedule. For many there also arises a necessity to play this or that role that can often run contrary to the individual's personal qualities.

These and other conditions make necessary a repression of emotionality and the rejection of spontaneity and especially of impulsiveness, which has always been a means of self-expression, a means of discharging tension and that lies at the source of all creativity. Alcohol is capable of creating the illusion that the chains of the conventional have been broken and that one's spirit is in "free flight", a feeling everyone has strong need of. It was the free "flight of the drunk's spirit" and the "metaphysic" of drunkenness, together with its discovery of the theme of alcohol and its "depths", that made Moskva-Petushki, by Erofeev, so special and important beyond its actual literary merits.

In the course of the last 150–200 years, changes in life have occurred much faster than changes in psychology, in the consciousness of people formed over millennia in conditions of patriarchal labor and customs. It is possible that, over the millennia, there was a selection from generation to generation of psychological types best suited to patriarchal-communitarian forms of existence and relatively slow rhythms. For millennia contacts between individuals were few, largely with neighbors, and profoundly personal and took place in a context of resolving concrete, often vital, tasks through individual labor that provided space for daily creativity. This is not an idealization of the past but only a way of underlining its significant difference from contemporary life and its requiring quite different psychological traits and methods of adaptation.

Some processes, long underway in civilization, probably reached a critical level in the second half of the 1900s, contradicting the psychological nature of a large portion of human beings. This is why today's individuals are weary of overcrowding and hurry, of the multiplicity but superficiality of human contacts, of informational overload and excessive standardization. The adaptive powers of many people appear to be limited. And here comes alcohol "to the rescue" playing the role of the adaptive gene.

The concerns that used to fill life lost vital significance. The concepts of "daily life" and "being" grow farther and farther apart. An "existential vacuum" (Frankl, 1985), filled with a complex of negative phenomena, has formed. One of these is the increase of drunkenness.

In a crude way, one can describe the consumption of alcohol as a measure that "all is not well" in the social sphere. The constituent elements of what is not well may vary: the poverty and humiliating position of some and the important social status of others, the lack of goods for some and the lack of time for others despite an abundance of goods.

Naturally, an equal measure of dissatisfaction does not signify equality in alcohol consumption. Individual choices are at work here. This selectivity is a function of, in addition to social factors, the psychological characteristics of individuals, their personalities and particular biological traits.

Many attempts have been made to draw a general psychological portrait of the heavy drinker or alcoholic, to bring into focus a typology of persons inclined to the abuse of alcohol. But the effort has failed. Only the most general features of the disposition to alcohol consumption have been clarified. These include personal difficulties beyond the individual's capacity, with resultant irritability or depressed mood, feelings of inadequacy, a lack of self-confidence and immaturity of the personality manifesting itself as egocentricity, a need for external approval and unrealistic plans. Finally, these also include a primitiveness arising from basic intellectual incapacity or defects in rearing and education. All of these can cause difficulties in socialization and a resultant need for alcohol as a means, albeit very incomplete, of adapting. In speaking of the psychological typology of alcoholics, one must not overlook social factors that may influence the emergence and actualization of psychological characteristics.

Discussion of alcohol in terms of need must include mention of the psychoanalytic understanding of alcoholism as an unconscious form of self-destruction and seeking of death, as a kind of "chronic suicide", the chosen weapon for which is alcohol (Menninger, 1938).

The starting point of the psychoanalytic hypothesis cannot be denied: the shortening of life by means of chronic alcoholic intoxication. Moreover, alcoholics' direct expressions of attitudes of indifference toward their own lives and early deaths are sometimes in agreement with the hypotheses of Freud. Alcoholism not infrequently ends in suicide. Nonetheless, acceptance of Freud and his followers' theory is made difficult by the absence of empirical evidence and the speculative character of their conclusions (Fromm, 1973).

However, even from a non-psychoanalytic standpoint it is easy to see that simpler factors predominate in the lives of alcoholics. These include alcohol dependency, psychological or physical, and related frequent and severe periods of intoxication, increases in the dosage of alcohol required and increasing degeneration of the personality and depression. Along with this as a rule goes a substantial somatic pathology. It is these processes and conditions that lead alcoholics to an early death. However, long before the tragic finale, the awareness of the alcoholic narrows radically; their psychic life is extremely reduced and their intellectual and volitional reserves for overcoming life's difficulties disappear. The alcoholic's self-destructive behavior suggests a striving for death, although almost nothing remains to the ailing individual other than a deliberate striving after alcohol.

Obviously, the definition of what is central to alcoholism depends very much on the scientific world-view with which the researcher starts out and how free he is to draw conclusions. The interpretational method of psychoanalysis does not accord with contemporary scientific methods and their insistence on proof. Its justification and strength lie in its healing power, not in its theoretical standing. This mention of the psychoanalytic conceptions of alcoholism is merely a tribute to the memory of this only recently blooming branch of psychiatry that has already become an "intellectual antique" (Menzhulin, 2002).

This is all I will say concerning psychoanalytic theory's contribution to the understanding of alcoholism. However, adherents of psychoanalysis have made many observations of value for understanding the psychology of alcohol consumption and alcohol-related behavior. It was, in fact, psychoanalysis that first drew attention to the importance of the symbolic function of alcohol, specifically as a symbol of adulthood for adolescents, as a symbol for adolescents and adults of belonging to a meaningful group and, finally, as a symbol of friendship. Adler, as part of his teachings on the complexes of inadequacy, saw alcohol as a means of trying to overcome psychological difficulties. Hence, later the idea of alcohol as an adaptive gene was arrived at. Moreover, psychoanalysts have made interesting contributions as regards understanding the motivations of alcohol consumption.

* * *

In summing up the findings of this chapter, I find it necessary to underline that society's need for alcohol will never be zero. There will always be a base level of use determined by the pleasure-seeking inclinations of some individuals or the psychological imperfections of others. This more or less permanent base level will sometimes grow in the face of rising social tensions or conflicting social interests. For these there is no end in sight. This is a fundamental given of the alcohol situation and of all the problems of alcohol consumption. However, a need for alcohol and realizing that need are not the same thing. Factors exist that can swing alcohol consumption in either direction (Fig. 1-1). Several of these factors will be described in the chapters that follow.

The idea of this chapter has been to demonstrate that drunkenness is not merely due to a lack of discipline and dissoluteness, although this can be encountered. Drunkenness and the alcoholism that may succeed it have their social, psychological and biological reasons; at their base lie individual and/or social flaws that are as worthy of understanding and sympathy as are physical flaws or somatic illnesses. This is not to absolve the alcoholic of the responsibility for his life and for the welfare of those close to him.

The picture is not a simple one nor does it suggest a single answer. But the situation could not be otherwise in the increasingly complex world in which we live. However, vagueness about morality cannot be endless. The limits have been known at least as long as the Ten Commandments, or at least five of the final six.

Chapter 2-2
The epidemiology of alcohol consumption in the World

Epidemiological studies are, as a rule, expensive. Some of them are based on surveys or other methods of gathering information about many groups within a country or the country's entire population. They require the utilization of a large number of highly trained and thus highly paid specialists. This is why the overwhelming majority of such studies are conducted in the industrially developed countries of Europe and America, which have the material resources to support such massive undertakings.

But the matter goes beyond resources. The study of alcohol problems in the leading capitalist countries has also been encouraged by the high level of democratic development in these countries and the resultant interest of the government and society in the health of the nation, which to a significant extent depends on the level of alcohol consumption. That is why, for example, Sweden with its relatively safe average per capita alcohol consumption (5.3 liters of pure alcohol per person per year, 1994), on its entrance into the European Economic Community (EEC or Common Market), devoted considerable effort to preserving its state monopoly (which EEC rules forbid) on the sale of alcoholic beverages and thus control over consumption. For the same reason, the Swedish Council for Information on Alcohol and other Drugs annually issues a book of one hundred-plus-pages - an epidemiological report on the condition of alcohol problems in the country as a whole and in its separate regions (total population 9 million people).

Another example is the United States, where the powerful National Institute on Alcohol Abuse and Alcoholism was founded in 1957. The large and productive epidemiological department of this institute annually publishes several extensive compilations of detailed information on the alcohol situation in the country and in each of its states. It is important to note that the institute was organized at a time when alcohol consumption in the U.S., although then slowly rising, stood at less than 5 liters per person annually (in 1965 the figure was 5.6 liters). But this sparked concern on the part of the government.

A natural consequence of the uneven distribution of material resources and the inequality in various governments' interest in alcohol problems is unevenness in the epidemiological coverage of the world. For many years, Western researchers hardly carried out any epidemiological work beyond the borders of the industrially developed nations. It is only towards the end of the 1990s that large-scale research has been done, under the aegis of the World Health Organization, on the level and character of alcohol consumption worldwide, with special attention to developing countries (Chapter 1-2). During this time such studies have been conducted in Russia by Western researchers in connection with the unique alcohol situation that has developed there (Chapter 2-3). Nonetheless, the main body of work on the epidemiology of alcohol use still relates to the materially advanced capitalist countries.

The majority of studies can be divided into two groups. The first is made up of works dealing with the condition of, or trends in, the general indexes of alcohol consumption and alcohol-related problems (for example, average per capita consumption of alcohol) and to the factors that affect these average indexes. Studies of this kind deliberately avoid personal or group details in order to present alcohol problems in the most general form possible.

The second group are made up of studies of particular problems, in summary form, however, describing the entire spectrum of separate alcohol problems (the distribution of users by frequency of drinking and dosages of alcohol, as well as the consumption of alcohol by specific cohorts of the population such as, for example, adolescents, young adults, women). Works on the epidemiology of alcoholism belong in this group.

2-2A. General characteristics of consumption

In Chapter 1-2 descriptive data was presented on the alcohol situation in the world, in its various regions and, of special importance, in individual countries using, as a rule, their most general and average characteristics. These data serve as a background against which to compare the alcohol situation in Russia (Chapter 1-3). They will also be used for the purposes of this chapter, with some supplementation of several general points.

The 58th session of the World Health Organization, held on 7 April 2005, was devoted to "problems of public health caused by harmful alcohol consumption". The report of the Secretariat asserted that such problems "had reached threatening proportions, and alcohol has become one of the most serious risk factors for health throughout the world; its use is one of the leading risk factors in developing countries ... and holds third place in developed countries...." In 2000 consumption of alcohol bore responsibility for 4 percent of the illness burden of the world, on a par with the use of tobacco (4.1 percent) and high blood pressure (4.4 percent).

In the developed countries, alcohol abuse accounts for 9.2 percent of the total number of lives lost per year, the largest portion of which occurs from nervous-psychiatric ailments (dependency, psychoses and depression) and accidental injury (road traffic accidents, burns, drowning, falls and others). Estimates show that, for the world as a whole, alcohol consumption was the reason for 3.2 percent of the total number of such incidents in 2000.

This is the most general picture of the consequences of alcohol consumption in the world. Thanks to the vast amount of work undertaken in recent years under the aegis of the WHO (Global Status Report on Alcohol, 1999; Global Status Report: Alcohol and Young People, 2001; Global Status Report on Alcohol, 2004), we can now add that, over the course of the past 40 years, average alcohol consumption in the world for adult individuals (from age 15) has been 5.1 liters, of which 1.9 liters has been beer, 1.3 wine and 1.7 liters hard liquor.

The distribution of alcohol consumption by continents presented in Fig. 2-1, shows that the European region has had, and continues to have, the highest level of consumption. In Europe, America and Africa consumption was at its highest level at the end of the 1970s or the beginning of the 1980s, after which several countries witnessed the start of a decline in consumption. The eastern Mediterranean region shows consistently low figures. An increase in consumption in the course of the last 40 years has been seen in Southeast Asia, while growth in consumption has been especially sharp in the western Pacific region. The WHO includes China and Japan in this region and it was these countries which underpinned the growth in this region.

Fig. 2-1: Alcohol consumption by regions of the World, age 15+. Europe (1), America (2), Western Pacific Region (3), Africa (4), Southeast Asia (5), Central Asia (6). Source: Global Status Report on Alcohol, 2004.

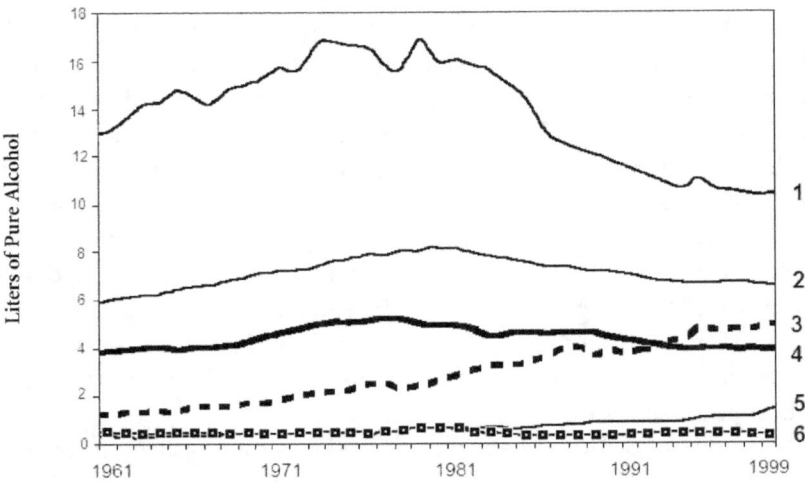

With the exception of the eastern Mediterranean region, where a Muslim population is predominant, the general rule is that for continents with high levels of consumption a decline is underway and that where consumption was low 40 years ago it is now increasing. This picture agrees with the model according to which developing countries increase consumption in proportion to their economic growth.

These measures as well as those presented in Chapter 1-2 are drawn from the 1980s onwards. The analysis of a longer period shows consumption changing in a wave-like fashion. In the middle and especially toward the end of the 1800s, the level of consumption in Europe, in contrast to Russia, was very high. However, at the turn of the 1900s, consumption began to decline, then was relatively low in the period between the two world wars, but rose rapidly after World War II in the majority of countries in Europe and in America (Mäkelä et al., 1981). The second high point was reached at the end of the 1970s–early 1980s, as was the case, for example, in Great Britain (Fig. 1-2), for which there were two high points for consumption across the century. Similar long-wave changes in consumption occurred in the majority of other countries with reliable statistics. Of course, there were several exceptions.

Earlier (in Chapter 1-2), economic factors were primarily offered as explanation for particular portions of this wave. Such explanations are difficult to rebut. However, if one excludes the hypothesis of the wave nature of consumption, it is difficult to explain why an increase in consumption began soon after the end of World War II, but not after the less destructive World War I.

As Mäkelä et al. (1981) see it, the long-wave nature of consumption cannot be explained by changes in purchasing power, leisure time, poverty or riches, industrialization or urbanization. Room (1991) postulated that the decline in consumption at the beginning of the 1900s and the low level of the mid-1900s might be linked to "a dialectical process of social learning" in periods of high consumption; as a result of the serious and often fatal consequences of such consumption, the population's attitude toward drinking and drunkenness change and there are stepped-up controls on consumption. This ends, in Room's view, when consumption declines. Such a speculative scheme has a right to exist, especially in the absence of other alternatives. However, it does not settle the problem of the nature of the long-wave cyclicity of consumption. It does not explain the synchronicity of the process in many countries, including developing countries (Smart, 1991) and Russia (Chapter 1-3), which for so long was behind the "Iron Curtain" and, most importantly, had not experienced the significant rise in consumption of the late-1800s–early-1900s that occurred in many European countries.

The difficulty of defining the nature of the long-wave cyclicity in consumption is also evident in the fact that it still cannot be said, in the early 2000s, whether the first century-long wave has ended and a new one has started. In a significant number of countries (Chapter 1-2), there was a start to or continuation of a decline in alcohol consumption as the 1970s turned into the 1980s

(France, Italy, U.S., Canada, Australia). At the same time, in other countries consumption stabilized (Norway, Sweden, Switzerland, Austria), while in a third group the increase in consumption continued (Denmark, Finland, Germany, Japan). Thus, at the end of the 1900s, there was a breakdown in the synchronized dynamics of consumption in various countries, and is it not known how long this may continue for, or what it is connected to. One can only presume that the variety in trends at the close of the 1900s reflected the variety of alcohol policies in various countries.

It would be easier to resolve this problem if we knew the condition of the countries of Europe at the peak of their alcohol consumption in the second half of the 1800s. However, at that time records of consumption existed in far from all the (modern) European states, while an absence of alcohol policies meant that alcohol processes would have manifested themselves spontaneously. It is feasible that the answer to the question concerning the start of the new cycle will appear in the next two or three decades. But it is also possible that the century-long cycle has been broken as a result of political interventions.

Unable to deal with the question of the nature of the long-term processes that underlie alcohol consumption, alcohology has accumulated much material on the factors that determine short-term and medium-term changes. They play the role of modulators in relation to what is principal and decisive in alcohol consumption – the desire for alcohol on the part of the individual and the population as a whole (Chapter 2-1). This factor is basic and is more than long-term, having been active now for four millennia.

The short- and medium-term factors affecting consumption include economic, social and political causes that, to a significant degree, overlap each other. Among the notable economic factors that affect consumption levels are the prices of alcoholic beverages, on the one hand, and the income of the population and thus its purchasing power, on the other. These two factors – prices and incomes – are interrelated, although the influence of prices of alcoholic beverages on alcohol consumption has been studied in greater detail and more persuasively.

Based on a large number of countries and a great quantity of research, the following general rule has been formulated for industrially developed countries: when other factors are held constant, price increases for alcohol lead to a cut in consumption, while lower prices are accompanied by increased consumption. In exactly the same way, when other factors are constant, an increase in the income of the population leads to increased consumption, and decreases in income are accompanied by decreased consumption. In other words, alcoholic beverages in market conditions behave like other commodities and obey the law of supply and demand or, in the final analysis, on the basis of what is most advantageous for the consumer.

This is the picture in its most general character. However, consumption of various alcoholic beverages (hard liquor, wine, and beer) varies differently in its relation to price changes, especially if the specifics of geography, traditions, time period and several other secondary factors are taken into account. Thus, if demand for a particular beverage is high and the portion of the family budget for it considerable, even minor changes in price greatly affect consumption, as was the case, for instance, with hard liquor in Canada in 1949–1969 (Lau, 1975). Another example is France from 1954 through to 1971, when lower prices on wine had no effect on the consumption of this beverage, as the wine portion of the family budget was small (Labys, 1976). Thus, without altering the main thesis that consumption of alcoholic beverages has an inverse relationship to prices, there remains great variety in the response of consumers to changes in the prices of various beverages in various economic conditions.

This and much other data exists about the countries of Europe and North America. Unfortunately, our knowledge about other regions is very limited. There may be quite different relationships between prices and consumption there. Thus, Partanen (1991) demonstrated that in Kenya in the period 1963–1985 the consumption of bottled beer was highly sensitive to price, and that this sensitivity was much greater than in the industrially developed countries. Partanen holds the view that this is not specific to Kenya but merely reflects the lower social significance of legally produced beer for a population which produces this beverage at home in large quantities illegally.

The dependence of alcohol consumption on price, makes prices (and tax policies) important and perhaps the most powerful regulator of consumption that the state possesses. An already classic example of this is Denmark during World War I, when the wartime blockade had the effect of lowering imports and production of alcohol and, as a result, triggered a 1000 percent increase in the price of hard liquor and a doubling of the beer price. The result was a 75 percent decline in average alcohol consumption in a period of two years, largely due to a reduction in the consumption of hard liquor. Naturally, there was also an accompanying sharp decline in the incidence of alcohol psychoses (Nielsen, 1965).

The world has other examples of this dynamic at work. In Sweden in 1955 the rationing system on alcoholic beverages was abolished, and this led to an increase in consumption. To stop the latter, prices were raised by 30 percent in 1957–1958. This brought consumption down from 0.8 liters per capita per month in 1956 to 0.6 liters in 1958 (Österberg, 1995; by the same token, from 9.6 to 7.2 liters of alcohol per year). This may be considered a substantial reduction in consumption and an example of an effective state alcohol policy.

Österberg believes that the real price of alcoholic drinks has fallen significantly in many Western countries in recent decades in connection with the growth in income. At the same time, price has been used either very weakly or not at all as an instrument of control over consumption.

There is also the problem of the crossover influence of changes in price for one kind of beverage on the consumption of other types of beverage. The problem comes down to the fact that increased prices on some drinks result in their substitution by other drinks. Johnson and Oksanen (1974) found that an increase in beer prices in the U.S. was met by an easy shift to wine, although a move in the other direction was difficult. There have been other studies of this kind. However, later with the use of a more refined methodology, the crossover effect, when prices rise, was found to be negligible in Great Britain (Godfrey, 1989). This has also been found to be the case in Russia (Andrienko & Nemtsov, 2005).

Prices, independent of taxes, are only one regulator of consumption; another is the income of the population. It should be noted that, unlike in the case of tobacco, alcohol is very "responsive" to changes in income, especially among that part of the population with low incomes. However, the relationship between income and price is not a simple one. For example, Godfrey and Maynard (1992) predicted that an annual hypothetical 5 percent increase in the price of alcoholic beverages in Great Britain could lower consumption by 31 percent by the year 2000 but that this reduction would be cut to 20 percent in case of a 2 percent annual increase in incomes. And if the income gain was 3 percent, consumption would actually rise by 14 percent.

One regrets that there are so few studies of this kind in Russia. However, it is known that demand for strong beverages (vodka, samogon) in Russia falls at a time of rising incomes, while demand for lighter drinks (beer, wine) rises. With increased prices on vodka, the substitution effect is observed: consumption of vodka falls while that of beer and samogon rises. With a simultaneous increase in incomes and prices of alcoholic drinks, the frequency of alcohol consumption has been increasing, but overall there has been a positive social effect – the consumption of ethanol falls because of the smaller quantity consumed per single drink (Andrienko & Nemtsov, 2005). The strength of this effect depends on the relationship between prices and incomes.

2-2 B. Personal characteristics of consumption

In the preceding chapters, average per capita consumption features as the principal, but not the sole index of the alcohol situation and as the main criterion for the success or failure of alcohol policy, with a high level of consumption acting as a signal to activate an anti-alcohol policy. However, this and other generalized indexes, as well as the factors that influence them provide only the most general picture, one that minimizes both individual consumers and the groups they are a part of. Some of these are very large and differ in their attitudes towards alcohol and alcohol consumption.

For a long time, interest in alcohol problems in the West was fueled by their association with crime. At the center of attention were extreme forms of alcoholization, that is, alcoholics, drunk-debauchees and those who commit crimes while drunk. In other words, the social paradigm was dominant. However, as part of the policy of banning alcohol in the United States (Prohibition, 1919–1933), a significant role was also played by physicians who had become concerned early in the 1900s about the negative effects of alcohol abuse on the health of the population. However, until the late 1930s and early 1940s the medical paradigm that dominated was that which linked disease with infections, poor nutrition and hormonal inadequacies. In this connection, the overall incidence of disease, specifically somatic illnesses, was in no way linked with alcohol consumption; the physical ill-health of alcoholics was explained by their poor nutrition. The level of consumption held no significance for alcohol policy or for medical practice (Katcher, 1993).

A widening and deepening of interest in problems relating to the consumption of alcoholic beverages took place from the mid-1950s through to the early 1960s in connection with a sharp rise in consumption. By this time a new medical paradigm termed the ecological or epidemiological had come into being. It linked morbidity with causes found in the environment and, later, with the lifestyles of individuals. This was a time of decline in infectious diseases in the West and their retreat from center stage. Instead, social factors came to the fore, including sedentary lifestyles (hypodynamia), poor nutrition and smoking. Abuse of alcohol was also part of this group of factors. At the same time, there occurred a shift in public and scientific interest away from general problems toward a more differentiated attitude to those with alcohol problems. Interest now extended beyond alcoholism to embrace other groups of users.

The first work of this kind was the book by the French demographer Sully Ledermann (1956) that for a long time defined the path of development of epidemiological alcohology. Ledermann's principal hypothesis asserted the existence of a strong link between average per capita consumption and serious drunkenness. He was the first to uncover the fact that there is no moment of sharp conversion from moderate to heavy consumption of alcohol. Until he did so, the approach to the problem had been dualistic, an assumption that these two groups of users could be clearly distinguished. Ledermann expressed his new understanding in mathematical terms as the distribution of users by quantity of alcohol consumed (monomodal, log-normal distribution; Fig. 2-2). From this it followed that the distribution of serious drunkenness can be determined by working merely from average per capita consumption. Using features of his model, Ledermann (1964) reached the conclusion that the basis for the prevention of illnesses associated with alcohol was to reduce all types of consumption, not just excessive, or drunken, consumption. He believed that the chief instrument of prevention should be controlling access to alcoholic beverages.

Fig. 2-2: The theoretical distribution of consumers by alcohol use following Ledermann Hypothesis (diagram; details in text).

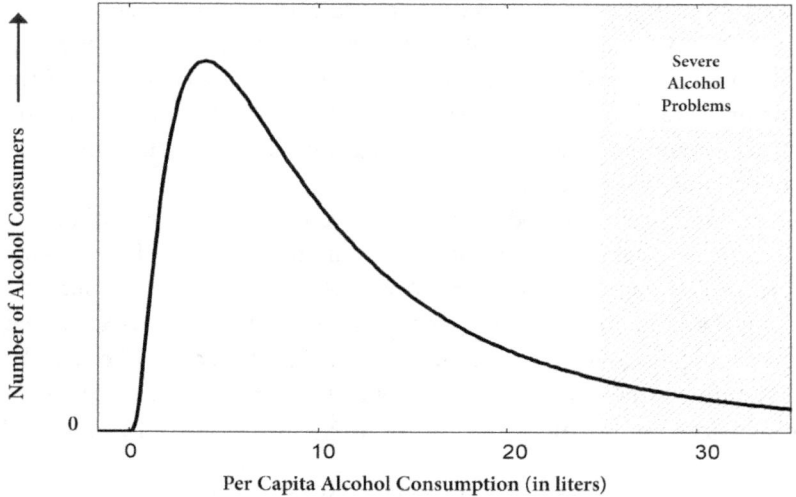

Ledermann's activity coincided with an important stage in the development of the science – the widespread introduction of mathematical methods into its arsenal of tools. Hence much effort was subsequently devoted to testing the accuracy of Ledermann's mathematical model (de Lint & Schmidt, 1968; Smart & Schmidt, 1970, as well as two international conferences under the name "The Ledermann Curve"). The strict form of the log-normal distribution of users was not confirmed. And description of the new empirical data characterizing users and employing an exponential distribution also encountered difficulties at times. However, this protracted testing of the Ledermann model, as part of the general trend towards the mathematizing science, for a time pushed into the background the deep and practical significance of the conclusions of this French researcher as regards the consistent patterns in population consumption.

The start of renewed interest in this aspect of the matter and in Ledermann's findings was the large collective work of Brunn et al. (1975), which formulated a new, broader paradigm that was, nonetheless, close to Ledermann's conclusions. Its basic points were that alcohol consumption affects public health (this idea was at that time still new!), that control over the accessibility of alcohol is required and that there is a correlation between average per capita consumption, abusive consumption and the serious consequences of these phenomena. The authors stressed the importance of the index of average per capita consumption as making possible approximate determinations of the dimensions of alcohol-related problems, although not in a strictly mathematical form. The work of Brunn et al. (1975) imparted a degree of relativity to Ledermann's rigid conclusions.

Further work was undertaken to clarify Ledermann's ideas on the relationship between average per capita consumption and the dimensions of serious drunkenness. It was demonstrated for example (Duffy & Cohen, 1978) that two populations with identical average per capita consumption could be very different in terms of the number of alcoholics each contained, if the distributions of users showed slight differences in the type of their consumption. Even more surprising were the results of Lemmens (1991), who found an increase in the share of serious alcoholics against a background of a reduction in overall consumption in the Netherlands.

These and other works led away from the unequivocal nature of Ledermann's original ideas, especially as regards determining the extent of alcohol abuse on the basis of average consumption. Skog (1985a) offered a softer formulation: a doubling of average per capita consumption leads to a fourfold increase in the population of heavy users who imbibe more than 100 milliliters of pure alcohol daily.

A significant stage in the development of Ledermann's concepts came with Skog's theory of social interaction (Skog 1980, 1985b), according to which:

- the alcohol-related behavior of some individuals is explained by interactions among them, an exchange of relevant experience ("diffusion", according to Skog; "by social infection", according to Ledermann),
- changes in consumption reflect the multiplicative action of factors in the surrounding society on the individual or group.

Skog's system of proofs (Skog, 1985a) was built on a base of studies of the alcohol consumption in 21 cohorts, each of which had its own, distinct average consumption (x-axis in Fig. 2-3) and with a wide overall range of averages (from 2 to 50 liters). All of the cohorts were divided into five subgroups reflecting the seriousness of the consumption (y-axis). It transpired that each of the five subgroups from all of the cohorts comprised a kind of entity. Expressed logarithmically, these results took the form of five inclined straight lines almost parallel to each other (Fig. 2-3).

From these relationships, Skog drew an important conclusion: the cause of a change in individual consumption is the pressure felt by the individual from his surroundings, most often from his own cohort whose consumption has changed for one or more reasons. This occurs because of the "diffusion of influence" or "social interaction" with the aim of equalizing consumption so that the consumption of one does not differ greatly from that of the remaining members of the group in question. As a result, the individual and his cohort "move" up or down along the same line, proportional to the "peer pressure" and together with this the degree of dependence (Fig. 2-3). The speed at which various factors (prices, for example) exert influence, the speed and degree of "diffusion", is defined by the

Fig. 2-3: The relationship of average consumption in 21 groups of consumers (abscissa) with 5 subgroups (ordinate) rated by seriousness of consumption, from "heavy" to "light". Straight lines are lines of regression for the 5 subgroups. Source: Skog, 1985.

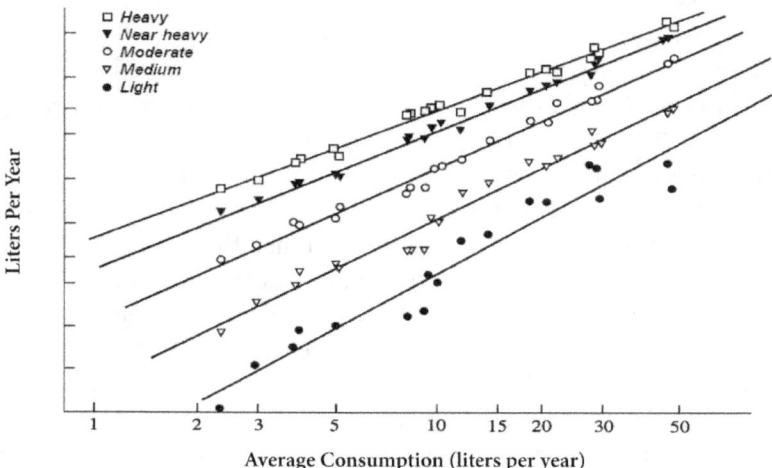

characteristics of the population, the particularities and structure of its "human network" (all quoted words and phrases are expressions in Skog's article).

The multiplicative (that is, based on the multiplication of factors, not on their addition) model of Skog, now a classic, is essentially a generalized Ledermann model. It preserves the link between the average consumption of a population and the consumption of its separate members, but now the links are more varied and dynamic. At the same time, Skog's model has no need for strict links between the form of the distribution of users and average per capita consumption.

Lemmens et al. (1990) supported the basic ideas of Ledermann-Skog using the example of large samples of consumers of alcohol in Holland, the United States, Great Britain, Germany and Switzerland. At the same time, they went further, demonstrating that the correctness of the theory of social interaction does not depend only on the form of the distribution of users. Distributions may take various forms (gamma, Weibull, log-normal).

The further movement of these ideas concerning the distribution of consumers was in the direction of an increasingly differentiated attitude toward drinkers and their particular groups. This reflected general trends in the post-war Western world of greater acceptance of different points of view and interests, i.e., of movement along the path of greater freedom. Specialists researching the epidemiology of consumption were with increasing frequency calling attention to the heterogeneity of the population, to the specific and distinctive alcohol behavior of cohorts, interaction between which was sometimes absent or showed a negative correlation. This is linked to the fact that in the contemporary Western world, separate (and sometimes quite large) groups of the population, may reflect the influence of various and sometimes contradictory stimuli in their consumption of alcohol. If the effects of general factors are dominant over the majority of users, we will have an alcohol situation which agrees with the theory of Ledermann-Skog.

The question may be posed this way: do all groups present within the population always lower (or increase) their consumption when average per capita consumption declines (or rises), as Ledermann and Skog believed, and as is the case, in all likelihood, most of the time? At the time of writing, there is an accumulation of findings that do not fit into these schemes. Attention has been turned toward characteristics of consumption other than quantity. Thus, in connection with the observation of large samples of users over the course of 10 years (1979-1989), a positive but weak link has been found between average per capita consumption and the average frequency of consumption (Duffy, 1991). However, the correlation between daily, i.e., serious drunkenness, and overall consumption may be negative, although also weak. Duffy interpreted these results as showing that the change in average consumption to a large extent is due to the change in the frequency of consumption of relatively moderate users, who make up the largest portion of the population.

It should be noted that Duffy's research (1991) was conducted in the U.S. against a background of relatively moderate and declining average per capita consumption (7.5-8 liters) and a spreading negative attitude toward drunkenness in the population. These two circumstances, especially the latter, limit the full freedom to choose an alcohol lifestyle, which is probably necessary for the Ledermann-Skog patterns to be realized.

As time has passed, exceptions to these patterns have been more frequent. Knibbe et al. (1985) conducted a longitudinal study (observation of the same individuals over a period of many years) in the Netherlands in 1958-1981. At the end of the 24 years, average consumption had tripled. Most of the groups studied increased their consumption in line with the overall increase and in such a way that the relative rankings of groups within the series did not change, as per the model of Skog (1985a). However, in those instances when general consumption temporarily declined or remained stable, the number of serious alcoholics in groups of young and/or non-religious men continued to increase. In Sweden, with declining alcohol consumption in 1976-1984, it was shown that the decline moved at a faster pace than that for average consumption in several groups of the population. These groups were: the top layers of society, younger people and men in general (Romelsjö, 1987).

Fillmore et al. (1994) conducted a meta-analysis of 25 randomized studies carried out in 14 countries and showed that the various groups in a society make differing contributions to changes in average consumption. Women and younger people were more dynamic as regards consumption. Moreover, according to these authors, for average consumption the frequency of consumption held greater significance than the quantity of consumed alcohol, a finding already remarked on in connection with the work of Duffy (1991).

A vivid example of the fact that consumption changes for various population groups are not always homogenous is provided by the findings of Norström (1987). He described the situation in Sweden when the rationing system for alcoholic beverages was ended in 1955. The end of rationing had various consequences for different groups of the population, in part, because the end of rationing was accompanied by an increase in prices for alcoholic beverages. Moderate drinkers cut back on their consumption, but heavy drinkers, with the limits removed, increased their drinking. The result of the action of merely two of the factors (the end of rationing and the rise in prices) that affect alcohol behavior dramatically increased the spread in consumption. In other words, political action is capable of eliciting various, sometimes contradictory responses in various population groups. This example shows how important it is to try to envisage all of the possible consequences of a broad political measure that affects the entire population of a country.

In concluding this topic, one must return to its sources in the persons of Ledermann and Skog, who discovered the most general patterns relating to the alcohol behavior of most of a population in terms of the distribution of consumption. The further development of these ideas consisted of adding detail, describing particulars, some of them, it is true, have been very important for predictions of the alcohol situation and the behavior of particular cohorts of drinkers.

At the same time, it is important to note that deviation from the alcohol behavior conceived by Ledermann-Skog has been observed most often in instances where there has been a change in the availability of alcoholic beverages, after which the alcohol situation over the course of time returns to the patterns described by Ledermann and Skog.

It should also be noted that the development of the ideas of epidemiological alcohology on the character of and factors affecting alcohol consumption has not taken place in isolation, but has moved hand-in-hand with the development and deepening of interest in the fate of the individual. Moreover, these new, more deeply humanitarian views and approaches have stimulated alcohology to make its theories more complex and thus make it possible for every consumer to find his or her place in the theoretical schemes. There have been and continue to be a large number of studies of particular, often very narrow, groups of users, such as, for example, 9th-grade high school pupils in Los Angeles. It is difficult to find a place for such specific studies in a review of the general ideas of Western alcohology. And only one narrow topic demands attention in connection with the alcohol situation in Russia. Moreover, the topic, while urgent, has not yet been addressed in Russia.

The topic is "beer and adolescents", which was broached in Chapter 1-9 in connection with a description of the "anti-beer campaign". It may be remembered that the campaign began in late 2000 on the initiative of Chief Public Health Physician G. Onishchenko. His resolution and the media responses to it reflected concerns about young adults and adolescents acquiring the habit of beer consumption. One of the grounds for such concern was the assertion that beer consumption was increasing among adolescents and that "beer alcoholism" was spreading. However, the assertion was based entirely on "impressions", for no serious analysis of "beer and adolescents" had then been conducted in Russia. While "impressions" may be sufficient for statements in the press, they are hardly sufficient for a state policy proclaimed by the first deputy minister of health. It should be noted, too, that at the time of the anti-beer campaign a scientific foundation on which policy might be based already existed, but it lay outside of Russia's borders in the form of a large group of publications that went unnoticed by both the media and the Chief Public Health Physician in their "crusade" against beer.

Thus, Bjarnason et al. (2003), on the basis of research involving 34,000 pupils in 11 European countries (Great Britain, France, Sweden, Hungary and others), reached the conclusion that a higher level of sales of beer in a country was associated with a greater frequency of serious drunkenness among adolescents. However, it was but one factor and not the main one; the authors uncovered many other causes of frequent intoxication, including, in the first instance, living in a broken home. Yu and Perrine (1997) studied the link between the alcohol consumption of parents and their children. Besides much else, this work showed that early beer consumption more "effectively" influenced future alcohol consumption than the early use of wine or hard liquor. In addition, it has been shown (Smart & Walsh, 1995) that antisocial adolescent behavior is more often observed when the adolescents regularly consume not just beer but mix two (beer and hard liquor) or three types of alcoholic beverage, including wine, in conjunction. In the view of these authors, frequency of consumption and overall quantity are more significant for adolescent antisocial behavior than the types of beverage consumed.

The influence of advertising in relation to adolescent consumption of alcoholic beverages has also been a major focus for Western research. Thus, Wyllie et al. (1998), on the basis of a survey of 500 pupils aged 10–17 years, concerning their attitudes toward the television advertising of alcoholic beverages, found that a more positive response to beer advertisements was linked with the more frequent consumption of this beverage. In addition to that; boys aged 10–13 perceived the advertising as a real event and experienced a desire to drink as the advertisement was being shown. Finally, Connolly et al. (1994) studied the quantitative indexes of consumption of alcoholic beverages among 18-year-olds in connection with their recollections of beverage advertisements that they had seen at the ages of 13 and 15. It was demonstrated that young people who were better able to recall beer advertisements that they had seen, when aged 15, consumed more beer aged 18.

Almost all of the researchers mentioned have called for caution in interpreting their results because the data were obtained from surveys. But, if a summation is made of the cited results, it can be construed that the early socialization of adolescents to beer can have undesirable consequences for their alcohol futures and that beer advertising negatively affects the extent of their consumption of alcoholic beverages. In connection with this and aside from the obvious decisions (a ban on sales before the age of 18), there is also the question of the education of adolescents, i.e., it has been shown that knowledge relative to alcohol, drugs and tobacco lowers the intensity of their consumption of beer (Lundborg, 2002).

Finally, an internet search (PubMed, 1990–2002) produced not a single work in response to the keywords "adolescents-alcoholism-beer" and only two for "adolescents-alcoholism" (Tarter et al., 1994; Cornelius et al., 2001). Both works tell of how adolescent alcoholics have no preferences among alcoholic drinks; their alcohol behavior is marked by a lack of order as regards choice of drink. To give some idea of the size of the sample, it may be noted that for the years 1990–2000 inclusive for the keyword "alcoholism" the internet yields almost 10,000 articles, for "adolescents" more than 35,000 and for "beer" more than 600.

Chapter 2-3
Epidemiological studies of Russian alcohol problems

Praiseworthy epidemiological study of alcohol consumption was underway in Russia in the period 1860–1970. In the mid-1930s it came under attack for political reasons, as did many other socially oriented sciences. Statistics on the production and consumption of alcoholic beverages, as well as relating to spending on alcohol and on other measures relevant to the alcohol situation, continued to be published until the early to mid-1960s, after which secrecy was imposed. Relatively more information was available about the incidence of alcoholism, but this, too, was very limited, the data often stamped "DSP" (for staff use only).

As a result, epidemiological alcohology in Russia suffered irreparably and has not yet regained its former strength. A 50-year-plus interruption is almost lethal for a modern science. There was a sharp drop in the number of publications, for example. Until the start of the anti-alcohol campaign in 1985, it was only the sporadic work on very partial problems that ever saw the light of day (Fig. 2-4).

Fig. 2-4: The annual number of epidemiological publications on alcohol problems in Russia (1968–2002). Light columns represent Russian publications; dark columns represent non-Russian publications.

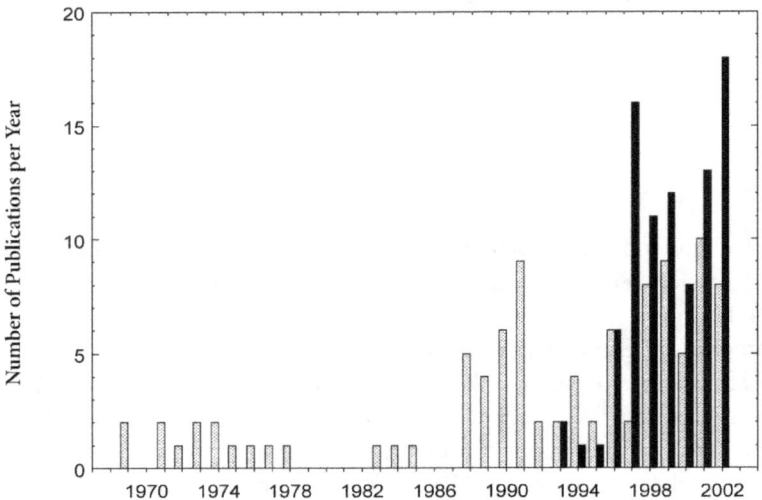

The number of scientific publications in the open press increased, beginning in 1988. The campaign had opened the sluices of information slightly, but the main reason was the state's need to have non-specialist medical-science institutions conduct research on alcohol problems. In connection with this, the leadership of the country and the leaders of scientific institutions often censored publications to serve the interests of the campaign. The result is that many works published in the second half of the 1980s and in the early 1990s sin against truth, making the seriousness of the alcohol problems in the preceding period seem worse and inflating the effectiveness of the government's anti-alcohol measures and the degree of popular support for them.

It is of interest that a Russian author (Segal, 1990) who had moved to the United States and published a long book there about Russia's alcohol problems, by depending on the countless media articles in these years, substantially overestimated Russia's alcohol-related ills, although these were enormous. It would appear that only a single book (Bechtel, 1986), that was written before 1985 and had been prevented from being printed for a considerable period of time but which was finally published at the start of the campaign, was uninfluenced by political considerations.

The second half of the 1980s saw the appearance, in the press, of much epidemiological and statistical data that can hardly be termed strictly truthful, even in cases where the authors were widely known and respected scholars (for example, see the article, "Black Plague of the 1900s", *Nedelya*, 1987, No. 33, p.21).

A propagandistic flavor was even more evident in the articles by a group of scholars with extremist views headed by F. G. Uglov, an Academician of the USSR Academy of Medical Sciences, who wrote from a nationalist point of view and, even before the start of the campaign, was calling for the introduction of "prohibition" in the country.

That is the most general presentation of the pre-history of Russian alcohology in its epidemiological form. How did it develop in the succeeding years? What population research was undertaken to fill in the gaps? And how did this filling-in process develop?

To answer these questions, an internet search was undertaken using the PubMed search engine using the following descriptive words (all in combination with "alcohol in Russia"): consumption, mortality, morbidity, violent death, liver cirrhosis, poisoning and intoxication, psychosis, suicide, homicide, Moscow and several others. The search continued through 2002. Publications from a date later than 2000 were taken into account only in cases where they analyzed material collected before the end of 2000. The nationality of the researchers was noted. Publications by Russian-nationals were considered Russian whether published in Russian or English. Articles by more than one author and a combination of nationalities were considered as belonging to the nationality of the first listed author.

Not all of the articles unearthed by PubMed when using these search terms could be considered epidemiological. As criteria for such research, two definitions were applied:

- "For epidemiological studies observation is made of groups within a population in which these or other illnesses are encountered" (Barker, 1973).
- "Epidemiology may be defined as a science that studies the most general aspects of human illnesses" (Plant, 1991).

Two basic points relating specifically to alcohology must be added:

- The epidemiology of alcohol consumption and its consequences extend beyond the range of pathology. The sphere of interest of this branch of epidemiology includes not only, for example, those ill with alcoholism or alcohol cirrhosis of the liver but all users of alcohol including teetotalers (whose consumption equals zero);
- Insofar as all epidemiological research in the field of alcohology is selective, those works have been chosen for review which are more or less representative of the population or its particular cohorts.

PubMed's responses contained, along with summaries of articles and a small number of complete texts, the electronic contact or institutional addresses of authors, and requests were subsequently sent to these authors for copies of any articles not in the author's library. Russian publications and a few foreign articles were found in journals. PubMed summaries constituted about one-third of the material analyzed. While the results from most of the author's own publications will be examined in the chapters that follow, they are also included in the general list.

PubMed is not the sole internet source of information and contains records of far from all of the works that have been published on the subject of this review. This is because, first, many Russian journals are not referenced or available on the internet; second, books are not referenced in PubMed; and third, there can be no assurance that the search terms used encompass the entirety of the topic. In addition, PubMed does not reference publications on the economic problems of alcohology, specifically several articles by Treml. Yet he is one of the leading specialists studying the alcohol problems of Russia and actively published in the period 1975–1997. It has also been reported (Davis, 2006) that in 1978 John Dutton of Duke University (U.S.) studied the influence of serious drunkenness on mortality in the USSR. His work (Dutton, 1979) is not referenced in PubMed. It is possible that there are other omissions of this kind. Nonetheless, this sole source of information, despite its incompleteness, has made it possible to perform a quantitative analysis of publications over time selected by uniform criteria.

The incompleteness of the review is, of course, regrettable. However, it should be borne in mind that publications not on the internet are available to only a limited circle of researchers and thus, are not part of ordinary scientific exchanges and lose any value that they might have had.

The analysis included 75 foreign and 92 Russian articles. The distribution of publications by time period is presented in Fig. 2-4, which shows the number of publications rising, at first for Russian (from 1988) and later for foreign (from 1993) articles. Beyond the declassification of statistical data and the ending of censorship, a number of other factors have contributed to this growth.

- The almost experimental conditions, with sharp fluctuations in levels of consumption in Russia, made it easier to study alcohol problems.
- The uniqueness of such conditions for the 1900s. Other anti-alcohol campaigns of the 1900s were small in scale (Canada, Finland, the Netherlands, Gdansk in Poland) or so fully documented and described (for example, the U.S. "dry law", Prohibition, 1919).
- Many researchers, in particular those in Finland and Sweden, sought to find in Russia solutions to their own national concerns in the alcohol arena. In these cases Russia served as the battlefield where it was possible to study super-high alcohol consumption, as the "horrible example" with which to frighten the populations of countries much

- more concerned about their own alcohol problems, however much smaller these problems were than those of the Russians.
- Foreign researchers felt that Russia's alcohol problems were the most obvious and more easily dealt with than other crisis phenomena of the post-Soviet period.

All this has evoked and continues to evoke unwavering scientific interest in Russia's alcohol problems.

* * *

For content analysis, the journals *Voprosy Narkologii* and *Sotsialnaya i Klinicheskaya Psikhiatriya* were reviewed in addition to the publications found in PubMed (the S. S. Korsakov Journal of Neurology and Psychiatry is in PubMed). Works dealing with partial and otherwise ignored topics as well as methodologically weak articles are not included in the content review. Collections of articles but not collections of abstracts are taken into account along with journal publications.

It is not the task of this chapter to offer an exhaustive review of the literature; its main function is to make clear the more active directions of epidemiological research into Russia's alcohol problems during 1990 and 2000. Older works have, as a rule, become outdated. Moreover, by 1991 (Fig. 2-4), the series of Russian publications, administratively stimulated at the start of the anti-alcohol campaign, had come to an end. In large part, this series of works set for itself partial tasks and consisted of works based on surveys, for example, of school pupils, students, workers in oil-refining and forestry, girls suffering from gonorrhea and so on for the purpose of clarifying the character of alcohol consumption and with respect to several other alcohol problems. As a rule, these works were scientifically poor and so most of them have been excluded from the review. The end of the series essentially marked the finish of the anti-alcohol campaign, which had ended a year or two earlier.

Among the articles chosen on the basis of these selection criteria, attention should be turned first – because of its fatal implications for the population and because the topic has been so actively developed – to the body of publications on mortality linked to alcohol consumption in Russia. One astounding thing about the topic is that, since the mid-1990s it has been dealt with largely by non-Russian researchers. However, the earliest works in this field were by Russian authors.

The first study was undertaken by a researcher from Novosibirsk who examined data on 7,000 cases of sudden death from ischemic heart disease (Solomatin, 1988) and discovered that 30 percent of the victims had traces of alcohol in their blood. In 1990 Markov and coauthors published the results of an eight-year-long observational study (from 1978) of 5,500 workers at six industrial plants in the city of Cheboksary, which investigated various causes of death. Accidents, poisonings, traumas and suicides accounted for 35 percent of all the deaths, of which 77 percent were linked to alcohol use. The second most frequent cause of death was a diagnosis of cardiovascular disease, where one-fifth of these deaths were sudden and linked to alcohol abuse. Similar results were reported by Kalinina and Chazova (1991), who studied the male population between the ages of 40 and 50 years in the city of Moscow. They found that alcohol abuse increased the mortality of this cohort by 1.5 times, largely as a result of accidents.

An article by Anderson and Hibis published in 1992 noted that abuse of alcohol was a powerful factor in the rise of mortality in the USSR. In 1995 Ryan, using data from official sources as well as the estimates by Nemtsov and Shkolnikov that were published in *Izvestiya* (1994), described the basic features of the demographic situation in Russia with respect to alcohol: a decline in consumption and mortality in the mid-1980s, a rise in these indexes beginning in 1987, and all of this to a large degree for the male population and from "non-natural" causes of death. Ryan drew attention to an important attribute of Russian drunkenness – the episodic consumption of alcohol in large doses, which he labeled the "macho manner" of consumption or "doses which deliver a punch". This kind of consumption came to be known as "binge drinking", a phrase widely used in the English-language literature and now established as a term.

Remarkably, these works, although referenced on the internet, elicited no response in the scientific press. Probably that is because there was an insufficiency of facts for broad generalization in the late 1980s and early 1990s. Moreover, the works of the early 1990s were not only insufficient in facts or as regards the standing of the journals publishing them, they also did not address fundamental questions. The article by Leon et al. (1997) however was fundamental in character and included new data on the realm of the interaction of alcohol problems.

The authors studied the age and cause components of deaths in Russia between 1984 and 1994 and showed that the level of mortality from all principal causes, excluding neoplasms, dropped in 1985–1987 and increased in 1988–1994. The changes were mostly in the group aged 40–44, for men and women, although the changes were significantly greater for men. The article importantly noted the similarity in the dynamics of mortality from alcohol poisoning and diseases of the circulatory system. The authors did not exclude the possibility that the character of nutrition and the quality of medical services might have significance for the change in the level of mortality. However, the detailed analysis of these and other possible causes of the oscillations in the mortality level showed that the major cause was fluctuations in the level of alcohol consumption.

The article by D. A. Leon et al. appeared in the 9 August edition of the *Lancet*, and by 27 September the same journal had already published three commentaries on it. Another one appeared in the 21 August edition of *Nature*.

By this time a large group of researchers were active in London at the European Centre on Health of Societies in Transition (Adamets, Andreev, Britton, Chenet, Deev, Leon, McKee, Sanderson, Shkolnikov, Vassin, & Walberg). In addition to other problems, they were interested in the relation between mortality and alcohol consumption in Russia. The group began to study this problem systematically from various angles. As early as 1998, this collective had already been highly productive in terms of its publications.

An article by McKee et al. (1998) looked at mortality in Moscow in the period 1993–1995. It showed that there was an increase in mortality in the summer period, which was unusual for European countries, that this growth occurred especially among young people and that it was principally from accidents and other causes linked to alcohol consumption. This underlined the important role of alcohol consumption in Russia's mortality crisis.

Walberg et al. (1998), in comparing regions in the European part of Russia, showed that the fall in life expectancy was not the same in all regions and that some of the largest changes in mortality were found in several of the richest regions. This, in the authors' view, ruled out linking the drop in life expectancy with poverty. They demonstrated that, among the many factors operating to reduce life expectancy, the main one was alcohol consumption which they suggested may be more important than the effects of crime, inequalities in income and other factors.

Another approach used by the London group when studying the role of alcohol in Russian mortality was to examine the educational level of those who had died (Shkolnikov et al., 1998). It was shown that, among the various groups of the Russian population, mortality was greater where the educational level of the deceased was lower, especially among men. And this brings Russia closer to Western countries, and especially to the countries of the former Soviet bloc (the Czech Republic, Estonia and Hungary). The dependence of the type of death on the level of education increases in the following order: accidents, violent deaths, alcohol cirrhosis and alcohol poisoning. The authors linked these results with the fact that increased alcohol consumption in Russia in the 1990s was especially sharp among men with low levels of education.

The article by Chenet et al. (1998a) probably made use of the same material that was used in the article by McKee et al. (1998), but in this instance the authors studied the distribution of deaths by days of the week and demonstrated a significant increase in several types of death on Saturdays, Sundays and Mondays. While paying particular attention to the increase in mortality from cardiovascular disease on these days, they revealed a similarity in the dynamics of mortality from cardiovascular disease with that of alcohol poisoning, other accidents and violence, in all of which alcohol plays a very large role. The increase in cardiovascular deaths on days off stood out with particular clarity in the analysis of sudden deaths. The authors linked all of these facts to the dynamic of alcohol consumption in the course of the week, as variations in the other risk factors for cardiovascular disease mortality (smoking or fatty food consumption) are distributed evenly throughout the course of the week and could not explain the observed pattern of mortality. In this work the authors especially emphasized the character of alcohol consumption in Russia (*kutezhnoye p'yanstvo* or "binge drinking"), which is unlike the consumption in many other countries, where alcohol is taken in smaller doses and in a more moderate manner which may make it cardiac protective.

Unfortunately, Chenet et al. (1998b), who had to rely on indirect data, were unaware of the studies conducted in Novosibirsk (Solomatin, 1988) that had demonstrated the direct connection to alcohol of a significant portion of sudden death cases where ischemic heart disease was present.

The discussion of alcohol mortality increasingly diverged from general problems and concentrated on the part of it that was connected to cardiovascular pathology. This was a function of the fact that, in the period from the late 1960s until the early 1990s, a great deal of work was done in a number of Western countries on the dependence of cardiovascular mortality on the level of alcohol consumption. It had been demonstrated that this relation is expressed by a J-shaped curve at the individual level: in comparison with abstainers, the risk of death falls with small doses of alcohol but rises with large doses (see the review by Anderson, 1995). At the population level however, the correlation between cardiovascular mortality and the level of average per capita alcohol consumption was negative: with greater consumption, mortality falls. This is because there are relatively few serious alcoholics in Western countries, and with moderate consumers in numerical dominance they are thus to a significant degree determinative of the average level of consumption for the population as a whole as well as for the cardio-protective effect of alcohol.

By the mid-1990s, this conception of the role of alcohol was a scientific fixture. Yet the same pattern was not reproduced in Russia: cardiovascular mortality fell with a lowering of alcohol consumption at the start of the anti-alcohol campaign and rose toward its end with the rise in consumption. It was necessary to explain the "Russian paradox".

In their review, McKee and Britton (1998) presented data on the pathological physiological consequences of binge drinking in the form of changes in the composition of blood lipids, the elevation of coagulability and episodes of cardiac arrhythmia. The authors cited work done in Russia (Deev et al., 1998), which demonstrated that those who were found to have died with a low content of cholesterol in their blood (hypocholesterolemia) were distinguished by severe alcohol consumption during their lives. In these cases, a change in the proportion of cholesterol of different densities in the direction of more "bad" cholesterol of high density was also observed. The special importance of these findings lay in the fact that Western investigators had frequently demonstrated the increasing risk of coronary pathology with increases in the cholesterol content of blood. As in the case of cardiovascular mortality, in Russia, a pattern was not evident (Deev et al., 1998).

But the topic of alcohol mortality in Russia did not get beyond this point so easily. Bobak and Marmot (1999) considered the lowered mortality of 1985 as only an indirect testimony that alcohol had played a role. They believed that the lowering of cardiovascular mortality belied this role, since the already mentioned cardio-protective role of alcohol had by now been demonstrated. Another line of objection that they advanced was based on the fact that the data on consumption were "too low"; they were relying on official figures (5 liters of alcohol per capita per year) and on the results of several surveys (Simpura et al., 1997). Bobak and Marmot paid no attention to the fact that Simpura et al. had in the same book expressed strong doubts about the accuracy of Russians' answers and advised at least doubling the survey data on consumption in order to obtain a truer representation of alcohol consumption in Russia. Naturally, with such an approach, Bobak and Marmot did not obtain confirmation of the hypothesis from previous researchers and expressed their doubts about it.

The Bobak and Marmot article quickly evoked commentaries. In one of them, a French researcher, Balkau (1999), laid out in a logical fashion all of the evidence against the hypothesis of the London group and called for further study of Russian mortality and its connections with alcohol.

As a result of the great dynamism of the alcohol situation in Russia, new facts accumulated rapidly. Accordingly, the discussion of alcohol mortality continued, in a very keen manner with respect to alcohol as a risk factor in cardiovascular pathology and death. Britton and McKee (2000) put forward the proposition that the link between consumption and mortality is defined less by the average quantity of drunk alcohol than by the character of the single-drinking occasion. Most Western investigators in works of this kind took into account the average consumption in a week or month. In that light, the cardio-protective role of alcohol predominated, even in the presence of relatively large, by Western standards, average doses. In works that looked at the frequency of hangovers and other serious effects of drinking, it was found that the risk of cardiovascular death, especially sudden death, rose with a rise in frequency. Britton and McKee concluded that regular drunkenness and binge drinking are different types of intoxication with different consequences, specifically in relation to cardiovascular pathology and death.

In the course of 1998–2000, the London group published studies of similar problems in the countries of the Baltic region and Eastern Europe. It was only in 2001 that Shkolnikov, McKee and Leon returned to the subject matter of Russia in the middle of the 1990s. They demonstrated that between 1994 and 1998 the level of mortality in Russia fell and returned to the level of the early 1980s. The authors noted an important feature of Russian mortality: over the entire period of the 1990s, the mortality of the most vulnerable groups of the population either fell steadily (children) or did not change (elderly people) but that the reduction in mortality in 1994–1998 was chiefly a function of a decrease among middle-aged people.

The same group was responsible for the rise in mortality before 1994. Among the causes of death, the main ones were linked to alcohol consumption. The investigators again concluded that alcohol had played an important role in the fluctuations in Russian mortality in the 1990s.

And again, as in 1997, the authors were subjected to almost immediate criticism for their staunch adherence to the hypothesis of the alcohol provenance of oscillations of mortality in Russia in the 1980s and 1990s. The first to make the case were Vlassov and Gafarov (2001), who saw the weakness in the hypothesis of the London group in the fact that from an overall increase in the rate of mortality of 718 per 100,000 of the population (from 1981 to 1994), only 56 of these deaths were attributable to alcohol poisoning (it is unclear where the authors obtained this statistic from). They regarded the assumption of Shkolnikov et al. (2001) that the majority of cases of cirrhosis of the liver were linked to alcohol abuse as being doubtful. Meanwhile, Voinova (1999) using the results from the autopsies of more than 6,000 bodies found this to be exactly the case. She concluded that in Russia alcohol is the main etiological factor in the development of diseases of the liver with fatal outcomes.

Vlassov and Gafarov while finding fault with Shkolnikov et al.'s results made a number of errors. One of them was linking alcohol mortality exclusively with alcohol poisoning. The very merit of the London group was that it had moved alcohol mortality in Russia beyond the limits of direct losses to alcohol to include such "non-alcohol" causes as some portion of cardiovascular pathologies.

Unlike Vlassov and Gafarov (2001), Wasserman and Värnik (2001) found much agreement between the data of Shkolnikov et al. (2001) and the results of their own investigations of the dynamics of suicide in Russia. However, they considered it an error to limit the analysis of mortality in Russia to a single factor – alcohol consumption. Wasserman and Värnik wrote that, among the causes of Russia's very high mortality level, it was wrong to exclude social, economic and political factors, especially the loss of "a feeling of hope". They postulated that alcohol consumption in Russia is a "defense mechanism in a situation where faith in the future is inadequate". One cannot entirely reject Wasserman and Värnik's arguments (on the causes of Russia's high mortality level). But it is also difficult to accept them because the authors presented no evidence, and there has been no scientific study of mortality and non-alcohol, specifically, social factors.

In fairness, it should be noted that the non-scientific, "literary", development of the topic of Russian mortality as linked with "psychosocial stress" is found not only in the works of Wasserman and Värnik but also in that of other investigators, always, it should be said, in a declarative form, as being something self-evident. Later (Chapter 2-5) it will be shown that in the period 1995–1998 mortality declined in Russia, against a background of a substantial increase in social tension. This episode in Russia's alcohol history shows the need for great care in interpreting mortality with respect to psychological concepts or in connection with stress.

The third commentary on the article by Shkolnikov et al. (2001) was by Ogurtsov et al. (2001). These authors called attention to the disjunction between the level of alcohol mortality in Russia and the level of alcohol consumption, which is only slightly higher than the level of consumption in several European countries, including France and Germany. The level of alcohol mortality in these same European countries however is between a quarter and a fifth of that in Russia. In explaining these differences, Ogurtsov et al. relied on the results of their studies of the special genetic features of the Russian population, which were later not confirmed (Marusin et al., 2004; Borinskaya et al., 2005). However, the disjunction between consumption and mortality in Russia and several other countries to which Ogurtsov et al. drew attention deserves special consideration. It will be discussed in more detail in Chapter 2-5.

It is surprising that all of this intensive discussion went unremarked by a group of St Petersburg researchers (Plavinski et al., 2003). They concluded that alcohol had played a small role in the rise in Russian mortality in the 1990s and that the main cause was social factors, which the authors saw as being expressed by the level of education. On the basis of a single study, the authors concluded that alcohol consumption does not depend on educational level, although by 2003 studies had already been conducted that proved the opposite. And again (for the umpteenth time) the increase in cardiovascular mortality was put forward as an argument against alcohol as a factor in the increase in mortality in the 1990s.

In a commentary on this article, Ronellenfitsch (2003) expressed justifiable doubt about the propriety of the methodological approach of the authors, who did not take into account the difference in alcohol consumption during and after the anti-alcohol campaign.

It is important to note, among alcohol problems and concepts, the very important understanding of alcohol-related illness that took shape in Russia in the late 1980s and early 1990s. This is linked to the fact that the alcohol damage done to different organs and systems is often connected, and includes somatic illnesses and alcoholism, which are ordinarily thought of as covering all alcohol problems. However, the larger portion of people whose deaths are alcohol related die of somatic ailments linked to drunkenness before the onset of the psychological ailment, alcoholism. Moiseev and Ogurtsov (1997) defined alcoholic disease as "a complex of psychological and/or somato-neurological disorders of health linked to regular consumption of alcohol in doses dangerous to health (with chronic alcohol intoxication)".

Unfortunately, no one in Russia has defined the doses of alcohol that are "dangerous to health". However, it is possible to use foreign data that define the risks of negative medical consequences. There have been many such studies, and their results are quite similar. Generalizing the view of many researchers, Kendell (1987) believes that the danger line, "if such a point exists" can be considered as the regular consumption of 80–90 milliliters of vodka a day for healthy men and 50–60 milliliters for healthy women. Another example is found in the recommendations of the Council on National Health and Medical Research (1987) for daily consumption (Table 8).

Table 8: Safe, dangerous and harmful daily consumption of alcohol (vodka equivalent, 40 percent ABV, in parentheses; calculations by author).

	Safe consumption	Dangerous consumption	Harmful consumption
Men	≤39 gr.(125ml)	40–60gr. (130–190 ml)	≥61gr. (≥190 ml)
Women	≤19gr. (60 ml)	20–40gr. (65–130 ml)	≥41gr. (≥130 ml)

Source: *National Health and Medical Research Council, 1987.*

It is important to note that the indicated consumption doses are only safe in the absence of other risk factors. These individual risk factors are given as follows:

- Consumption of medicines, especially those with psychotropic or sedative effects
- Men with a family history linked to alcohol problems or alcoholism
- Previously infected with hepatitis B
- An elevated susceptibility to alcohol that is genetically based
- Smoking
- surgery on the gastrointestinal tract,
- Poor nutrition
- A number of physical and psychiatric illnesses (diabetes, stomach ulcers, psychosis and others)

Increased risk situations were also given:

- During pregnancy
- Driving a car
- Working with machines and mechanisms
- Dangerous situations including swimming, cold environments, domestic conflicts, low mood or depression, and any potential danger in one's immediate surroundings

Also important in defining a safe dose is the character of consumption – episodic or regular, which was discussed by Babor et al. (1987, Table 9). To many in Russia the indicated doses of alcohol (vodka) would seem naive or laughable. For these "laughers", one can cite the recommendation of the father of English alcohology:

> Having gauged the whole circle of effects of alcohol consumption, one must assume that any entirely risk-free consumption of alcohol is a figment of the imagination. The basic recommendation for safe consumption of alcohol is 'the less the better'. (Edwards, 1994)

Table 9: Limits of episodic and regular alcohol consumption (vodka equivalent in parentheses; calculations by author).

	Episodic consumption	Regular consumption
Men	~ 50 gr. (160 ml)	~ 40 gr./day (130 ml)
Women	~ 35 gr. (110 ml)	~ 25 gr./day (80 ml)

Source: Babor et al., 1987.

In the opinion of World Health Organization experts, relatively safe can be considered, for men, as a single drink of 20–40 grams of alcohol a day (about 40–80 milliliters of vodka a day) and, for women, 20 grams (or 40 milliliters of vodka). Consumption of alcohol in single doses exceeding these limits substantially increases the risk of a whole spectrum of ailments.

The topic of the serious consequences of the alcoholization of the Northern Peoples is widely known in Russia. The idea persists that this is linked to the special genetic makeup of the Mongolic people of Northern Russia (Chukchens, Eskimo-Inuits, Yakuts, Udegeitsy, Nenets, Khanty, Mansi). However, it may now be asserted with confidence that this idea is fundamentally incorrect. Interest in this question was spurred by studies of the native peoples of the northern regions of Alaska, who, although being a Mongolic race, nevertheless differed in their reaction to alcohol when compared with people of the Mongolic race from continental areas of Asia (for example, the Chinese and Japanese). The topic seems to have "jumped" across the Bering Strait (Segal et al., 1991). In this connection, it was also demonstrated (Kurilovich et al., 1998; Avksentyuk et al., 1995) that the Northern Peoples of Russia differed from continental Mongolics in terms of the "reddening reaction" of the face in response to imbibing alcohol as an outward manifestation of an accumulation of acetaldehyde in the blood. Even earlier, this difference was confirmed in studies of ferments used in the deactivation of alcohol (Kurilovich, 1994). Only the Nenets were an exception, demonstrating a typical "reddening reaction" where related metabolic processes made the intake of large quantities of alcohol impossible. As regards the other peoples of the Russian North it was concluded that the effects of drunkenness (very high mortality and thus short life expectancy: 48 years for men and 60 for women; Khanty-Mansiysk Autonomous Region) were conditioned not by genetic but social causes. This led to the emergence of so-called "modernization stress". This is taken to mean the psychological tension occasioned by abrupt changes in preconceptions about life and difficulties in adapting to new conditions of existence (Kozlov & Vkshubskaya, 2001). This leads to massive alcoholization and the subsequent mortality linked to it, especially among men.

Among the important problems linked to the epidemiology of alcohol consumption in Russia, it is necessary to remember the incomplete nature of the recording of deaths from alcohol poisoning and the frequent treatment of this pathology as cardiovascular disease either by mistake or as a result of intentionally false diagnoses. The first person to draw attention to this was Tishuk (1997). He showed that 9 percent of men and 3 percent of women who died suddenly in Kursk in 1991 and who were diagnosed with diseases of the circulatory system had lethal concentrations of alcohol in their blood. In other words, these people died of alcohol poisoning, but in the official mortality statistics they were entered with a diagnosis of cardiovascular disease. The author linked this to "the undesirability of the moral-ethical, social and material consequences of a diagnosis of accidental alcohol poisoning for the relatives of the deceased". One can take this psychological trait as having broader meaning: in the presence of a very high level of alcohol consumption, there is a strongly expressed psychologically defensive attitude and a displacement of alcohol problems by the people of Russia. This manifests itself, in particular, through "pressure on experts to remove alcohol diagnoses from information about deaths" (Tishuk, 1997), although such information serves as the main source for the register of mortality in the country.

Analogous work was conducted in Izhevsk (Shkolnikov et al., 2002), where similar errors were not found, but the authors reported that 13.5 percent of the deaths with cardiovascular diagnoses had occurred while the person was highly intoxicated. Moreover, the blood alcohol concentration of the deceased was not indicated, thus reducing the significance of the results, especially in light of the fact that for the attribution of deaths to alcohol poisoning the authors elected to use an absolutely lethal blood alcohol concentration (0.4 percent). However, actual mistakes and intentional "mistakes" occur within the limits of relatively lethal blood alcohol concentrations (0.25–0.35 percent), which are often encountered in Russia (Naubatov, 1990; Khotimskaya & Lukash, 1989) as well as abroad (Veljkovic et al., 1989). In the first work, blood alcohol concentrations of less than 0.4 percent were found in 20 percent of the deceased; in the second, in half of the deceased, and in the third the scatter of measures among those dead from alcohol poisoning was 2.66–7.19 g/l (average concentration - 4g/l, which is almost exactly 0.4 percent). It is worth noting the opinion of Nordum et al. (2000) that concentrations of alcohol in the blood of deceased persons beginning with readings of 0.5 g/l should be considered as an accompanying cause of death. This is very far from the Russian practice in diagnosing deaths linked to alcohol. One more difficulty in Russia with respect to the recording of alcohol mortality is linked to the diagnosis of alcohol cirrhosis of the liver, which was mentioned earlier.

Mistakes are also encountered in other regions and affect not only deaths attributed to cardiovascular disease. In 2000, according to data from the Regional Statistical Administration of Krasnodar Region, 9.3 percent of those who died from external causes were found to have alcohol in their blood, but according to the data of the Forensic-Medical Review Bureau, the percentage was 53.9 percent (Redko & Sakharova, 2006), that is, almost six times more. Thus, for a single year and merely in the Krasnodar Region, the undercount of those who died from external causes found to have alcohol in their blood amounted to 3,771 cases.

All this bears witness to the fact that postmortem diagnosis in Russia, as an important indicator of the health of the population and of the seriousness of the alcohol situation, is significantly degraded. Zaratyants (2001) offers quantitative data. In 1996–2000 autopsies were performed on only 43–48 percent of Moscow's deceased and 23–25 percent in Russia overall, while there was a failure of agreement between clinical and postmortem diagnoses in 16–17 percent of cases in hospitals and 48–56 percent of cases for non-hospitalized patients. Moreover, it is difficult to ascertain the exact selection criteria that determined which of the deceased would be autopsied, the choice of which, was most likely, not made by accident.

The low quality of Russian statistical data on mortality was noted by Semyonova and coauthors (2004), who highlighted the fact that, in the period 1989–2000, mortality "from imprecisely indicated conditions" and from "injuries (with specification)" grew by 6–8 and 2–3 times, respectively. The authors suggested that such increases in these indexes took place as a way of hiding a portion of "unnatural and violent deaths" under these rubrics. It is possible a role in this was played by changes in the rules for registering death diagnoses at this time and by the careless attitude of physicians to the changes. Whatever the reason, however, for the paradoxical increase in these types of mortality, the statistics became less accurate as a result: some violent deaths "exited" the register. Semyonova and coauthors correctly noted that statistics of this quality are a hindrance to the development of public health and make it impossible to determine real priorities or to judge the actual dimensions of the losses from one or another cause.

Unfortunately, Semyonova and coauthors (2004) used relatively brief runs of data (1989–2000). Increasing the time-span analyzed makes more evident the decline in the quality of the postmortem diagnosis of mortality in Russia (Fig. 2-5). For comparison, the diagram shows deaths from suicide, the level of which since 1990 has been substantially lower than that of "unspecified" diagnoses of death. It is important to note that the "unspecified" death diagnosis reflects the fluctuations in alcohol consumption. The sharp rise in mortality from "unspecified conditions" and from "injuries (unspecified)" began in 1990 and continues today to serve as an indicator of the collapse of the Expert Pathological-Anatomical and Forensic Medical service in Russia. These local changes in medical indexes vividly reflect the general deterioration of social institutions in Russia – inaccuracy in postmortem diagnosis increasingly trends from a matter of insufficiently qualified personnel to outright careless and ethical breakdowns.

Fig. 2-5: Mortalities of "inexactly designated states" together with "from injuries (without specification)" (1965–2003). For comparison, mortalities from suicides and estimate of alcohol consumption.

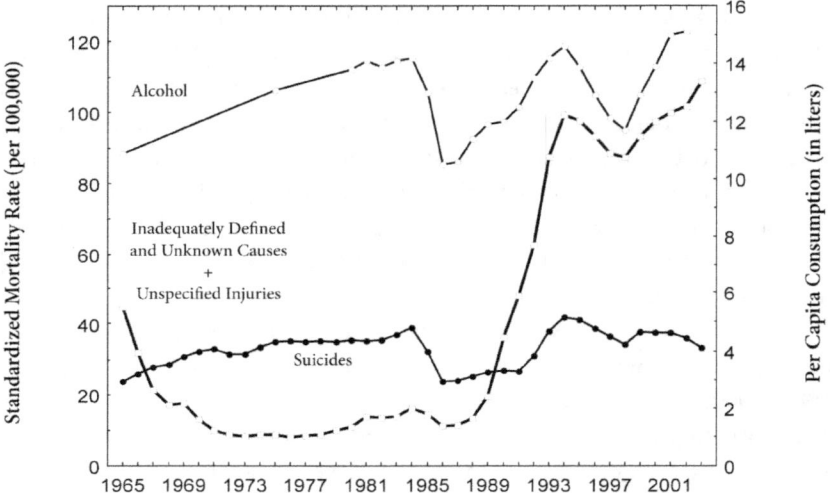

Several studies have looked at the link between suicide and alcohol consumption. Mäkinen (2000) studied suicide in 28 countries of the former Eastern Bloc in 1984–1989 and 1989–1994. He was interested in the dependence of the suicide level on economic conditions (overall industrial production was used as the index), on political changes (for this a whole range of indexes were used, including the possibility of free elections), on social tensions, about which the author made judgments from projected life expectancy, and on the level of alcohol consumption using the WHO figures, which in the case of Russia reproduce very incomplete official statistics.

The indexes chosen by Mäkinen (2000) cannot be considered as valid and completely adequate for the purposes of the study. As a result, the author's findings should be treated with caution. The analysis of specific phenomena on the basis of the multifactor model showed that in 16 of the 28 countries, including Russia, the level of suicide was well forecast by such measures as general tension, the level of democratization, alcohol consumption and social disorganization. At the same time, none of the factors, including alcohol consumption, taken in isolation, could explain changes in the levels of suicide. This is not surprising given the fact that the alcohol statistics kept in almost all the countries of the former Eastern Bloc are far from accurate. Russian figures are approximately half of what they should be (Chapter 2-4).

Somewhat more definite results about the link between suicide and alcohol consumption were obtained by Wasserman, Värnik, Eklund (1994, 1998). They demonstrated that a positive correlation existed between these two phenomena and that half of suicides by men and 27 percent of those committed by women involved significant alcohol consumption. However, it is necessary to keep in mind that these authors also used official measures that poorly reflect the realities of consumption in the country.

Studies about alcohol mortality also include publications that examine alcohol consumption in relation to the risk of cancer. The work done by a group of Russian researchers led by D. Zaridze serves as an example of this. These studies are based on large samples (1,000 or more persons) and are methodologically sound. In one of them (Zaridze et al., 2000), it was shown that abuse of alcohol, especially of vodka, increases the risk of developing cancer of the stomach. This largely affected men, for whom the risk was three times greater than it was for a control group. In another study, Zaridze et al. (1991) investigated risk factors for breast cancer and showed that alcohol consumption substantially increases this risk during menopause.

Hugo (1990) asserted that 45–70 percent of venereal infections occurred in conditions of alcohol intoxication, chiefly on Saturdays (19.8 percent) and Sundays or holidays (37.7 percent). Alcohol abuse has also been shown to play a very substantial role in the course (Floyd et al., 2006) and fatal outcomes of tuberculosis (Zamborov, 1999), while alcohol abuse was common among such patients (32–49 percent, Floyd et al., 2006).

It is too early to sum up the literature on the link between Russian mortality and alcohol consumption. As we have seen, the stream of literature is growing (Fig. 2-4). However, it is already possible to see that the link is not artefactual and that a significant share of mortality in Russia is due to alcohol. This is why, as regards mortality, there has been a predominance of deaths among men of working age (40–44 years; Leon et al., 1997), with relatively low levels of education (Shkolnikov et al., 1998), while these deaths occur most often at the end of the week. Among the causes of death in this cohort, accidents and other alcohol-related events predominate. The link between cardiovascular mortality and alcoholic beverages and the special danger of so-called *kutezh* (binge) drinking that is characteristic for Russian drinkers has been a discovery of the past seven or eight years.

It remains to be noted that a substantial contribution to working out the relationship between Russian mortality and dangerous alcohol consumption has been made by an international group of researchers led by Martin McKee and David Leon. The main characteristic of the works of this group is that most of them are undertaken from a strictly demographic point of view, without any admixture of material from the field of alcohology. As a result, in their studies, the link between Russia's extreme mortality levels and the abuse of alcohol has an indirect and qualitative character. The certainty of the link arises from the multifaceted approach and the large number of sound publications it has produced.

* * *

Recent years have produced a large number of works, most of them foreign, based on surveys of the Russian population. This research has clarified a wide range of questions about alcohol consumption. These works fall into groups of descending size (from 7 to 2 publications) around the following topics:

- the level and character of individual consumption,
- the same for adolescents and young adults,
- factors in individual consumption,
- the same for the *bomzh* (the economically and socially marginalized),
- the link between the health of the individual and his consumption.

The following topics have produced one publication each:

- alcohol consumption among the elderly,
- the determinants of alcoholism among the population,
- somatic pathologies associated with alcohol consumption,
- antisocial behavior and alcohol consumption,
- the influence of ideology on lifestyle and, in particular, on alcohol consumption,
- school pupils' assimilation of information about alcohol problems.

This list is based on a total of 31 articles. An analysis of a portion of them follows.

Among the works based on surveys of the population, the most voluminous is The Russian Longitudinal Monitoring Survey (RLMS: http://www.cpc.unc.edu/rlms; Zohoori et al., 1997a, 1997b), which was conducted from 1992 through to 2002 once a year (except in 1997 and 1999). The research is based on interviews with members of more than 4,000 households or 10,000 individuals in many regions of the country. Among the tasks that the RLMS set for itself, which included defining the character of nutrition and smoking and attitudes to health and medical services, was to obtain answers to a whole range of questions concerning alcohol consumption. According to RLMS data, in 1992 alcohol consumption for men, women and adolescents was 11.2, 2.4

and 1.3 liters per capita per year for the members of these respective groups. Based on these contingents' shares in the total population, it is possible to recalculate the three RLMS measures as a single measure of average per capita consumption, as is done in Russia and other countries. The result is 4.8 liters, which is lower than the official figure from the State Statistical Committee (5.01 liters), which does not include the consumption of illegal alcohol. Moreover, the RLMS level is almost only a third of the estimates of consumption for 1992 made while using other approaches, for example 13.81 liters (Treml, 1997).

According to the data compiled by the RLMS, maximum consumption occurred in 1993 (9.9 liters per capita per year; author's recalculation), while in 1994 there was the start of a steep decline in this measure (to 6.9 liters). This was nevertheless accompanied by the highest number of alcohol-related consequences in 1994–1995, which hardly seems credible in view of the steep reduction of consumption by almost one-third. Also suggestive of the need for caution when viewing these consumption figures is the RLMS finding of a six-fold difference in alcohol consumption between men and women.

An even larger difference between genders was found in a survey of 1,735 Moscow residents in 1994 (Simpura et al., 1997). At that time, consumption in the country was at the highest level in this period. Nonetheless, according to the answers provided by the surveyed women, their consumption was the lowest from among women in 12 European countries and America. The replies also showed that the share of serious (daily) drinkers in Moscow was very low when compared with most of the other industrialized countries. The authors justly attribute their results to the imprecision of the interview method, which was further compounded by "the particular difficulties of surveying women and men in Russia".

It is altogether likely that the lowered measures of alcohol consumption in Russia found in the RLMS data are linked with features of the methodology and specific attributes of the Russian population, although it is now known that representatives of other nations also lower their self-estimates of consumption. However, such errors are substantially smaller than those in Russia (Midanik, 1982, 1988).

The lowered RLMS estimates may be partly linked to the choice of "households" as the unit of study: the choice excludes large contingents of the population – members of the military, prisoners, refugees, migrants and an army of millions of economically and socially marginalized citizens (the *bomzhy*), all of whom together comprise 10 percent of the population. Moreover, one does not say of members of the Russian military that they drink little alcohol. It is also well known that new settlers and migrants drink more than long-established residents and that the *bomzhy* are heavy users of spirits and include about half of all alcoholics (Afanasyev et al., 1995). The exclusion of these population groups, along with the unaccounted-for population of "difficult" territories (4 percent), can distort the picture of the level of alcohol consumption in Russia.

However, the chief contribution to the problematic estimates emanating from the RLMS is made by the respondents themselves. It is easy to suppose that the "specific difficulties of the Russian population" (Simpura et al., 1997) were a function of the mental inheritance from Soviet and possibly, from even earlier Russian history. Deliberate or not, the underestimated dimensions of alcohol consumption can be explained by the "facade-like" psychology of the Russian population (the surveys were conducted under the aegis of U.S. researchers) and by fears "that something might happen". Interestingly, the other sections of the RLMS found Russians to be quite healthy overall, their nutrition quite satisfactory, except for a slight lag behind developed Western countries in terms of the intake of fruits and vegetables. These results were higher and sometimes much higher than the official figures from the State Statistical Committee of the Russian Federation. All of this suggests that in Russia surveys on the subject of alcohol consumption are more reflective of the psychology of the population than of the phenomenon itself.

Unfortunately, the same caveats apply to a large part of the work based on surveys of the topics already listed. Control and "hidden" questions in a framework that is wholly based on interviews are of little help, as in the case of the RLMS research and other works. Hence, there are frequent contradictions that appear in surveys of the population. For example, Malyutina et al., (2001), on the basis of a survey of 7,500 residents of Novosibirsk about the character of their consumption, found no difference in consumption between 1988–1989, when consumption was relatively low in Russia as a result of the anti-alcohol campaign, and 1994–1995, when it rose steeply and reached its highest level ever in the history of Russia.

Another example is offered by the work of Bobak et al. (1999), which analyzed data compiled by the All-Russia Center for the Study of Public Opinion (VTsIOM) in a survey of more than 1,500 persons in various regions of Russia and came to the conclusion that material deprivation had no effect on the level of consumption and that the level of alcohol consumption in Russia was uniform and does not depend on variations in the socioeconomic status of respondents. World experience bespeaks the opposite, although Russia may have its own specificities. It is most likely, however, that the crux of the matter lies in something else. A pivotal element in Bobak et al.'s ideas about the burden of drunkenness in Russia were the results of surveys conducted by Simpura et al. (1997) that showed a low level of alcohol consumption in Russia. The authors themselves (Simpura et al.) considered this an error arising from the interview method. But Bobak et al. paid no attention to these criticisms.

Table 10: Examining the quantity and frequency of alcohol consumption in Russia, using data from a number of studies.

Source, region, sampling, year of research		No	Sex	Consumption; gr./day	Prevalence rate (%) (extreme parameters only)	
					Daily	<1 time per month or never
RLMS *, >10 000	Round 6, 1995	1	M	27.7	2.3	32.8
			F	3.6	0.3	56.5
	Round 11, 2002	2	M	27.4	3.3	30.5
			F	4.9	0.5	51.2
Simpura et al., 1997; Moscow, >900, 1994		3	M	Per capita	1.0	74
			F		–	
Bobak et al., 1999 *, >1500, 1996		4	M	Single dose	–	29
			F			71
Malyutina et al., 2001; Novosibirsk, >4500	1985–1986	5	M	17.4	–	
			F	4.4		
	1994–1995	6	M	26.3		
			F	5.9		
Malyutina et al., 2002, >6300, 1984–95		7	M	Single dose	–	12
Laatkainen et al., 2002, Karelia, >1500	1992	8	M	6.2	–	
			F	1.0		
	1997	9	M	10.1		
			F	1.3		
Bobak et al., 2003*, >2000, 2001		10	M	–	–	41
			F			83
Bobak et al., 2004, >900, 1999–2000		11	M	12.9	5.0	14
			F	1.6	0.6	26
Zaigraev, 2004b, Villages in 3 provinces, >200, 2001		12	M	85.5	65.0	0
			F	35.1	23.0	0
NOBUS, 2003*, >100 000, 2003, vodka only		13	M	–	3.1	29.8
			F		0.4	47.3
FOM, www.fom.ru, Moscow, 1500, 2002		14	M	Per capita	6.0	12
			F		0.0	20
CINDI, 2000–2001, >1600, Moscow (Frequency for spirits only)		15	M	Per capita	1 time per 6.5 days	
			F		1 time per 40 days	
ROMIR-monitoring*, 2004, 1600		16	M	–	3.6	31.9
			F		0.2	67.3

Sampling of the Russian population

The results from many surveys of the population on alcohol consumption are summarized in Table 10, which shows the quantity of consumed alcohol and the extent of frequency for drinking by men and women.

Creating this table was quite difficult because of the variety in the frequencies of consumption and in their quantitative characteristics. This necessitated the recalculation of the results of various authors into a single quantitative form. The data of the majority of authors, expressed in grams of pure alcohol per week (Table 10) have been recalculated into liters per capita per year, and are represented in Fig. 2-6. It was also necessary to take into account the difference in starting ages (which ranged from 16 to 35 years) used by different surveys.

Fig. 2-6: Figures from various authors on alcohol consumption, based on surveys (RLMS – Russian Longitudinal Monitoring Survey, FOM – Public Opinion Foundation, CINDI – Countrywide Integrated Noncommunicable Disease Intervention).

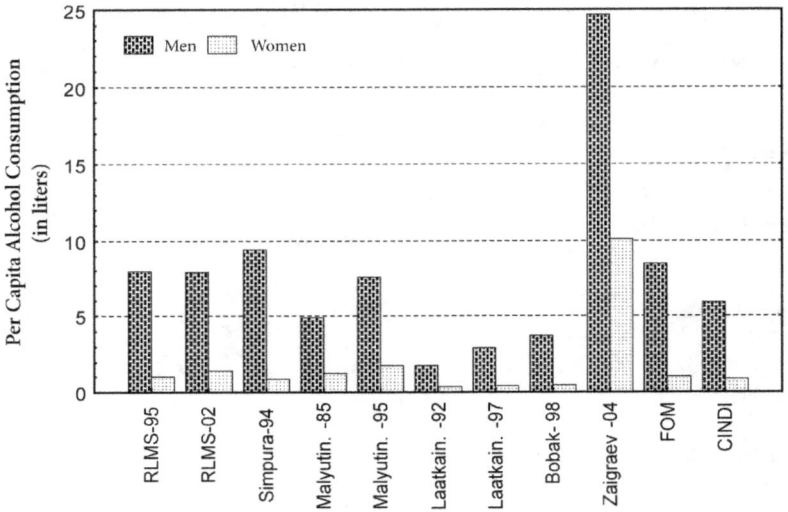

With all of this taken into account, the average per capita consumption found in various studies showed a spread from 1.1 (Laatkainen et al., 2002) to 16 liters of pure alcohol (Zaigraev, 2004b; Fig. 2-6). The remaining measures varied, from 2.1 to 6.5 liters, i.e., they were, as a rule, lower than the very incomplete data of the State Statistical Committee of the Russian Federation. They were also lower or even much lower than indexes of alcohol consumption for most of the countries of Europe and America (Chapter 1-2).

Similarly, the indexes for the frequency of drinking are also of doubtful standing, as the differences in frequencies reported by respondents in various studies are very large. Thus, the share of men reporting a frequency of drinking sprees of less than once a month or never varied from 0 percent (Zaigraev, 2004b) to 81 percent (Simpura et al., 1997). It was much the same for women: from 0 percent (Zaigraev, 2004b) to 83 percent (Bobak et al., 2003).

Two survey-based studies are of great interest because of the particulars of their methodologies. In the first (Laatkainen et al., 2002), the data on self-estimates of consumption were, for the first time, placed in conjunction with the biochemical markers of alcohol consumption for the same person – residents of Finland and Russian Karelia in 1997. The results from surveys conducted in the two regions showed that the consumption of alcohol was identical. But this was not borne out by the biochemical studies. The levels of the markers were 10 percent higher for Finnish men and 9 percent higher for Finnish women, which is in accord with average European data. The Russian indexes were much higher than the European: by 37 percent and 18 percent, respectively. At the individual level, the information given by Russian respondents about their consumption did not at all agree with the results found in the biochemical studies. Laatkainen et al. (2002) concluded, as had Simpura et al. (1997), that it was difficult to judge consumption in Russia on the basis of self-estimates. The same group of researchers in another work (Laatkainen et al., 2002) was more categorical, writing: "self-reports on alcohol consumption in Russia are extremely unreliable".

The second study (Zaigraev, 2004b) was conducted in rural areas of three typical regions: Voronezh, Nizhny Novgorod and Omsk (February-May 2001). Unlike all the other surveys, which were based on single conversations (for the RLMS, it was once a year), this survey was conducted over the course of 32 days in a four-month span. Each researcher was responsible for observing five families in one village. The researchers then completed forms on the daily quantities and types of alcoholic beverages drunk.

The methodological thoroughness of the study led, for the first time in a population survey, to deriving measures of the actual consumption of alcohol (16 liters per capita per year) that were close to other independent estimates (Nemtsov, 2000) obtained by means other than surveys. In addition to the high level of consumption, the work also revealed that in rural areas the consumption of samogon far outweighs that of vodka (4.8:1), that women consume only two fifths the amount alcohol men do and that among the respondents, who ranged from 16 to 102 years of age, there was not a single teetotaler! The work by Zaigraev (2004b) contains much other interesting information about alcohol consumption in Russia. And it is the only work which shows that reliable information on alcohol consumption can be obtained in Russia when using surveys. Nor was it necessary to use large numbers of respondents, as was done in the other studies, which have used from 900 to 10,000 individuals.

Carlson (2001) studied yet another large sample, when he conducted a health survey of 1,009 residents of Taganrog in 1993–1994 and in 1998. Respondents linked their poor physical condition primarily with the economic difficulties of the period of transition but not with drinking. And it is difficult to disagree, since this is the way the respondents did think. However, Carlson provided no proof that people's psychological perceptions are entirely reliable about the realities of their lives. He unqualifiedly accepts the psychological as the social.

Carlson (2001), relying on his earlier work, undertaken in 1993 (Carlson & Vågerö, 1998), became yet another critic of the "pioneering" work of Leon et al. (1997). He maintained that Leon et al. devoted too much attention to the alcohol-specific causes of the extremely high mortality in Russia at the expense of the socio-economic and psychological consequences of "Russia's transition" from socialism to capitalism.

In passing, one should note that other Western researchers (for example, McKee & Leon, 2005) also saw something of heightened interest in the social transition. Some investigators attributed to it almost exclusively the collapse of the value structure (Durkheim's anomie), the negative health situation and the mortality crisis. One might be mistaken in thinking that all had been well in these spheres before 1985! Such a bias in scholarly perspectives can be explained by the fact that foreign specialists gained access to Russia to conduct their own research only after 1988–1989; what they saw stunned them, but they had no materials with which to compare it to the preceding period, nor were there any such in the arsenal of Soviet science. The collapse of the USSR and the change in the political system had great significance for the inclination of scholarly investigators to focus on the social aspects of life in Russia. These changes could not but affect the social life of Russia. But proof is required if one is to assert that the changes had a relation not only to life but to mortality.

Returning to Carlson's work (2001), it should be noted that it repeats the errors of other works that are based on surveys of Russians. Using RLMS data on alcohol consumption in Russia, the author considered high consumption to be 0.5 liters of vodka a week. That would make the defining daily dose 70 grams of vodka. Thus all the extensive detail of this work in its section on consumption of alcohol breaks down. Those who live in Russia would disagree with the idea that 70–80 grams of vodka a day constitutes a large dose ("high consumption of alcohol", according to Carlson). Yet, according to Carlson's data, this tiny dose, in Russian eyes, was consumed by only by 29 percent of men and 2.5 percent of women in 1993–1994 and by 14 percent and 1 percent, respectively in 1998. It is hard to imagine how such moderate intake might lead to serious consequences.

The situation is better in those instances where surveys of those close to the respondents are used to check their information. Thus, for example, Williams et al. (2001) checked information obtained from school pupils with their parents. Moreover, the authors were interested less in alcohol consumption than in how Moscow schoolchildren were assimilating an anti-alcohol educational program that had been developed in Minnesota (U.S.). After three years of work, involving 1,212 fifth-grade pupils from 20 Moscow schools, the authors noted the pupils' high level of participation in the program and substantial gains in their knowledge of alcohol problems. In addition, the authors also highlighted an important circumstance: Russian schoolchildren begin to use alcohol earlier than their Americans counterparts and, unlike the situation in the U.S., there is inadequate resistance to this use on the part of parents and schools.

Elgarov and Elgarova (1994) came to similar conclusions earlier, finding that the reason for early and frequent use of spirits by Russian schoolchildren (594 individuals in the city of Nalchik were studied) was their extremely limited knowledge about the harmful effects of alcohol on the body and the widespread nature of drunkenness among adults.

Another example of the successful use of population surveys is a cycle of works by researchers led by Debora Hasin (1999, Rahav et al., 1999). The investigators were not interested in absolute doses but in the relative indexes of consumption for three groups in the population of Israel, two made up of immigrants from Russia who had settled in the country before and after 1989 and a third made up of "other" Israelis, without a connection to Russia. The three groups were equivalent in age, gender distribution and level of education, differing only in their level of religious belief – arrivals in Israel after 1989 were less religious.

The work was premised on the large difference in alcohol consumption between Israel and Russia. It transpired that the "new" immigrants drank more often, in larger quantities and got drunk more often than the "old" immigrants and the "other" Israelis. The authors attributed the difference between the two Russian groups to the "old" immigrants having "grown into the culture" and had assimilated the lifestyle of those around them, while the "new" immigrants had not yet succeeded in doing so. Hasin et al.'s conclusions are very important; they again show the significance of the social environment for drunkenness and the possibility of non-physically-punitive pressure on drinkers resulting in lowering their consumption.

Cockerham et al. (2002), using the data from the 1999 RLMS survey broached an interesting topic. The authors wished to learn about respondents' attitudes toward their own health and, specifically, toward their own consumption of alcohol and how that depended on their attitude toward socialist ideology ("pro-socialists" and "anti-socialists", i.e. those who would like to return to the socialism of the pre-Gorbachev period, and those who were favorably inclined to the changes and hoped for substantive political and economic reforms). Comparison of these two groups found that among drinkers the "pro-socialists" were 1.5 times more likely to be frequent drinkers than the "anti-socialists". The typical "pro-socialist" was an elderly man who drank heavily often. In terms of level of education, income, employment and family situation, the groups did not differ from each other.

In connection with the low self-estimates of alcohol consumption in the RLMS studies, the question may arise, were the "pro-socialists" exactly as far off in their answers as the "anti-socialists"? It is entirely possible that the "anti-socialists," being more oriented toward the future, have other value standards beyond the political. As a result there might be an actual lowering of consumption or an elevated "filtering" of what was said about consumption.

The data presented by the authors on their comparison of the two groups of respondents in terms of their attitude toward their own health offer clearer results. The "pro-socialists" evinced less interest in this aspect of their lives than did the "anti-socialists". And this seems to be in line with the greater frequency of alcohol consumption by the "pro-socialists". However, it is important to note that both groups were equally poor when it came to living healthy lives. Moreover, this group of questions can be rated the most neutral, and on them no difference appears between the two groups of respondents. In this connection, one may speculate that the difference found in the answers to other questions reflected not an essential difference but only the mind-sets of the two groups.

As distinct from the RLMS and the authors who followed in its wake, every time surveys about alcohol consumption approached the subject obliquely the results were more productive. Korolenko and Kensin (2001) focused less on alcohol behavior than on the psychological difficulties of residents who had recently come to live in the North. These people often feel uncomfortable, experience difficulties in socializing, despondency or depression. Questions on these topics made it easier for these respondents to go on to discuss their alcohol problems, as did the fact that the investigators were seeking a qualitative description of these problems. They demonstrated that alcohol consumption was a typical means of overcoming psychological difficulties and led to the rapid development of psychological dependence on the part of the new arrivals.

On the other hand, direct questions about consumption guarantee that the investigators will get paradoxical results. Thus, Palosuo (2000) conducted a survey of residents of Moscow and Helsinki in 1991 regarding their alcohol behavior. In this instance, the residents of the Finnish capital offered information about their serious consumption of alcohol significantly more often than did the residents of the capital of Russia. Taking into account that estimates of alcohol consumption in Moscow are much higher (Nemtsov, 1998a) than in Helsinki (Simpura et al., 1997), Palosuo's (2000) results mostly pertain to the fact that Muscovites are less open and frank and substantially reduced the dimensions of their own alcoholization.

The work of P. P. Ogurtsov (2002) also belongs among works based on population surveys. It showed that only one-third of patients entering hospitals in connection with somatic alcohol pathology admitted to abusing alcohol. Sometimes denials of abuse were made by patients transferred because of somatic complications to therapeutic wards from narcological hospitals where they had been treated for alcoholism. This work shows, better than others, the "specific difficulties of surveys of women and men in Russia" (Simpura et al., 1997).

It follows that most of the works based on population surveys asking about alcohol consumption tell us less about consumption than, indirectly, about the psychology of "Homo Soveticus". At the same time, there are significantly more works based on surveys than on other kinds of data collection. However, almost all of the authors mentioned so far have failed to take into account issues surrounding the reliability and validity of their surveys. There reliability, or lack there of, is evidenced by the fact that principles relating to the grading of the "quantity" or "frequency" scales of consumption are hardly ever mentioned. Yet it is well known that the distribution of consumers by consumption is distinctly asymmetrical, with a shift of the maximum in the direction of relatively small differences (Skog, 1985b). This is the source of the great inconsistency in classification among different authors (Table 10).

Studies of alcohol consumption in Russia have never raised and thus never resolved the problem of internal validity, i.e., the issue of the agreement of the survey results with the task in hand. Insofar as this applies to works already mentioned, it means that two questions have been left unresolved: the degree to which the answers of respondents accord with actual consumption and what besides consumption do their answers reflect. It is most likely that the results of the majority of such surveys reflect not only and, perhaps, not so much the dimensions of consumption as the attitude of respondents to the survey itself and to the interviewers, as well as the mind-set of their society towards the consumption of alcoholic drinks and so on. Almost all of the authors mentioned above ignored the question of how to distinguish these essentially psychological constituents of the situation. A number of Finnish authors (Simpura et al., 1997, Laatikainen et al., 2002) have expressed serious doubts about the reliability of the results obtained from surveys conducted in Russia. Remarkably, these authors are cited by many investigators but only in connection with confirming their own conclusions about the relatively low level of alcohol consumption in Russia.

After what has been said about the methodology of these adult surveys of Russians, it is difficult to judge the value of the quantitative findings from the many studies conducted on the alcohol consumption of Russian adolescents. Here, as distinct from the situation with adults, one lacks such basic data as the average alcohol consumption for the country as a whole, or quantitative measures of the consequences of alcohol abuse. One can only hypothesize that adolescents are less encumbered with preconceptions than adults and thus give more accurate information about themselves, although it is impossible to exclude the possibility that adolescents' answers may be skewed by the special psychology of their transitional period of life or the circumstances surrounding the interview. Thus, for example, Koshkina and coauthors (2004) found that pupils interviewed on the street, when asked about alcohol consumption, gave positive answers 1.5 times more often than pupils interviewed in the school where the basic research was done. Possibly because of this, the measures of alcohol consumption for Moscow pupils did not differ from those for pupils in Western countries, unlike the findings of other researchers who used repeated surveys (Grechanaya & Romanova, 1997; Williams et al., 2001). There is yet another difficulty: Elgarov and Elgarova (1994) found that 20 percent of 4,500 pupils (in the city of Nalchik) had difficulty understanding the simple questions put to them on paper. This finding, made in connection with research on the topic of alcohol, is in accord with a broader study conducted by the Institute of Age Physiology (Bezrukikh, 2000). There it was shown that 27 percent of 15-year-old pupils in Russia are unable to interpret, retell or analyze what they have read. Critical remarks about this issue have been absent from other works on adolescents, although almost all of them were conducted in Moscow, where one might expect a higher level of development among pupils. However, not a single one of the Moscow-based studies indicates if there was any attempt to check the adolescents' understanding of the questions.

Very detailed work has been done beyond the limits of Moscow and St Petersburg. In 1991–1992 E. S. Skvortsova (1997) conducted an anonymous survey of 30,000 ninth- and tenth-grade students (15-17 years old) in 21 cities, including Arkhangelsk in the North-West and Khabarovsk in the Far East. The author found a very high level of widespread alcoholization: approximately 70 percent of adolescents said they drank alcoholic beverages at least episodically, and one-fifth of them said they did so twice or more per month. Alarmingly, half of the pupils inherited their drinking habits at home during family occasions. The alcoholization of adolescents was distributed substantially more widely than smoking (approximately 30 percent of boys and approximately 20 percent of girls) and drug use (approximately 2 percent of boys and 1 percent of girls). It is important to note that these forms of abuse are interrelated but that alcoholization not only predominates but is one of the factors leading to smoking and drug use. Unfortunately, the problem of the validation of results was not taken up even in this very large study.

* * *

It is easy to see why there is such an abundance of studies based on surveys – sociological studies of this type are relatively simple to execute and appeal to most of those studied. Moreover, they yield results quickly, especially when conducted without control groups or means of objectively checking self-estimates, trusting the respondents and taking no account of the particularities of their mind-sets. As a result, the facts stand "naked", unsupported by validation and isolated from competing approaches or from being juxtaposed with the results from works that go beyond the limitations of the sociological. Yet these results are then taken as facts and made part of the discourse of science. The majority of such works have not been justified by their achievements, and some of them are simply worthless in scientific terms. However, the general interest in Russian alcohol problems and the already well-worn path followed by Western sociology on Russian soil probably means that there will still be, for some time, more works based on "head-to-head" surveys of Russian citizens and the increasingly few "dry remainder".

Nothing of this kind can be said of the many works devoted to alcohol mortality in Russia, although they are, for the most part, based on indirect proofs. However, thanks to the intensive efforts of British, French, Finnish and Russian researchers and to the variety of their approaches and the accumulation of evidence, it may now be considered as proved that alcohol makes a substantial contribution to Russia's negative demographics and that, when taken in large doses, alcohol loses its cardio-protective potential and becomes cardio-pathological.

Several authors who have studied Russian mortality link its extremely high level with other factors besides alcohol: with poverty, the collapse of forms of thought hitherto taken for granted, with psychosocial tensions, with the effects of the radical reforms, inadequate nutrition, environmental pollution and poor medical services (all items mentioned after the colon are taken from scientific publications). What is characteristic, however, is that these causes, unlike alcohol, are regarded as being obvious. It is difficult entirely to exclude these factors, but declarative statements alone are insufficient in the contemporary world of science; evidence is needed. Among the other factors underpinning Russia's extreme mortality levels, smoking, which is a major contributor to mortality, has been better studied. It remains, however, to establish the hierarchy of the causes of Russia's super-high mortality and to find alcohol's place in this series, along with the other listed factors (all of them hypothetical except smoking).

Chapter 2-4
An estimate of actual alcohol consumption in Russia

By far the simplest and most general indicator of a country's alcohol situation is the quantity of alcohol consumed by the population per capita. However, for the period 1961–1968 in the USSR, a period of very rapid growth in the consumption of alcoholic beverages, data on production, per capita consumption and spending for alcohol were kept secret. Much other data connected to alcohol consumption were also classified. All foreign publications, including the large study by Treml (Alcohol in the USSR, 1982), were kept in closed sections of libraries (the so-called *spetskhran*) and not generally available. They did not become part of Soviet scientific discourse.

Not until 1987–1988 did the State Statistical Committee of the USSR and Russia again begin to publish current and past data on consumption of alcohol produced by state factories and industrial cooperatives (*promkooperatsya*). These data were denoted as "consumption of alcoholic beverages from state resources of the RSFSR [registered alcohol] as calculated on a per capita basis for the population". It became public knowledge that the index for 1958 was double that of 1950, that 1965 had tripled the 1950 level and that the index had continued to rise right up to 1979 (Table 1, Fig. 1-4). The period 1980–1984 and through the first half of 1985 can be seen as a period of stability in alcohol consumption in Russia (Table 1).

It should be noted that the official data of the USSR and Russia State Statistical Committee do not tell the whole story of alcohol consumption in the country. A significant portion of consumed alcohol was and still is made up of illegal (unregistered) alcohol, an accurate estimate of which has always presented great difficulties. As a task set by the party leadership beginning in 1980 (and kept under secrecy until 1988), Russian State Statistics began doing this on the basis of reviews of family budgets and higher than normal purchases of sugar – the key ingredient of samogon in Russia. In 1997 Treml offered an estimate of alcohol consumption in Russia for 1960–1993. According to him, actual consumption rose by almost 1.5 times between 1960 and 1980 (Table 1). The data of Treml and Russian State Statistics show that overall consumption in Russia at the beginning of the 1980s stood at 13–14 liters per capita per year. This is more than 30–37 percent higher than the figure for registered consumption. The data on illegal alcohol also reflect the fact of stabilization in overall consumption in the early 1980s.

As a result of the anti-alcohol campaign, which began on June 1, 1985, state sales of alcoholic beverages dropped in the course of 2.5 years (1985–1987) by 62.9 percent (registered alcohol; Table 1 and Fig. 2-7). Accordingly, the income portion of country's budget was sharply reduced. Along with the reduction in state sales of alcohol, there was a steep increase in the production of illegal samogon in the country. Toward the end of 1987, the Soviet leadership realized it had "gone too far", and from January 1, 1988, state sales of alcoholic beverages began to rise (Chapter 1-6).

Fig. 2-7: Indexes of alcohol consumption in Russia (1970–2003): RussStat (registered alcohol – 1 and unregistered alcohol – 2), Treml (1997) and Nemtsov (Chapter 2-4).

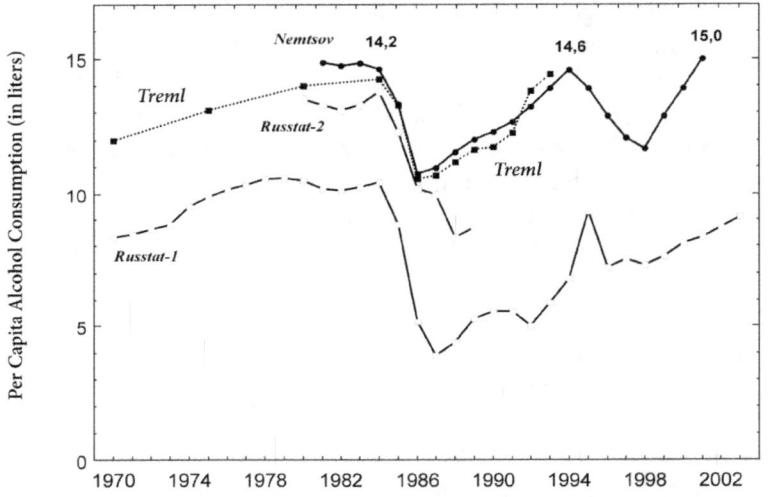

Even earlier, in late 1985–early 1986, purchases of sugar for the production of samogon began to rise. The increase was so significant that as early as late 1987 there were interruptions in supplies of sugar to the population that led to the "sugar panic" in the following year. The public began buying up large quantities of sugar and storing them at home. Thus, in Moscow in June 1988 sales of sugar were double sales of the preceding June (Chapter 1-6, Fig. 2-8). This made Russian State Statistics calculations of samogon production for 1988–1989 very inexact (Table 1 and Fig. 2-5). They were discontinued for this reason, beginning in 1990.

The anti-alcohol campaign may provisionally be considered to have ended in 1991. Market reforms went into effect as of January 1, 1992. With galloping inflation affecting prices on all commodities, the alcohol situation in Russia grew even tenser However, the prices of alcoholic beverages rose significantly slower

Fig. 2-8: Monthly sales of sugar in Moscow (1984–1988).

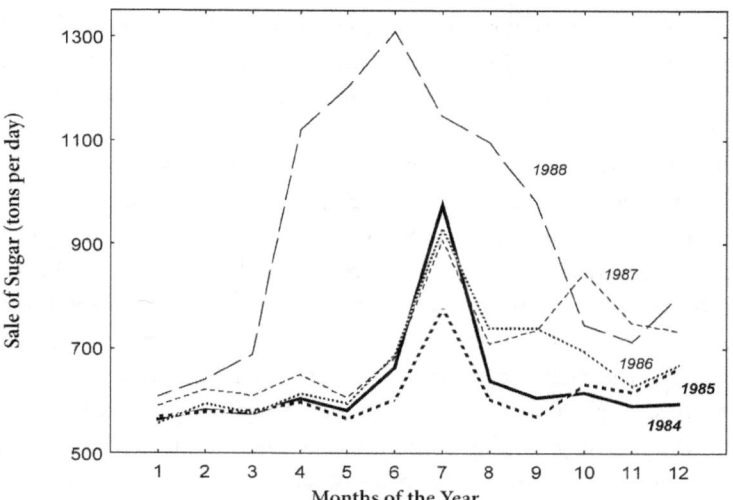

than other prices (Chapter 1-7, Fig. 1-8). This bifurcation in prices reflected the further criminalization of the alcohol market, manufacture of large quantities of cheap alcohol surrogate beverages and the non-payment of at least half of the taxes due on alcoholic beverages. The upshot was a new and sharp increase in consumption (Fig. 2-7).

In such circumstances, the estimate of actual consumption of alcohol, the principal indicator of a country's alcohol problems, was of great significance. However, because of the "sugar panic", Russian State Statistics' calculations of this index had stopped in 1990. Treml carried on his calculations up to 1993. Data based on numerous surveys of the population in the second half of the 1990s (Chapter 2-3; Table 10, Fig. 2-6) do not reflect actual consumption, except for the data compiled by Zaigraev for the single year 2002 (Zaigraev, 2004b).

But all this became known quite late. The data on actual consumption of alcohol as calculated by Russian State Statistics were declassified in 1988 and became available in 1990, Treml's figures were published in 1997 and the survey data in the late 1990s. The absence of any kind of estimate at the start of the campaign, or even information about their existence, made it necessary for me to work out my own method of defining the actual consumption of alcohol.

Today there are many estimates of consumption. However, solution of the problem depends on estimates. One more method for providing an estimate can only be helpful: the similarity of estimates reached independently by different methods is the sole way of verifying them.

Work on the method began in 1986–1987. The idea for it arose during the study of non-alcohol dependent medical and demographic phenomena in Moscow. Detailed explanation of the method of calculating alcohol consumption in Moscow and Russia is given in a series of articles (Nemtsov, 1992a, 1992b, 1995, 1997, 1998b, 2000). This chapter offers only the premises that underlie the calculations and a revised diagram of the overall method, while the time period covered by the analysis is enlarged and the results and some commentary about them are presented.

As a result of the processes, described in detail in Chapters 1-4, 1-5 and 1-6, the start of the anti-alcohol campaign saw the emergence in Moscow and in the country as a whole of almost experimental conditions, including a rapid and significant decline followed by a rapid return of alcohol-specific medical and demographic phenomena. This alternation of medical and demographic trends could be helpful in arriving at the actual level of consumption. For consumption of alcohol as an etiological factor in these phenomena changed, beginning in 1985, significantly more strongly and more rapidly than many other possible factors.

The task for the first stage of the research was to develop an estimate of actual alcohol consumption in Moscow on the basis of data on sales of alcoholic beverages and sugar. The task for the second stage was to pinpoint the medical and/or demographic phenomena that most dynamically respond to changes in alcohol consumption and thus reflect the level of alcohol consumption. However, after 1986, the chaos of the market reforms made it impossible to estimate actual consumption on the basis of statistics on trade. As a result, the task of the third stage was to define the actual level of alcohol consumption in Moscow on the basis of selected alcohol-related changes. Finally, the fourth stage was to take the patterns discovered for Moscow and apply them to the country as a whole.

Moscow was selected as the target area, most of all, because this is where the author and his coauthor, Dr Nechaev, were living. This is not as laughable as at first appears. One should not forget that the indexes connected to alcohol consumption were still classified as secret when our work began. In those circumstances, it took great effort to compile the needed data on sales of alcoholic beverages and sugar and, even more, data on mortality. It was very fortunate that Dr Nechaev was then on the staff of Moscow's emergency medical service. This organization had data on the number of persons suffering from alcohol psychoses who the emergency service hospitalized each day. These persons constituted 59.4 percent of all such hospitalizations in Moscow (Nemtsov & Nechaev, 1996; the others entered hospital from the dispensaries). By chance, it had not occurred to anyone to classify this valuable information, although the analogous summary data for the country and regions was classified as secret.

It was extremely important that the population of Moscow constituted a very large sample (more than 8 million people at the time). It was important, too, that Moscow record-keeping was better than record-keeping in many other regions of Russia. Moreover, Moscow's status as the capital city meant that agencies of the Interior Ministry were more active there. This made it impossible, before and during the anti-alcohol campaign, to bring into the city any large quantities of samogon. Some must be allowed for, but it can be assumed that the traffic in samogon went both ways.

During the anti-alcohol campaign, various base products were used for samogon production, including, for example, tomato juice. These were, however, mere novelties; for a large city like Moscow, the principal base ingredient of samogon could only have been sugar. Sugar sales were well documented by state trading organizations, as were state sales of alcoholic beverages. Of the latter, state sales of spirits in Moscow were higher on the eve of the campaign (11.3 liters for 1984) than in other regions of the country (9.3 liters for the Moscow region, an average of 10.5 liters for the country). This allows one to assume a relatively low level of samogon consumption in Moscow.

As the chief alcohol-specific consequences to be used as measures, those most tightly linked to consumption were chosen: incidence of alcohol psychoses, deaths from cirrhosis of the liver and pancreatitis and deaths from external causes, including alcohol poisoning and poisoning from other substances, automobile accidents, homicides, suicides, falls from heights, drowning and many others. It was important for the research that the Moscow Bureau of Judicial Expertise collected information on the presence or absence of alcohol in the blood of those whose deaths had external causes.

It has earlier been shown that the alcohol psychoses demonstrate a tight connection with consumption when consumption is abruptly decreased (data from Nielsen, 1965), but a less clearly defined dependence when consumption rises, as in Poland (a linear relationship, Wald & Jaroszewski, 1983, and a square relationship, Jaroszewski et al., 1989). The difference found in the two latter works may be because consumption of samogon was not taken into account, although samogon consumption in Poland is very high.

As for violent deaths, Skog (1986) has shown that intoxication with alcohol plays a significant role in them. The link between alcohol consumption and cirrhosis of the liver was studied earlier and in more detail than the other chosen indicators (Schmidt, 1977; Whitlock, 1974). In particular, a lag was demonstrated between mortality from this disease and consumption changes (Skog, 1980, 1984, 1985b). In the period since these basic epidemiological studies of mortality and cirrhosis of the liver were conducted, ideas about the etiological role of alcohol in this disease have changed substantially. The viral nature of an overwhelming number of the forms of hepatitis that are precursors of cirrhosis has been established (Nalpas et al., 1998; Pessione et al., 1998). Alcohol is now generally accorded a pathogenetic role, although the role remains very important: alcohol acts as a factor in the dissemination of the viruses of the liver parenchyma (Ohta et al., 1988).

The anti-alcohol campaign of 1985, for all its humanitarian and other ugliness, created unique opportunities for scientific inquiries into alcohol problems.

It made it possible to simultaneously track the sharp changes in the dynamics of these chosen indicators and come to a quantitative estimate of actual alcohol consumption, including unregistered alcohol, for Moscow and for Russia as a whole.

Most of the medical statistical data used in this work are expressed in annual terms, as is the sale of alcohol. Unlike for the indicators of medical phenomena, which are largely of the year in which they turn up on a register, alcoholic beverages may be purchased in one year and used in the next. However, the Russian tradition of alcohol consumption virtually excludes the possibility of any substantial delay from the time of purchase of spirits and their being downed, and even less chance of significant reserves of alcoholic beverages accumulating from one year to the next. It is conceivable that the sole exceptions to this are the New Year holidays. However, monthly data on sales of spirits in Moscow before the anti-alcohol campaign show purchases rising from January through April, falling in the summer months (the low point is July), followed by another increase that begins in August and reaches its peak in December. The immediately following January, in both 1984 and 1985, showed a steep drop in purchases of spirits (Fig. 2-9). The same pattern repeated itself just after the campaign (1989–1990). In other words, the increase in sales that climaxes in December is a five-month trend, possibly related to weather, but not in order to accumulate supplies for the New Year holiday. If we take incidence of the alcohol psychoses as indicator of consumption, the indicator reaches its maximum on Jan. 5, 6 or 7 of the next year, after which a decline sets in (Fig. 2-10). This gives us a basis for asserting that, in Moscow and probably the rest of the country, the level of purchases of alcoholic beverages through the year reflects their consumption.

We can now proceed to how the alcohol situation in Moscow developed before and during the anti-alcohol campaign. Over the course of the decade preceding the campaign (1975–1984), state sales of spirits fluctuated insignificantly – from 12 liters of pure alcohol per capita per year (1975) to 12.5 liters (1979 and 1980) and 11.3 liters in 1984.

A sharp decline in state sales of alcoholic beverages began in June 1985 (Fig. 2-9). Sales in August of that same year were at 64.2 percent of sales for August 1984. Thereafter the rate of decrease slowed. Beginning with 1988, increased state sales of alcohol took place in Moscow and the country as a whole (Fig. 2-7), an increase that continued through 1989, for which year the level of state sales stood at 77.1 percent of the 1984 level.

Sales of registered alcohol again declined in 1990–1991. Several causes explain the decline. Until 1992, there was a shortage of packing materials because the factories producing them had been reoriented to other work at the start of the anti-alcohol campaign. In addition, significant quantities of state-manufactured beverages had been stolen and thus were "lost" as far as official statistics were concerned. Trucks and rail cars loaded with vodka products were not reaching their destinations and were therefore not counted as sold.

As a result of the market reforms, beginning in 1992 the trade in spirits moved into private hands, and these entrepreneurs often concealed the actual size of their sales in order to reduce their tax payments. These problems led Russian State Statistics to stop calculations of registered alcohol, and move instead to estimating "volume of sales", thus supposedly taking into account sales of illegal alcoholic beverages.

Fig. 2-9: Monthly sales of alcoholic beverages in liters of pure alcohol (Moscow, 1984–1987; RussStat).

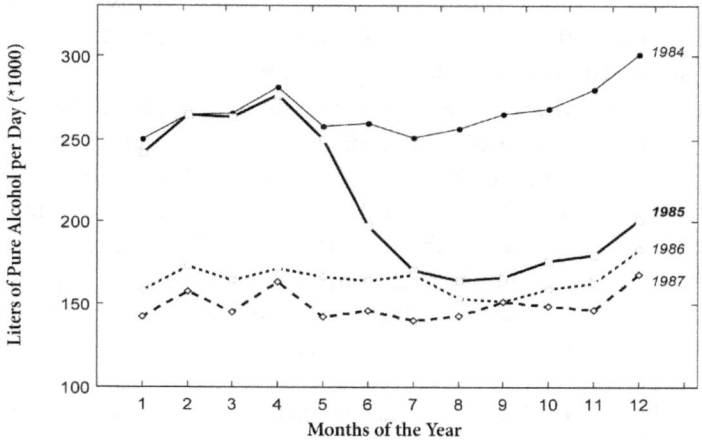

Fig. 2-10: Number of patients admitted per day with alcohol psychoses by Moscow emergency services from December 20, 1983 until January 14, 1984.

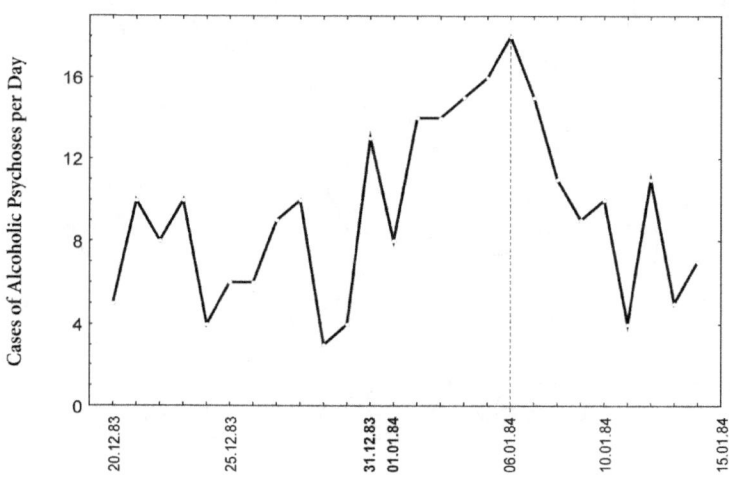

How did the alcohol-specific effects on health fare during this time? In 1976 a medically based narcological service was established in the USSR. Its efforts brought the incidence of alcohol psychosis in Moscow down from 112.4 (1976) to 86.6 per 100,000 of population in 1982, after which the rate remained stable (86.6 in 1984). Creation of the narcological service had no effect on mortalities from cirrhosis of the liver, which in 1981–1984 stood at 10.6–11.3 per 100,000. The level of deaths from external causes was very high into the early 1970s and continued a slow rise for the remainder of the decade. The indicator did not reach stability until the early 1980s (82.8 per 100,000 in 1984).

After the start of the campaign, all these indicators showed significant declines in 1985–1986 (Fig. 2-11). The largest was for alcohol psychoses (63.3 percent), and the least for deaths from external causes (32.5 percent). According to the data for Moscow, deaths of the latter type where the victim was found to have alcohol in their blood fell by 50.9 percent, while comparable deaths for sober individuals fell by 11.1 percent, as compared with the figures for 1984. Moreover, the decline in the latter index in 1985–1986 continued the trend of the preceding period (1981–1984, Fig. 2-12). In other words, the dynamic of mortality among sober individuals at the start of the anti-alcohol campaign did not change at the start of the campaign, as compared with the previous period, unlike the dynamic for those who died while intoxicated and thus accounted for the overall decline in mortalities from external causes.

Fig. 2-11: Mortality due to external causes (3) and cirrhosis of the liver (2) and morbidity by alcohol psychoses (1) (1980–2002).

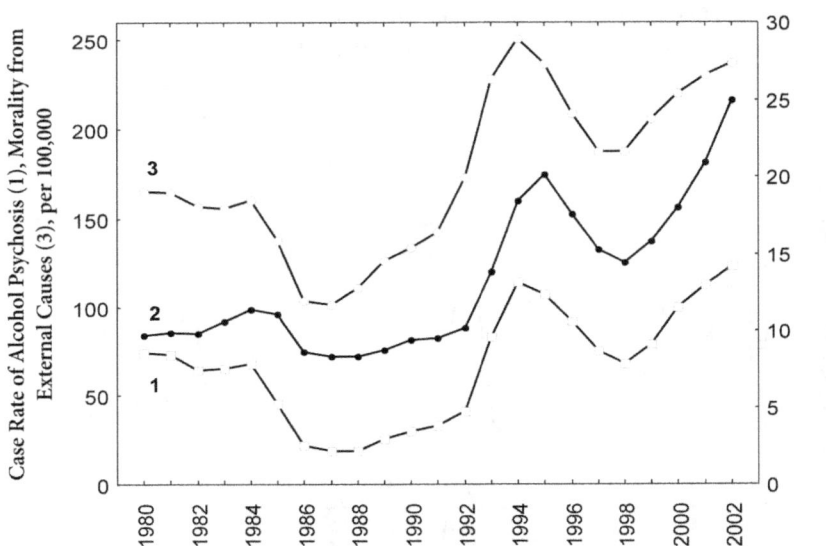

It is important to note that, after 1986, changes in the alcohol-specific phenomena were complicated. In Moscow overall deaths from external causes began to rise earlier than the other indicators (by 3.9 percent in 1987) due to an increase of 13.7 percent of deaths with alcohol found in the blood of the victims (excluding alcohol poisonings; Fig. 2-12). The change in deaths from external causes of sober individuals was insignificant. The number of alcohol poisonings continued to decline in 1987 and only began to rise again in 1988. That same year saw an increase in deaths connected to cirrhosis of the liver (by 23.4 percent) and incidence of alcohol psychoses (by 24.4 percent). In 1990–1991 almost all the indicators stabilized. The indicators for the whole country followed the same pattern as in Moscow (Fig. 2-11).

Fig. 2-12: Mortality by external causes (Moscow). Sober individuals (1), with alcohol in the blood (2), alcohol poisoning (3). Squares represent significant differences from relevant regressions (1981–1984).

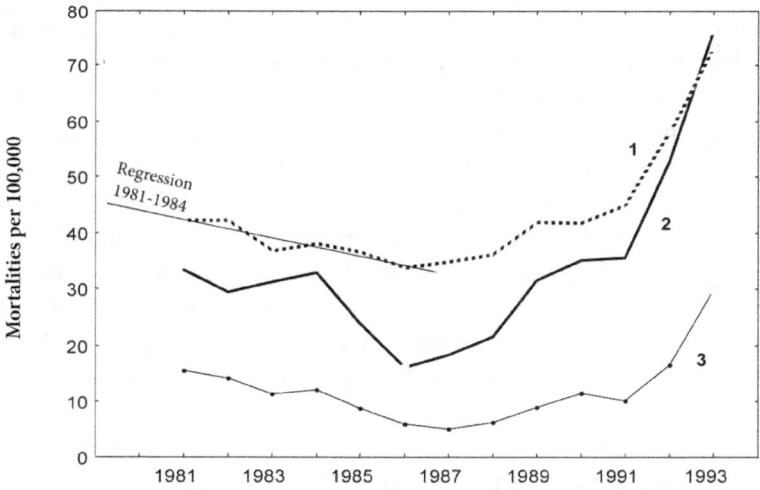

The events described in the preceding paragraph are essential to understanding the essence of the new method, which allows us to select measures on the basis of which it is possible to project an estimate of consumption. Here, then, we must take a hard look at what was occurring in these alcohol-specific areas after 1986. Obviously, 1987–1989 was a turning point for all of them; their previous declines were replaced in these years by inclines, thus signaling the start of an increase in alcohol consumption. The indicator, among those studied, that first began to rise however was deaths from external causes with alcohol found in the victim's blood and excluding cases of alcohol poisoning (Fig. 2-12). This tells us that this type of death has no lag in relation to alcohol consumption. Skog had described this earlier (1986). Thus, the level of this sort of death may be considered more sensitive to changes in consumption. That is why it works as the principal indicator of the level of alcohol consumption. The other alcohol-specific measures all appeared staggered in comparison with externally caused deaths and thus lag in relation to the onset of increased consumption.

Figure 2-11 shows there is a yearlong lag in the overall measures of Russian mortalities from external causes, behind the index of Moscow (Fig. 2-10). This is explained by the fact that it is impossible to distinguish between deaths of sober individuals and deaths of those with alcohol in their blood. The data from 25 regional Bureaus of Judicial-Medical Expertise is presented further on in the text. These data make distinctions between sober and intoxicated individuals, and are in line with the Moscow data.

1987 was a turning point as well for a whole series of non-medical phenomena. At the start of the campaign, as a result of steps taken against underground production of alcoholic beverages, a sharp increase took place in the number of individuals facing criminal charges for violations of the anti-alcohol laws – the numbers were up by 5 and 13 times, respectively, for 1985 and 1986 as compared with 1984. In 1987 this number declined by 37.4 percent from the number for 1986 and again dropped, this time, by 96.8 percent in 1988. This means that in 1987 there began a relaxation of anti-alcohol pressures and thus an opening of the floodgates of samogon distilling and, with it, a rise in alcohol consumption.

After this digression, we may now move on. With the onset of the market reforms of 1992, all the alcohol-specific measures began rising quickly, but deaths from external causes rose especially fast and with no lag (Fig. 2-11). Moreover, for Moscow, the increase in this kind of mortality with intoxication rose faster than for such deaths for sober individuals (for 1992–1993, the differences in increases were 57.5 percent and 31.4 percent a year on average; Fig. 2-12). This period of time also witnessed a steep increase in fatal alcohol poisonings (by 196 percent for the two years).

Unfortunately, in Moscow in 1995 due to errors in record keeping, there was a significant undercount (by 38 percent) of deaths from external causes of persons with alcohol in their blood, as a result of which the number of such deaths for sober individuals was inflated (by 45 percent). At the same time, the total number of such deaths changed by only 1.5 percent from the previous year. The next year saw a return in numbers for both intoxicated and sober mortalities to the original (higher) levels. This is why 1994 is used as the standard for calculations of alcohol consumption in Moscow.

Most important about the new method is the estimate of unregistered alcohol, which in combination with state sales of alcohol yields a good idea of actual consumption. For the estimate of unregistered alcohol, it is important to know about sales of sugar, one of the main materials necessary for the production of samogon in Russia and particularly in big-city environments, before and after the start of the anti-alcohol campaign. In 1984 (Fig. 2-8) as in 1983, there was a slight increase in sugar sales from January through to May, with some small deviations in the trend. A rather steep increase in sales took place in June (by 14 percent) and then, even more steeply, in July (by 45 percent), increases linked to the seasonal harvesting and treatment of berries and fruit. Beginning in August, sales declined, continuing steadily back to the starting level in December (Fig. 2-8).

A similar pattern of changes in sugar sales was observed for January-May 1985. From June through to September 1985, sales of sugar dipped as compared to the same months of 1984 in reaction to the launching of the anti-alcohol campaign (June 1, 1985). However, as early as October 1985 sales exceeded the index for October 1984 and the rising trend continued through December. Sugar sales in 1986 and 1987 exceeded sales in 1984 by 5.4 percent and 10.8 percent, respectively. Shortages of sugar in stores began to be experienced at the very end of 1987 and continued into 1988, triggering a steep increase in sugar purchases (Fig. 2-8). This ruled out further calculations of such sales as a way to measure samogon production. Theretofore, however, it was possible to figure the quantity of samogon produced by the quantity of supplemental sales of sugar in 1983–1986.

The decline in sales of sugar in the period June–September 1985 may be looked at as a result of the pressure exerted by the anti-alcohol campaign insofar as one of the campaign's aims in 1985 was to cut down production of samogon. The quantity of sugar sold in July, when people ordinarily buy large amounts of sugar for pickling and preserving their garden crops, must be excluded from the calculations. The minimal sales of September 1985 can be understood as the amounts needed to meet the food norms for the city of Moscow (24.3 kilograms per person per year). This amount is close to the norm for the population of the whole country (24 kilos), not including the sugar eaten in other products (Nutrition Institute of the Academy of Medical Sciences of the USSR). Amounts of sugar sold exceeding these norms, it is assumed, were used for the production of samogon.

We know that 1 kilo of sugar yields 1.3 liters of 40 percent ABV samogon. On this basis, we calculate production of samogon in Moscow for 1983, 1984, 1985 and 1986 as, respectively, 0.6, 0.6, 1.1 and 1.4 liters per capita per year. Adding these quantities to state sales of alcohol in those years (11.2, 11.3, 8.9 and 7.0 liters), we derive an estimate of the actual consumption of alcohol in Moscow for 1983–1986: 11.8, 11.9, 10 and 8.4 liters of pure alcohol per capita per year (Fig. 2-13).

We now have estimates of actual alcohol consumption for these four years and indexes of deaths from external causes, separated for intoxicated and sober individuals (Fig. 2-14a). As is evident, the estimates of consumption agree quite well with the change of cause of death away from: external causes of persons with alcohol in their blood; even with only four points, their correlation (Kendall Tau) is equal to 1.0 ($p=0.042$). Naturally, a correlation of alcohol consumption and deaths of sober individuals is non-significant.

Fig. 2-13: Official figures on sales of alcohol in Moscow and Russia (1970–1993). Estimate of actual consumption and of unregistered alcohol in Moscow (1982–1993).

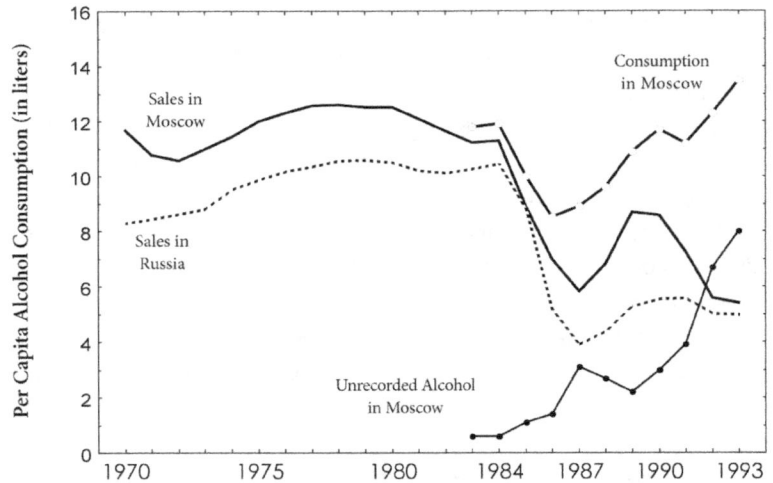

This result, first of all, makes evident that these estimates of consumption are meaningful and, secondly, they make it possible to express mathematically the level of deaths from external causes as a function of the level of consumption for 1983–1986. For construction of a regression model, one would prefer having more than four points (years), but the "sugar panic" made that wish impossible to realize. But it should be borne in mind as well that each of the points represents millions of liters of alcohol, hundreds of tons of sugar and thousands of human deaths. These considerations and the significance of the correlation make us think that four points are, at least, minimally sufficient.

Here it is appropriate to recall the three points made by Skog (1986). The first has already been mentioned: deaths from external causes, unlike other alcohol-specific changes, do not show a lag in relation to consumption. The second: between changes in consumption and deaths of this kind, there is a simultaneous link. The third and, at this place in our analysis, most important: among all the deaths of this type, the level of mortality among sober individuals reflects non-alcoholic factors of death that change from year to year. For example, in the case of automobile accidents, these factors are: the overall number of automobiles, the extent and quality of roads, weather conditions, the activity of the police service responsible for the roads and so on. Deaths linked to alcohol reflect both the non-alcoholic factors and factors conditioned by alcohol, adding them both, as it were. To represent the alcoholic factor in deaths ($x1$) in its "pure" form, i.e. without the non-alcoholic constituent, one can standardize (normalize) the number of deaths with alcohol in the blood ($n1$) by the number of deaths while sober ($n2$), assuming a relationship: $x1=n1/n2$.

One can with greater reason exclude deaths from alcohol poisoning (n3) from the number of deaths with alcohol in the blood (n1). This is because, first, these deaths cannot be standardized by analogous deaths of sober individuals (all other deaths from external causes may take place either while sober or intoxicated) and, second, the dynamic of deaths by alcohol poisoning after 1986 differs from the changes in other deaths from external causes with alcohol in the blood because of their lag (Fig. 2-12). Working from these assumptions, the alcohol factor in deaths from external causes (x2) is more precisely expressed in the relationship x2= (n1-n3)/n2.

This relationship is linked in linear fashion (directly proportional) with the estimate of actual alcohol consumption for 1983–1986 calculated above on the basis of the sum of state sales of alcohol and illegal alcohol (Fig. 2-14b).

The next important step in the formation of the method is correlation of the relation x2 for 1983–1986 with the indexes calculated above of actual consumption of alcohol in Moscow (y1) on the basis of equations of linear regression. The result is the equation y1=4.27 + 8.80 x2, but, for the population age 15 and older, the equation y2=5.08 + 10.97 x2.

For 1983–1986, we know both the left sides (y1 and y2, actual consumption of alcohol in Moscow) and right sides of these equations (x2), thanks to which we derive the constant terms (4.47 and 5.08) and the coefficients of the regression equation (8.80 and 10.97). For the following years, we know only the complex variables x2 (n1, n2 and n3), with which and with the help of equations y1 or y2 we can estimate actual consumption of alcohol after 1986. For 1987–1989, they are shown on Fig. 2-13. After subtracting the alcohol in state sales from the calculated alcohol consumption in Moscow, we have consumption of unregistered alcohol (Fig. 2-13).

These calculations can be checked by using areas where there is no consumption of unregistered alcohol and where there are data for the calculation of y1 and y2. Only one example has materialized. Haberman and Baden (1978) studied violent deaths in four areas of New York City and obtained data on the number of dead found to have alcohol in their blood and the number of dead sober individuals. Using these data and the formula y2, consumption of alcohol in New York came to 12.1 liters per capita per year. Data from the National Institute on Alcohol Abuse and Addiction show that in those years in the state of New York consumption stood at 2.91–2.89 gallons or 11 liters for persons 15 years old and up (U.S. Apparent Consumption, 1985). Such data for New York City are, unfortunately, not available.

The 10 percent difference between the actual and calculated consumption in New York may result from the geographical non-correspondence of the two figures (city versus state). Most likely, there is more drinking in New York City than in the rest of the state. With this in mind, the difference can be considered unsubstantial and the calculation by the formula, based on the relationship between

Fig. 2-14 (a/b): Deaths from external causes for sober individuals, individuals with alcohol in their blood (Fig. 2-14a) and their relationship with alcohol consumption (Fig. 2-14b) (Moscow, 1984–1986).

Fig. 2-14a

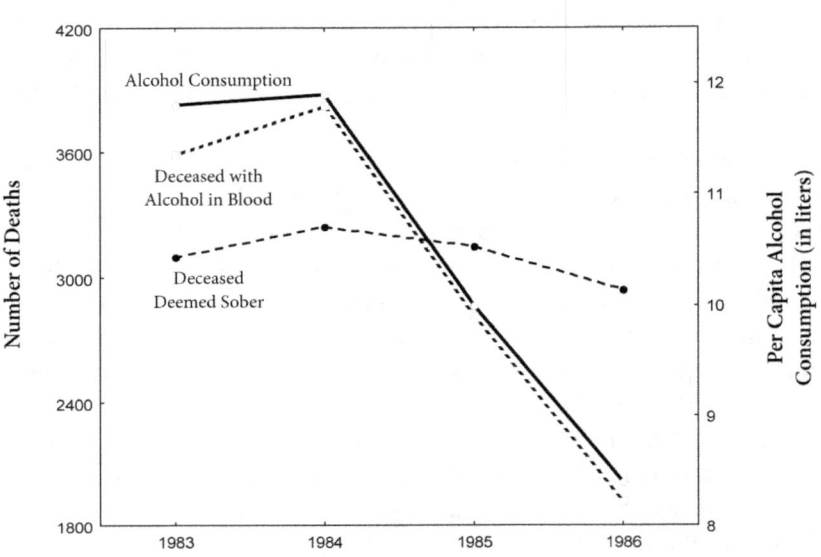

Fig. 2-14b

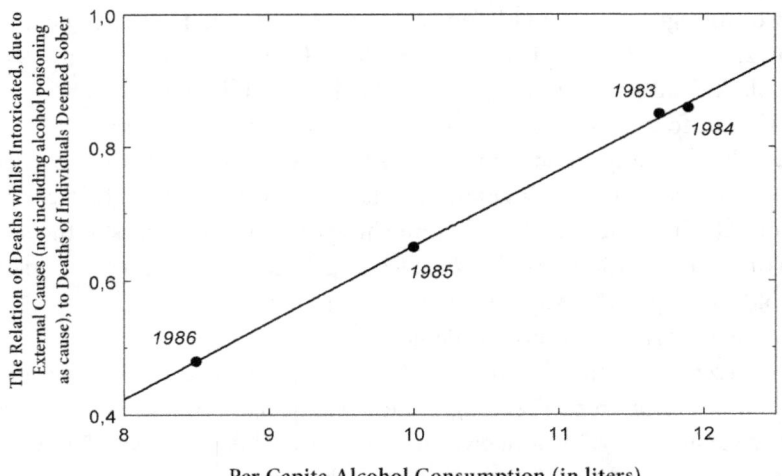

deaths from external causes in intoxicated and sober condition, applicable for estimating alcohol consumption in Russia .

But before turning to this, it must be noted that deaths from external causes in Russia are recorded in two kinds of medical documents. The first is the autopsy report, which lists all the pathologies present, a full diagnosis of the cause of death and information on the presence or absence of alcohol in the blood of the dead person. This is the basis for an information sheet on the death that serves as the main source for the official death statistics compiled by the State Statistical Committee of the Russian Federation. Unfortunately, the information sheet is required to show only the main causes of death and, specifically, need not include mention of accompanying intoxication. Moreover, the diagnosis of the cause of death in the information sheet may be deliberately tampered with to avoid unpleasant juridical, social or moral consequences, of which we have written earlier in connection with the work of Tishuk (1997). All this explains why the official statistics on deaths while intoxicated are obviously too low: 11.5 percent of the overall total of deaths from external causes. This 11.5 percent refers almost exclusively to deaths from alcohol poisoning, which constitute 84 percent of all deaths while intoxicated (1992; Table 11).

Table 11: Share of mortalities associated with alcohol (percentages based on figures from the Bureau of Forensic Medicine and RussStat).

Year	1984	1986	1990	1992	1994
Bureau of Forensic Medicine (25 regions)					
Alcohol in Blood (1)	59.3	47.3	52.3	57.3	62.7
Including alcohol poisoning (2)	13.2	9.0	9.5	14.1	18.7
(1) – (2)	46.1	38.3	42.8	43.2	44.0
RussStat					
Alcohol-related (3)	–	–	9.4	11.5	–
Including alcohol poisoning (4)	12.2	9.0	8.1	10.2	15.1
(3) – (4)	–	–	1.3	1.3	–

(–) data abs.

Because of the serious deficiencies of official statistics, data from the Bureaus of Judicial-Medical Expertise meant for internal use (autopsy reports) will be used as the basis for further work. These data are significantly different from the official statistics in that they show more deaths with alcohol in the blood of the dead (Table 11).

The discrepancy between the official and unofficial statistics as regards alcohol mortalities is striking (Table 11). Yet it is possible that the difference is actually even larger because the Bureaus of Judicial-Medical Expertise undercount a portion of deaths with alcohol in the blood. This can happen, for example, because of emergency room measures, taken before death occurs, that may remove alcohol from the body or because the body is found long after the occurrence of death. Other situations, too, can lead to undercounting the number of dead with alcohol in the blood (Chapter 2-3). In this regard, it is important to bear in mind that, as a result of the undercount, some alcohol deaths may be recorded as deaths of sober individuals. In this way, the size of x2 is reduced and, thus, the estimate of actual alcohol consumption. This is why the quantitative estimates of consumption in Russia by the new method should be understood as "not less than...."

These cautions noted, the autopsy reports are not subject to deliberate manipulation, that is, they remain in the archives of the Bureau of Judicial-Medical Expertise that conducted the examination of liquids in the corpse for the presence of alcohol. It is these documents, compiled as annual tables, which are the principal source for the calculations of alcohol consumption in Russia.

In 1991, when collecting data on deaths from external causes for the period 1981–1990, through the good offices of the Ministry of Health of the RSFSR, requests were sent to all 73 regional Bureaus of Judicial–Medical Expertise. They were asked for data on the overall number of deaths from external causes, including the number of deaths of persons in a drunken state and the number of deaths from alcohol poisoning. The same breakdown was asked for data on homicides, suicides and deaths as a result of road traffic accidents. Replies came from 39 regions. Refusals to give the needed information or very incomplete data came from nine regions (Vologda, Dagestan, Kaliningrad, Kirov, Krasnoyarsk, Stavropol, Tomsk, Tyumensk and the Chuvash ASSR).

For data to be selected for us, it was crucial that there be relative constancy in the basic indicators for 1981–1984. For both the Kaliningrad and Tula regions, significant year-to-year fluctuations of alcohol and non-alcohol mortalities were noted in years when the alcohol situation in the country was comparatively stable. This appeared as increases in alcohol deaths in tandem with fewer non-alcohol mortalities and the reverse, which, most likely, was the result of errors in the records. In Tambov region from 1981–1984 there was a very large increase in alcohol deaths, by 40 percent, with a 25 percent rise for sober individuals. In the Mari El Republic, there was a rise in violent deaths for sober individuals in 1984 of 22 percent. In the Udmurt Republic there was an unusual dominance of alcohol deaths over deaths of sober individuals (by 3.3 times in 1984). The data of these five regions were excluded from the research on the assumption of errors in the accounting of deaths with alcohol found in the blood of the dead or because of other anomalies.

The data from the remaining 25 regions (Table 12) are considered satisfactory. The regions are located geographically as follows: 6 regions of the former North-West Federal District, 7 regions of the Central Federal District, 1 region of the Southern Federal District, 3 regions of the Volga Federal District, 1 region of the Urals Federal District, 4 regions of the Siberian Federal District and 3 regions of the Far East Federal District. The population of the 25 regions in 1981 was 62.7 million, or 45.1 percent of the population of Russia. Registered alcohol in these districts and in Russia were analogous (Fig. 2-15). As is evident, the geographical extent of the areas under study is very large, registered alcohol is close to the indexes for the country as a whole, and the population makes up almost half the population of the country. This makes it possible to judge the researched areas as representative of the country.

Table 12: Regions from which data are used in the following text (+).

Regions	1981–1990	1991–1993	1994
Altai	+	+	+
Amur	+	+	+
Bashkortostan	+		
Yaroslavl	+	+	
Ivanovo	+	+	
Kaluga	+	+	+
Kareliya	+		+
Kemerovo	+	+	+
Khabarovsk	+	+	+
Kursk	+		
Leningrad	+	+	+
Moscow (city)	+	+	+
Moscow	+	+	+
Murmansk	+	+	
Novgorod	+	+	+
Novosibirsk	+		
Omsk	+		
Orel	+	+	+
Rostov	+	+	+
Ryazan	+	+	+
Samara	+	+	+
Saratov	+	+	+
Sakhalin	+		
St Petersburg (city)	+	+	+
Sverdlovsk	+	+	+
Total	25	19	17

In 1994 the same regional Bureaus were sent inquiries on deaths in the period 1991–1993. Twenty-four regions responded, of which the information from 19 was judged to be satisfactory. In 1995 satisfactory information on deaths in 1994 was received from 17 regions (Table 12). This is the point at which the collected data stops due to the fact that only nine regional Bureaus responded to requests in 1996 for information on 1995 mortalities. The others either did not reply to the inquiry or required large payments for the data.

Fig. 2-15: Sales of alcoholic beverages (liters alcohol per capita) in Russia and 25 Russian regions (1981–1994).

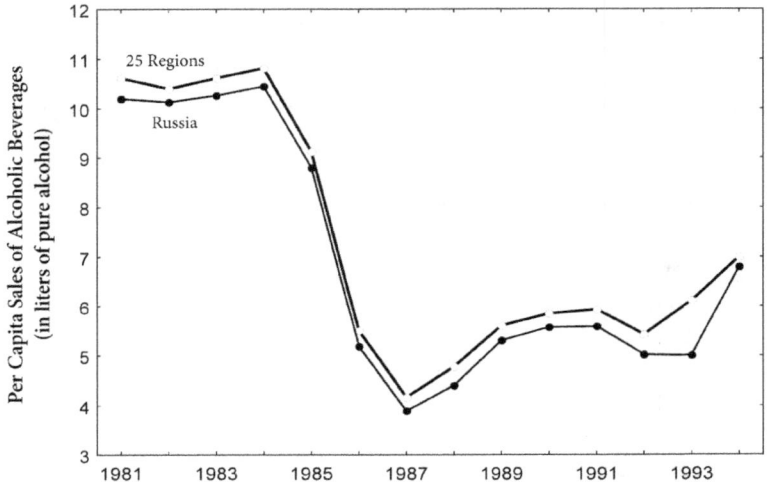

The total number of registered deaths from external causes in the 25 districts for 1981–1994 came to 1,182,015. In 1981–1984 for the 25 districts, deaths from external causes where alcohol was found in the blood of the victim came to 57.5–59.3 percent of all deaths from external causes. The low point of this measure was 1986 (47.3 percent, Table 11). As can be seen, official statistics reflect only one-fifth of these deaths from external causes with presence of alcohol. The errors in the official statistics are attributable, chiefly, to manipulations at the very bottom of the bureaucratic pyramid and are connected to the diagnoses of cause of death in the information sheets on deaths. Treml (1997; p 231) is probably wrong in supposing that errors of this kind arise from distortions of data performed at the top of the "statistical pyramid" – in order to create a more positive picture. Treml's discovery of deliberate falsifications of the indexes on national income cannot serve as proof of falsifications on mortality or incidence of disease at the governmental level.

Calculations of actual alcohol consumption for 1981–1984 in each of the 25 regions were performed in accord with the equation of linear regression (y1=4.27+8.80*x2). The dimensions x2 for the studied areas in 1984, 1985 and 1986 are presented in Fig. 2-16 in comparison with registered alcohol for those years. As can be seen, the main term of the new method, the variable member of the regression equation x2, clearly reacted to the drop in state sales in the studied regions in 1985 and 1986.

Fig. 2-16: Relationship of registered alcohol and deaths from external causes expressed in an equation 'times two' (explanation in text) in 25 provinces in 1984, 1985 and 1986. Separately indicated: Sakhalin Province (1), Novgorod Province (2), Karelian Republic (3) and Moscow (4; indexes for three years of separate regions are connected by straight line).

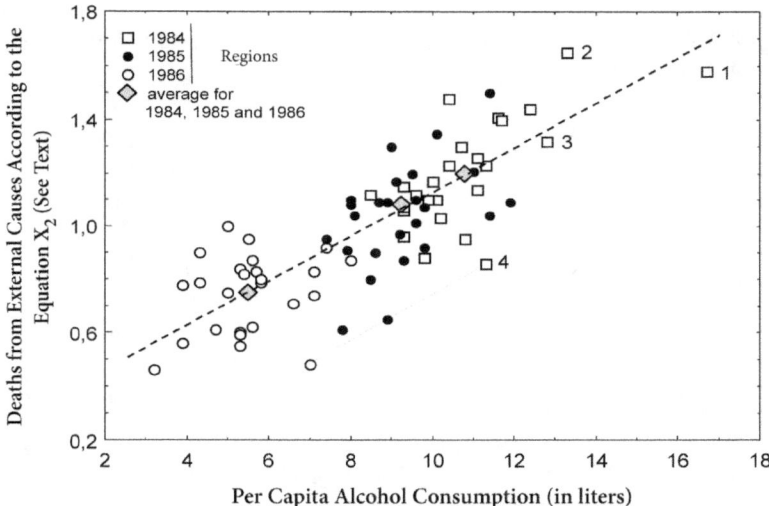

Among the 25 regions, the lowest amounts of x2 were observed in Moscow, where they move in linear dependence with registered alcohol. This was not the case in all the regions. This can be explained by the fact that the comparison is made in relation to state sales of alcohol (the x axis of Fig. 2-16), which in Moscow were the lion's share of consumption. The anti-alcohol efforts in several regions, as in Moscow, were predominantly aimed at state sales of alcoholic beverages; in others the predominant aim was underground production of samogon. However, the averaged function for 1984–1986 was linear in relation to registered alcohol (Fig. 2-16), which still predominated over samogon in these years.

The estimate of actual consumption reveals the start of a rise in alcohol consumption in Russia in 1987 (Table 1 and Fig. 2-7). It is important to stress that this estimate is based, not on the overall number of deaths from external causes, but on the relationship of the shares of deaths with alcohol in the blood and sober individuals. It must be stressed that this relationship is an entirely different index than mortality overall and is independent of the overall number of deaths. The calculations by Treml (1997) also show 1987 as a turning point for alcohol consumption in Russia. Moreover, the estimates by Treml and from the new (Nemtsov) method are quantitatively very close (Table 1 and Fig. 2-7).

Another way of judging the quality of calculations of consumption is comparison with alcohol-specific phenomena, for example, with incidence of alcohol psychoses (Fig. 2-17; after exclusion of the linear trend Rs=0.925; p=0.000002). As can be seen, the average measures of consumption and disease incidence correlate significantly; the small discrepancy in 1987–1992 is connected to the lag of psychoses behind consumption. Correlations with other alcohol-specific effects are similar. This allows us to believe that the estimate of consumption thus derived is valid and to use it for further calculations.

Fig. 2-17: Estimate of alcohol consumption and morbidity of alcohol psychoses in 25 Regions of Russia (1981–1994).

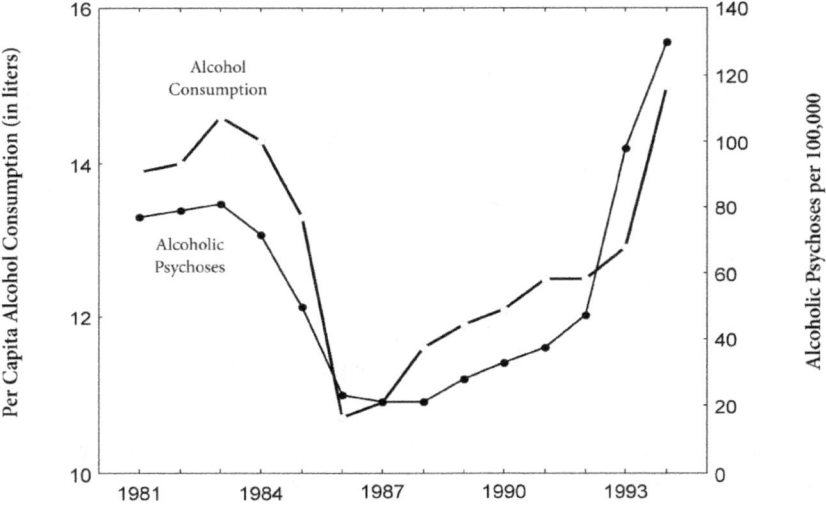

It is possible to consider the average estimate for the 25 regions as valid for the average for Russia as a whole (Shkolnikov & Nemtsov, 1997), in that the basic measures for the regions are representative for the country as a whole. However, it is also possible to go from the selective estimates to an all-Russia estimate by another route. For this, it is crucial that the dimension of consumption of unregistered alcohol in the regions studied is inversely related to sales of alcohol (a significant negative correlation). This is strong evidence of a predictive pattern: the higher the level of sales of legal alcoholic beverages, the less the consumption of illegal alcohol products and vice versa. This characteristic of Russian consumption makes it possible to use the estimates of consumption in the 25 studied regions to arrive at an estimate of actual consumption of alcohol for the country as a whole.

For this purpose, coefficients of linear regression for unregistered alcohol were calculated on the basis of registered alcohol in the studied regions for 1981–1994. Using the derived coefficients, a calculation was made of unregistered alcohol in Russia on the basis of registered alcohol. Thus, for 1990, the relationship of unregistered (y3) and registered alcohol (x3) in the 25 regions is expressed in the formula: y3=12.38 - 1.02 x3. In 1990 registered alcohol (x3) in Russia stood at 5.56 liters per capita per year (data from the State Statistical Committee of the Russian Federation). Solving the equation gives the dimensions of unregistered alcohol (y3) of 6.73 liters, and the sum (5.56+6.73) is 12.29 liters, the estimate of actual alcohol consumption for 1990. The results of calculations for 1981–1994 are presented in Table 1 and in Fig. 2-17.

Table 13: Distribution of consumption of registered and unregistered alcohol by regions of Russia (number of provinces studied in each region given in parentheses).

Region (n)	Estimation of Actual Consumption		Registered Alcohol		Unregistered Alcohol	
	1984	1990	1984	1990	1984	1990
Northern and North-west (n = 5)	15.6* ± 1.1**	12.3 ± 0.4	11.9 ± 0.5	6.3 ± 0.5	4.0 ± 0.8	6.0 ± 0.6
Central and Central – Chernozem (n = 8)	14.6 ± 0.7	12.2 ± 0.7	10.1 ± 0.3	6.0 ± 0.5	4.3 ± 1.8	6.2 ± 0.9
North Caucasus (n = 1)	12.7	10.7	9.3	4.8	3.5	5.8
Ural and Volga (n = 4)	13.9 ± 0.3	11.4 ± 0.7	9.6 ± 0.4	5.2 ± 0.3	4.4 ± 0.4	6.2 ± 1.2
Western Siberia (n = 4)	14.8 ± 1.0	12.8 ± 0.9	10.5 ± 0.4	5.6 ± 0.2	3.4 ± 1.0	6.8 ± 1.0
Far East (n = 3)	16.7 ± 0.9	13.3 ± 0.5	13.4 ± 1.6	6.2 ± 1.0	3.3 ± 0.9	7.2 ± 1.3

* per capita consumption of pure alcohol in liters; ** standard error of mean

The geographic distribution of alcohol consumption in Russia can be represented by combining the neighboring studied regions in conformity with the former division of Russia (Table 13). Before the start of the campaign, the increase of consumption moved in a south-to-north direction in the European part of Russia but moved from west to east in the Asian part of Russia. The "south-to-north" trend for the latter area was difficult to research because of the great north-to-south distances of several of the regions.

Among the 25 regions studied in 1984, the top consumers were the Sakhalin, Novgorod, Kaluga, Leningrad, Amur and Kemerovo regions (16–18 liters average per capita alcohol consumption). Next in line came the Moscow, Murmansk, Omsk and Rostov regions (11–13 liters). During the anti-alcohol campaign, the levels of consumption not only fell but converged. By 1994 the former hierarchy had been re-established, but at a higher level (about 20 liters for Kaluga and Novgorod regions; there are no data for the Sakhalin region, and consumption in the Leningrad region was 13.3 liters).

It is crucial for the new method that the new estimate of alcohol consumption in Russia (Table 1) is made independently of those used earlier (Treml, 1997; the State Statistical Committee of the Russian Federation). That said, the three estimates are close, and the largest exceeds the smallest on average by 7.9 percent (Fig. 2-7). Thus, we obtain one more testimony to the super-high level of Russian alcohol consumption, amounting, in the early 1980s, to 13.5–14.8 liters by the various estimates (Fig. 1). The level was close to this at the end of the anti-alcohol campaign. The agreement of the three estimates, derived by independent methods, may be considered indirect verification; direct verification, unfortunately, is not possible, given the conditions in Russia.

Calculations of consumption on the basis of the new method had to be halted in 1994, when it became practically impossible to obtain further data from the regional Bureaus of Judicial-Medical Expertise. Furthermore, there was a substantive collapse of the specialist review services in the country, including the pathological-anatomical and the judicial-medical (Zaratyants, 2001). At the same time, new data compiled by the State Statistical Committee of the Russian Federation now designated as "volume of sales" and supposedly taking account of illegal sales were approximately half of the actual consumption for 1984 as given in the figures of that same state organization (with samogon taken into account). Yet this was a time when the levels of all the alcohol-specific effects were much higher than in 1984 (Fig. 2-11). Thus, it can be seen that the official figures of the State Statistical Committee of the Russian Federation, new and old, do not agree with the actual consumption of alcohol in the country.

Such an undercount led, and still leads, to large impropriety in the estimation of the alcohol problems of our country. Thus, for example, the preamble of the draft of a federal law in 1999, states that "the legal manufacture of vodka and other liquor products in 1999 amounted to approximately 120–125 million decaliters as against a calculated production of more than 240 million decaliters. So, approximately 50 percent of vodka and other liquor products were illegally traded in 1999" ("On the Introduction of Amendments and Supplements to the Federal Law, 'On State Regulation of the Manufacture and Sale of Ethyl Spirits and Alcohol Products'"). Yet 120–125 million decaliters yields only 3.3 liters of pure alcohol per capita per year. If the alcohol in vodka is added to the alcohol in wine and beer, we find that consumption in 1999 was half what official figures give for consumption in 1984 (Table 1). But this is impossible if we judge by the alcohol-specific effects. It thus follows that while the government presumes that it controlled half of the alcohol market, which is hardly likely, it actually controlled only one-quarter of the market. Former Vice Premier B. E. Nemtsov in 1997, V. Berestovaya, chairperson of the Russian Federation's State Committee for Assuring the Monopoly on Alcohol Products, in 1998, and S. N. Almazov, director of the Federal Tax Police Service, also in 1998, spoke of the 50–60 percent control when the Accounting Chamber began to concern itself with the problem. By its data, illegal production of strong alcohol drinks amounted to 64 percent of the total, i.e. it accounted for two-thirds of consumption.

Besides the very approximate government estimates of alcohol consumption in the country in the second half of the 1990s, there are the estimates made by a large number of researchers, and based on selective interviews (Table 10) and ones that do not reflect actual consumption (Chapter 2-3).

All this pushed to the fore the need to estimate alcohol consumption in the country after 1994, the last year for which we have an estimate of actual consumption done by the new method. For this it is possible to relate in percentage terms the data of the State Statistical Committee of the Russian Federation on alcohol-specific effects after 1994 with the same effects for 1994, taking the latter as 100 percent. If we also take alcohol consumption in 1994 as 100 percent, one can calculate consumption after 1994 by using changes in the effects after 1994. At the same time, it is necessary to bear in mind that such measures as deaths from alcohol poisoning or incidence of alcohol psychoses are closely linked to alcoholism included those whose lives may have been saved during the anti-alcohol campaign and died after it ("doubling" of mortality and incidence of disease; see above). For this reason, these measures are not suitable for estimates of alcohol consumption. Nor are measures of deaths from cirrhosis of the liver, because of the long lag involved, suitable for accomplishing this task (Fig. 2-11). More suitable are measures of homicides, suicides and deaths from pancreatitis. Using them as the basis, indexes of consumption for 1995–2001 were calculated (Table 1).

There is no direct evidence of a decline in alcohol consumption in our country after 1994, but indirect evidence allows us to assume that the process began in 1995. Indicative of this is the drop in alcohol-specific effects beginning with 1995 (Fig. 2-11). Mortalities from cirrhosis of the liver began to drop with a year's lag, which is most likely linked to the greater rigidity of this index, especially in the face of a decline in consumption, as occurred at the start of the anti-alcohol campaign (Fig. 2-11). Possible causes of the drop in alcohol consumption in 1995–1998 are described in Chapter 1-8, and the factors behind the rise in consumption of 1999–2000 in Chapter 1-9.

The critical character of 1994 as a turning point is confirmed as well by Interior Ministry data: with a continuing growth in criminal cases, involving intoxicated and sober persons, the share of intoxicated accused began to decline in 1995, although until 1993 the trend for intoxicated had been rising (Fig. 2-18a). This is even more starkly evident in the case of homicides (Fig. 2-18b), among which the share of intoxicated persons began to fall as early as 1994.

One must be cautious about these indexes of alcohol consumption for 1995–2001 because they are only estimates. Caution is further advised because of the absence, after 1993, of other independent, carefully drawn estimates for comparison, as had been the case in the late 1980s and early 1990s. There exists one estimate, for 2001, of 16 liters of pure alcohol per capita per year (Zaigraev, 2004b). Its methodological thoroughness and the repeated contact between interviewers and respondents over a period of four months make this a unique work for Russia, and its results are believable. And they are close to our own calculations (15 liters). Unfortunately, it is the only study which offers solid basis for judging estimates of consumption after 1994.

* * *

On the basis of this multi-year analysis of alcohol consumption in Russia, it might be thought that the significant but relatively steady rise in consumption of the 1960s and 1970s was replaced by a strongly fluctuating index of consumption, the fluctuations caused by two powerful forces moving in different directions. The first was the anti-alcohol campaign, which sharply reduced consumption, and the other was the market reforms, which offered free access to alcoholic beverages. Although the reduction of alcohol consumption during the campaign was significant, almost one-third in 2.5 years, consumption remained very high (more than 10 liters per capita per year).

It is important to note that the rise in consumption in 1994 and 2001 lifted it to the level of the beginning of the 1980s (Fig. 2-7). Apparently, this level (14–15 liters) is the "ceiling" for the country. And only extraordinary political or economic factors lead to declines in consumption with subsequent returns to the "ceiling" level.

One supposed that, after 2001, fluctuations in the level of consumption will show a dampening trend. Unfortunately, one is forced to think that these fluctuations will occur around a very high level of average per capita consumption (13–15 liters).

2-4: AN ESTIMATE OF ACTUAL CONSUMPTION IN RUSSIA

Fig. 2-18 (a/b): Number of criminals (Fig- 2-18a) and number of murderers (Fig. 2-18b): overall number and number intoxicated by alcohol (figures from RussStat). Thick line represents percentage of those drunk in the total number of criminals.

Fig. 2-18a

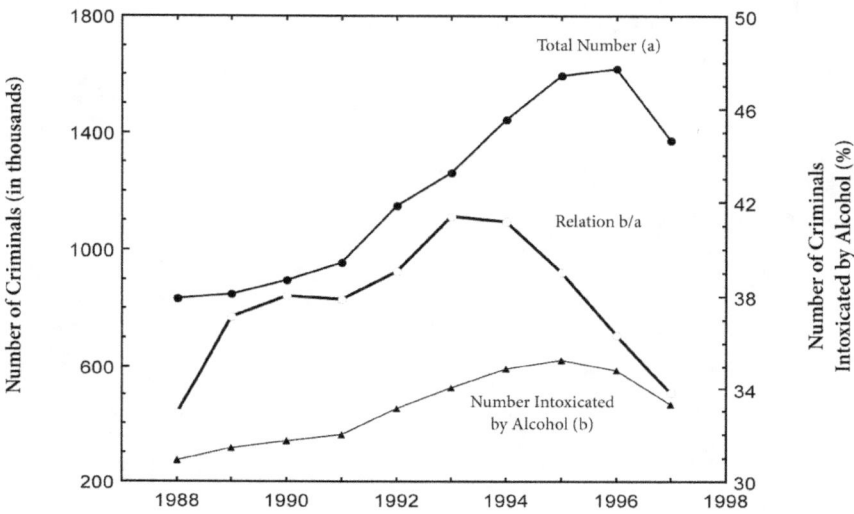

Fig. 2-18b

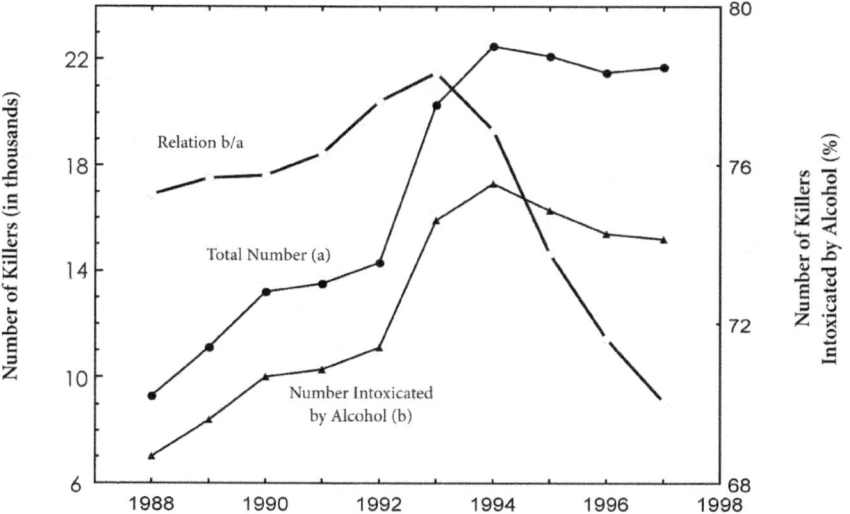

Chapter 2-5
Alcohol mortality before, during and after the anti-alcohol campaign

It is very difficult to determine the actual scale of alcohol-related mortality in Russia. As deaths "from causes associated with alcohol", official statistics include alcohol poisonings, alcohol-specific cirrhosis of the liver, alcoholism and alcohol psychoses. But these constitute only a portion of deaths due directly to alcohol, only about 3 percent of all deaths in some years, while alcohol consumption in Russia is probably the highest in Europe (up to 15 liters of pure alcohol per capita per year; Chapter 2-4 and Table 4). For purposes of comparison, alcohol mortality is about the same level in the countries of northern Europe, where, as in Russia, hard liquor predominates but consumption is lower and quality of life is higher. For example, with regard to mortality rate due to alcohol consumption Finland has Europe's highest (3.7 percent; Ramstedt, 2002), with a consumption average of 8.5 liters (Table 4) that, when illegal alcohol is taken into account as presumably 20 percent of legal, rises to 10.2 liters (Leifman, 2001).

The first error of our statistics is their undercount of direct alcohol deaths. Thus, despite the very high level of alcohol consumption in Russia, deaths from alcohol cirrhosis of the liver made up approximately 10 percent of all deaths from cirrhosis of the liver; only in 1998 did this measure begin to increase sharply (30.8 percent in 2005). Such an increase was probably the result of a change in the criteria of diagnosis. Worldwide, alcohol-cirrhosis diagnoses make up 30–80 percent of all cirrhosis deaths (Audigier et al., 1984). The second error is deliberate or accidental falsification of alcohol-specific deaths (Chapter 2-3), and the third is a complete disregard for indirect alcohol deaths, i.e., deaths for which alcohol is not the sole cause but is a substantial supplementary factor in shortening life.

Particularly poorly addressed in this regard, despite their social significance, are deaths from external causes. Before 1989, Central Statistical Administration Forms 5a and 5b, "Information about Deaths by Sex, Age and Causes of Death", did not call for the mentioning of intoxication as a circumstance of death. The form, S-51, that replaced these in 1989 included a section "deaths while intoxicated". Even so, Form S-51 reflected only one-fifth or one-sixth of such deaths.

Furthermore, for the years 1993–1997, the section on alcohol deaths was dropped from the form. That was just the period of time when alcohol mortality was at its highest in the country – and in the world.

A more complete estimate of alcohol mortalities in Russia became possible in connection with the sharp swings in levels of consumption of alcohol resulting from the anti-alcohol campaign of 1985 and the events in our alcohol history that followed it (Fig. 2-7, Chapter 2-4). It is best to make such estimates in light of the periodization used in the first part of this book, i.e., in connection with the phases of the country's alcohol consumption.

Alcohol mortality before 1985

By far the most commonly used index of mortality is number of deaths per 100,000 of population. This and other meaningful indexes will often be used in what follows. However, this way of characterizing mortality, while customary for specialists, may make it difficult for others to grasp the scale of mortalities. Therefore, we will use as our primary measure the overall number of deaths in the country by year.

Fig. 2-19: Number of deaths in Russia annually (1965–2005).

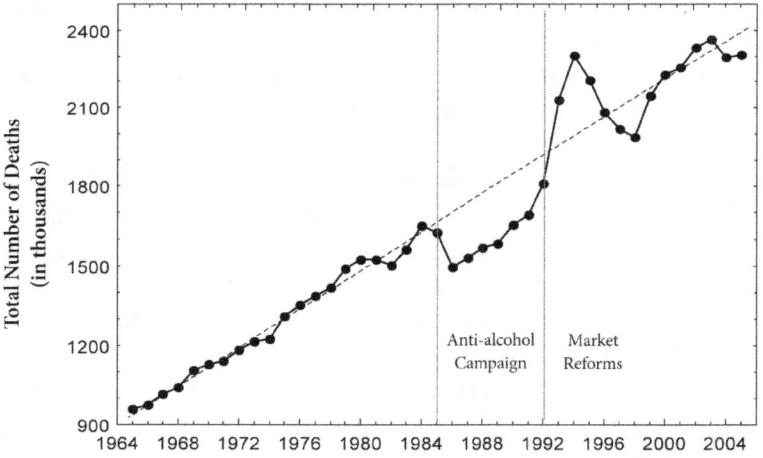

Figure 2-19 shows that the number of deaths steadily increased, beginning in 1965 and continuing until 1984. During the same period, the population increased, though proportionally the percentage increase in deaths was greater. This was reflected in the fact that, over the course of 20 years (1964–1984), life expectancy declined, significantly among men (by 2.5 years, from 64.5 years to 62 years; Vishnevsky and Shkolnikov, 1997a and 1997b). The gap between life expectancies for men and women increased substantially (from 8.7 years in 1964 to 11.3 years in 1984). The increased gap may be linked to the increase in alcohol consumption. This is suggested by the slightly more than doubling of state sales of alcohol (from 4.6 to 10.5 liters; the State Statistical Committee of the RSFSR). For this same period, actual consumption increased from 9.8 to 14 liters, according to estimates made by specialists (Treml, 1997; Fig. 1-4). Additional evidence of the dependence of mortality on consumption in this period may be the steady rise in the number of deaths from alcohol poisoning (Fig. 1-12): their share of overall mortalities doubled (from 1.1 percent in 1965 to 2.2 percent in 1979). This increase affected women as well as men beginning in 1965 (Fig. 2-20).

Fig. 2-20: Mortality from alcohol poisoning for men and women (Russia, 1965–2003). m/w – relationship of male and female mortality (numbers on diagram).

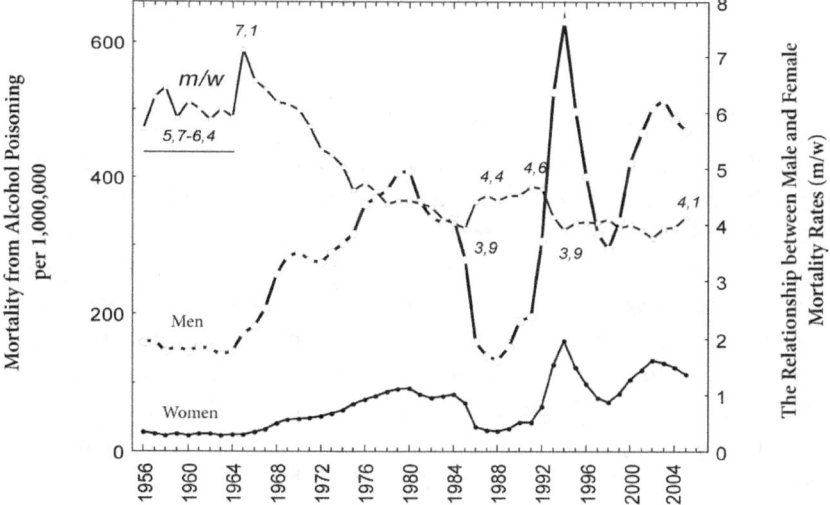

In 1981–1984 the level of deaths from alcohol poisoning declined slightly and shifted away from the preceding trend. This, along with a slight decline in the incidence of alcohol psychoses in these years (Fig. 2-21), was most likely due to the creation of three new services: medical-labor dispensaries (LTP; Decree of March 1, 1974) and the narcological and resuscitation services (resolution of December 1976). The impact of these measures showed up only after the passage of several years because of organizational difficulties.

The linear regression for 1965–1984 (the dotted line of Fig. 2-19) described in an averaged way the incremental increase in the number of deaths in this period: by 36,100 deaths a year. The increment is linked to the increase in population and its aging and to the effect of a whole series of negative factors. One of them might have been the increase in alcohol consumption.

Fig. 2-21: The overall number of deaths and cases with alcohol psychoses in Russia (1980–2003).

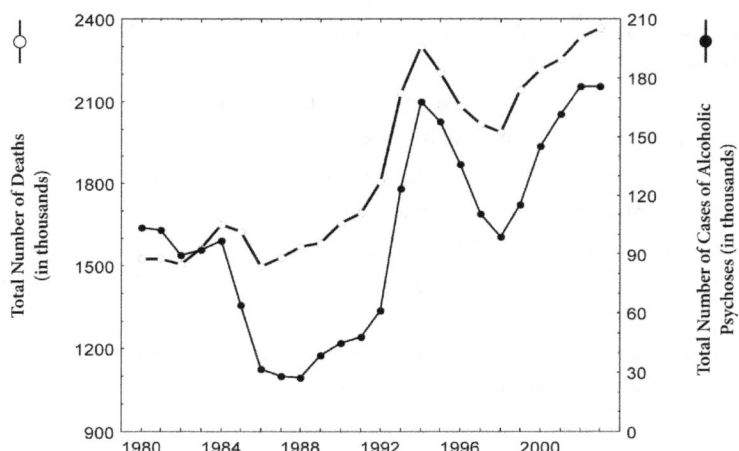

Gender aspects of alcohol mortality

An important feature of Russian mortalities from alcohol poisoning is the increase in the share of women, from 15.9 percent of these deaths in 1965 to 23.3 percent in 1984. Before 1970, then, one in six (to seven) deaths of this nature were women, but by 1984 the proportion was one in four (Fig. 2-20). During the anti-alcohol campaign, men began to make up lost ground (probably because of their greater role in the obtaining of spirits) in the mortality ratio vis-a-vis women (4.6:1; 1992). However, soon after the launching of the market reforms, and the greater accessibility of spirits, women brought the relationship back to the pre-anti-alcohol campaign position (1:4 in 1994), which has been maintained ever since.

It should be pointed out that, unlike the situation with respect to alcohol poisoning, the difference in the overall mortalities for men and women substantially declined during the anti-alcohol campaign (from 1.83 in 1984 to 1.72 in 1988; Fig. 2-22a). This is the result of in a large decline in male mortalities in contrast to female mortalities (by 16.6 percent and 14 percent, respectively, for 1988–1989; Fig. 2-22b). This is linked, most likely, to the fact that in groups of heavy users of alcohol, whose use often leads to death, there are substantially fewer women than men, and, thus, the decline in mortalities was less for women at the start of the campaign. This was evident, too, in later years – the fluctuations of overall mortalities among women are less pronounced than for men (after 1984 the coefficient of variation is 1.7 percent and 2.53 percent) except for mortalities from alcohol poisoning (9.71 percent and 9 percent, respectively).

Fig. 2.22a: The relationship of male and female mortality in Russia. Relationship of overall mortalities of men and women (m/w) as compared with alcohol consumption (1956–2003).

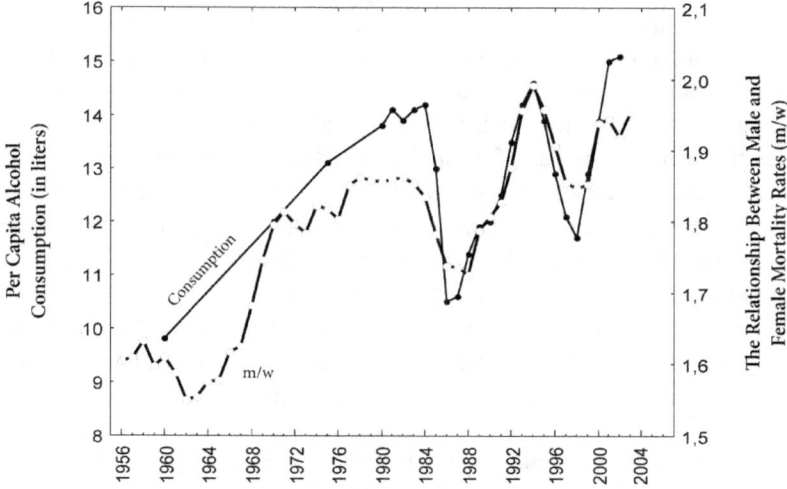

Fig. 2.22b: The relationship of overall mortalities and mortality from alcohol poisoning (1975–2005).

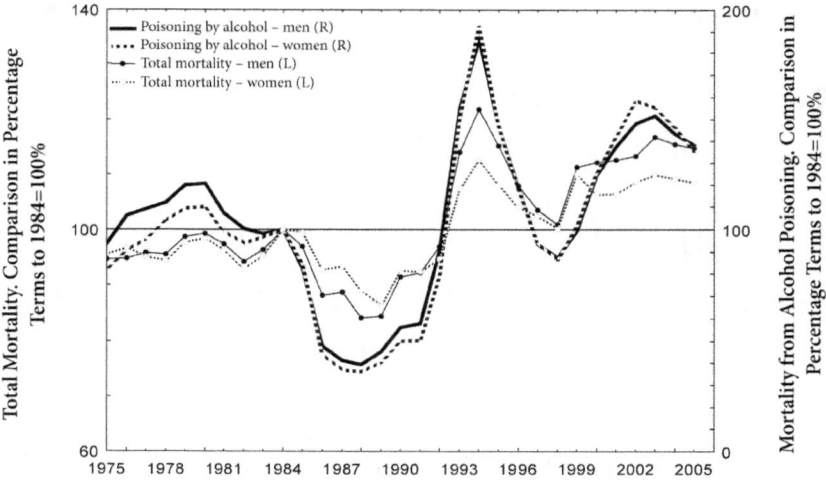

It also bears mentioning that, when overall mortality for men and women is compared with alcohol consumption, the gender relationship correlates rather well with consumption (Fig. 2-22a; Rs=0.802; p=0.000001) and reflects this level by the mechanism described in the preceding paragraph.

Alcohol mortality 1985–1992

The data for before the start of the anti-alcohol campaign do not allow us to separate the alcohol factor from other negative phenomena and, thus, estimate alcohol's contribution to deaths among the population of Russia. The anti-alcohol campaign, however, helped make this computation possible: the strictness with which it was run approximated experimental scientific conditions. An ignorant idea scandalously put into effect, the campaign offered a unique opportunity to measure the real dimensions of alcohol mortalities. This was because in the campaign's first years lowered alcoholization of the population was the sole or almost the sole cause of the decline in mortality. Also important was the fact that estimates of alcohol consumption before the start of the campaign were relatively stable: for 1980–1984, 13.8–14.2 liters per capita per year (Table 1).

A substantial decline in male mortalities took place in the first month of the campaign (Andreev, 2002; Fig. 2-23), which began on June 1, 1985. For women, the decrease reached a significant level after three months of the campaign.

Fig. 2-23: Number of male deaths per month in Russia from January 1983 to December 1988 (source: Andreev, 2002). Arrows mark the month before the start of the anti-alcohol campaign (May) and the first month after it (June 1985). Figures deviating significantly from earlier tendencies are marked by squares.

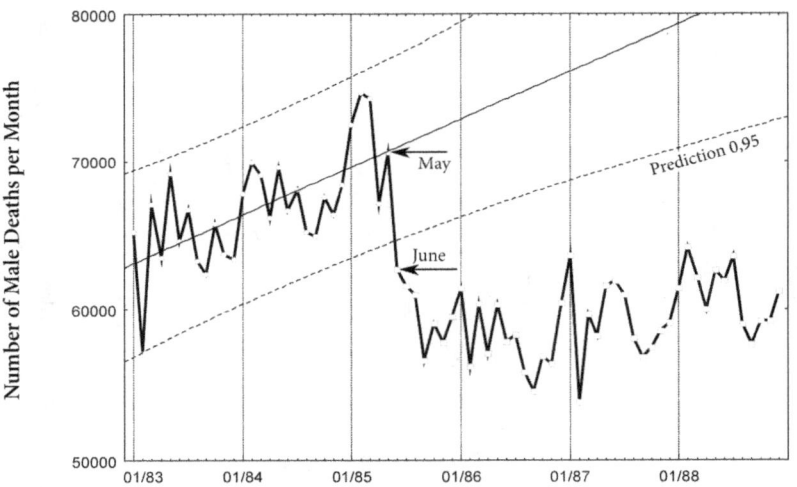

In the campaign's second year (1986), deaths were down by 203,500, or 12.3 percent of the overall number of deaths in 1984 (more precisely, from the level of regression for 1965–1984; Fig. 2-19). By this point, average per capita consumption had declined by 3.7 liters, but the dependence of mortality on consumption in 1984–1987 was a linear one (i.e., directly proportional; $p<0.01$). It follows from this that, at the start of the anti-alcohol campaign, for each liter of decline in per capita consumption, the overall number of deaths fell by 3.3 percent (12.3 percent: 3.7 liters). This figure rises steeply if the calculation is applied only to men between the ages of 35 and 59 years, for whom the number of deaths fell by 6.9 percent per liter of average per capita consumption of alcohol.

Norström and Skog (2001) have justly insisted that a large series of consistent data represent the most satisfactory method for estimating the influence of alcohol consumption on the combined health consequences related to alcohol. At the same time, it is necessary to keep in mind that the author's model is designed to highlight relatively weak and slow changes in consumption that have long-term consequences. Norström and Skog's method is therefore not well suited for Russia after 1984, after which year there ensued steep swings in the level of alcohol consumption. However, applying the Norström and Skog model to a long period (1980–1991), alcohol mortalities come to 3.6 percent according to the new World Health Organization standard (5.9 percent per liter of alcohol for men and 1.9 percent for women) and 3.9 percent per liter of alcohol if the calculations of mortality and consumption use 15-year-olds and up, as was done by Norström (2001). As can be seen, the result given using the Norström-Skog model and the result of arithmetic calculations are very close.

Norström (1996), using material from Germany and France, showed that an increase in per capita consumption of alcohol of 1 liter (in calculations using 15-year-olds as the age starting point) increases the mortality of men of middle age (35–59 years) by approximately 1 percent. Later the same author researched mortality and alcohol consumption in 14 European countries (Norström, 2001) and showed that the dependence might be even greater, up to 3 percent per liter of average per capita alcohol consumption, but only in countries of low consumption (in the range of 4.4–6.5 liters). In countries of medium consumption (7.6–11 liters) and countries of high consumption (more than 13.1 liters), the relationship is 1 percent mortality per liter per capita of consumed alcohol. Russia is a country of high consumption (13.6–18.5 liters). As is evident, European indexes of mortalities from one liter of alcohol are significantly lower than Russia's. Such a discrepancy can be explained by at least three factors.

The first is connected with the character by which the lowering of consumption was forcefully imposed during the anti-alcohol campaign in Russia. The slow and natural fluctuations in consumption in European countries may have been accompanied by a so-called "diffusion" effect (Skog, 1985a), i.e., the gradual increase or decrease of alcohol consumption by various groups in the population. As pointed out earlier (Chapter 2-2), consumption by some groups of the population can change at a pace quite different from the pace shown by the basic portion of users. This can lower the final result. What was specific to our country during the campaign was that anti-alcohol enforcement was powerful, went into effect suddenly and affected all layers of the population without exception, including serious alcoholics, judging by the decrease in alcohol psychoses (Fig. 2-11). This is why a substantial decrease in mortalities took place in the very first month of the campaign (Fig. 2-23).

The second explanation may be linked to the fact that alcoholic beverages consumed in Russia were more toxic. The important thing to remember here is that before the start of the campaign approximately one-quarter of alcohol consumption came in the form of samogon, containing very cheap oils – a mixture of ethers and other compounds – the toxicity of which is the same as the toxicity of ethyl alcohol (Nuzhny, 1995), and where the total content of cheap oils does not exceed 1 percent (Chapter 2-4). A portion of the beverages produced by state enterprises was also of low quality. These were fruit and berry wines (the famed *bormotukha*) and cheap port wines, which were consumed in large quantities but were "blended" in under the wide-ranging classification "grape wines". The principal source of added toxicity was technical spirits with high concentrations of substances of a non-alcoholic nature (acetone, aldehyde, sulfur compounds and denatured additives). This type of alcohol was stolen not only from places of production, whole tank carriers were stolen during shipment by rail (Chapter 1-3).

The third and final factor, which whilst not as obvious, may be the most significant. For estimates of mortality linked to alcohol in Russia, one must not overlook supplemental factors, the northern type of consumption, for example: large doses of strong spirits consumed in a short time. It was difficult to drink in that manner during the campaign. The high level of alcohol mortality in Russia may also be an expression of the relatively low quality of nutrition and medical services, the indifferent, even contemptuous attitude of citizens toward their own health and the contempt of Russian medicine for alcohol pathologies. All this may elevate the mortality per liter of alcohol consumed per capita of alcohol as compared with countries of Europe. In other words, the difference in the dimensions of alcohol mortality between Western countries and Russia during the campaign may be explicable not only by the character of alcohol consumption but also by special conditions of life. Taking this into account as well as the greater toxicity of beverages in Russia, this is the place to stipulate the following conditions before proceeding to calculations of the dimensions of alcohol mortality.

First: as it is impossible to distinguish the specific cause of death where alcohol is abused from secondary causes (extra toxicity, low quality of life), the whole group of causes associated with abuse should be taken to constitute alcohol mortalities.

Second: we will assume that the decrease in mortality at the start of the anti-alcohol campaign was primarily or solely caused by lower consumption of alcohol.

With these introductory points made, we may proceed to the work of estimating alcohol mortality during the anti-alcohol campaign. It is important in this connection that the linear regression of the number of deaths in 1965–1984 (dotted line of Fig. 2-19) can be used to predict what mortality would have been after 1984 if there had been no anti-alcohol campaign. It is crucial that the line should be said to "represent" all the causes of the increased numbers of deaths, including the increase, and aging of the population. Now all that remains is to determine how many male and female deaths after the start of the campaign fail to fit the linear regression. For the precision of the calculation, it is necessary as a preliminary to exclude the linear trend (Fig. 2-24a and 2-24b).

Fig. 2-24 (a/b): Change in the annual number of deaths for men (Fig. 2-24a.) and women (Fig. 2-24b) in 1965–2003 in relation to the line of regression for 1965–1984 after excluding a linear trend (equals "0"). Dotted line indicates a prediction 0.95.

Fig. 2-24a

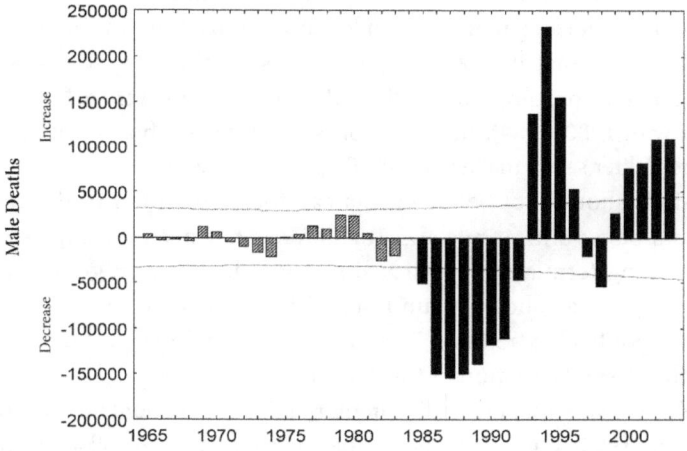

Fig. 2-24b

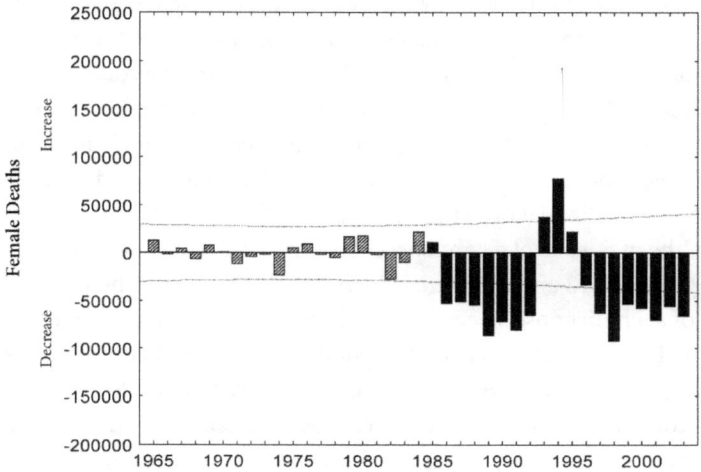

The number of deaths of men in 1985–1992 and of women in 1986–1992, having declined, significantly differs from what was the case in the preceding period (Figs. 2-24a and 2-24b). The numbers of people who might have but did not die during the anti-alcohol campaign are indicated by the deviation (difference) from the projected linear regression of 1965–1984 for men (Fig. 2-24a) and women (Fig. 2-24b) for the period of the anti-alcohol campaign. The sum of the deviations or, really, the number of lives saved amounts to 919,900 for men (115,000 on average; 1985–1992) and 463,600 for women (66,200; 1986–1992) – a total of 1,383,400 individuals or 181±16.5 thousands a year. But for the campaign, approximately 14.8 percent more men and 7.9 percent more women would have died.

Thus, more than a million lives were saved during and thanks to the anti-alcohol campaign. This is the main positive result of the campaign and points to lowered alcohol consumption as the essential factor in lowering mortalities in Russia.

It is important to note that the demographic success of the campaign was attributable to a lowering of consumption by all of 3.1±0.41 liters (on average for 1985–1992 as compared with 1980–1984). In other words, lowering alcohol consumption per capita by merely 1 liter saved the lives of 58,400 persons a year.

These conclusions should not be taken as a call for a repetition of the campaign, which would be a political mistake. Russia does not need a campaign. It needs a systematic, long-term alcohol policy aimed at a slow, steady, gradual and unremitting lowering of alcohol consumption. The campaign was a further demonstration that political extremism is incapable of bringing about a durable improvement in the alcohol situation of the country.

There is a widely held view that the decline in mortalities in our country (Russia) in the second half of the 1980s was a response to the euphoria of perestroika and new hopefulness in the society (for example, Värnik et al., 1998). It is difficult entirely to exclude this factor, but at this point there is no scientific evidence to support it. On the other hand, there are the incontrovertible facts of a steep drop in state sales of alcoholic beverages (Table 1), a decline in all the indexes that are highly dependent on alcohol, including the incidence of alcohol psychoses (Fig. 2-21), deaths from alcohol poisoning (Fig. 2-20), overall mortality, especially among men and particularly in the first month of the anti-alcohol campaign (Andreev, 2002; Fig. 2-23), deaths from cirrhosis of the liver (Fig. 2-11), violent deaths when intoxicated and crimes committed by persons intoxicated (Crime and Delinquency in the USSR, 1990).

The decline in the incidence of alcohol psychoses (Fig. 2-21) and mortalities from alcohol poisoning (Figs. 1-12 and 2-20) are evidence that alcoholics, who are the sole or chief subjects of such diagnoses, began to drink substantially less during the anti-alcohol campaign. This runs contrary to the persistent and often heard notion that during the campaign "alcoholics were drinking as they always drank".

The general conclusions about alcohol-related mortalities and lives saved during the anti-alcohol campaign, made on the basis of the total number of deaths during this period, are sound whether calculated on the basis of a simple index of mortalities per 100,000 individuals, or the new World Health Organization standard per 1,000,000 men and women (Fig. 2-25). The advantage of the index of total number of deaths is that it gives a clearer picture of the terrible dimensions of alcohol mortalities in Russia.

Fig. 2-25: Mortality in men and women (1965–2003, World Health Organization new standard).

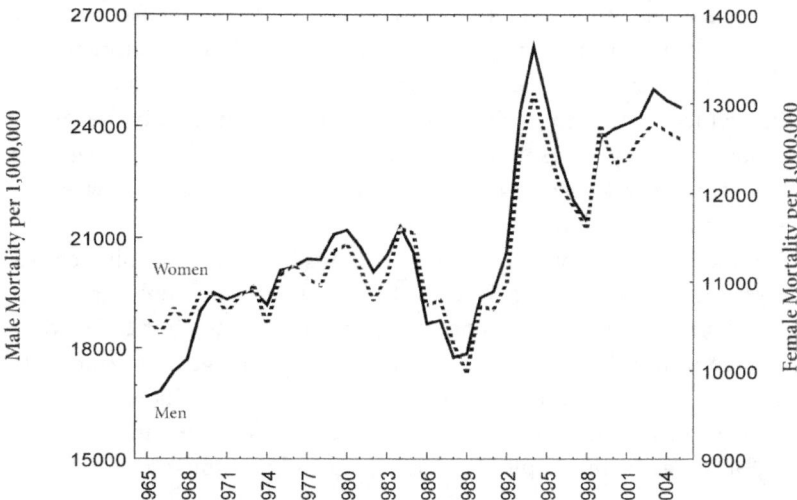

At the same time, it should be borne in mind that persons at risk from alcohol death would have perished had there been no campaign. This does not hold true for all of the alcohol mortalities, but only deaths of persons consuming 10.5–15 liters of alcohol per year. 10.5 liters of alcohol per year, however, is a very high level of consumption and contributes its share of mortalities. Thus, 181,000 alcohol deaths a year is not the entirety of alcohol mortalities but only a portion, as will be shown below.

Alcohol mortalities 1992–1994

After the steep decline in mortalities early in the anti-alcohol campaign, a bounce back in mortalities began in 1987 (Fig. 2-19), becoming a steep trend from 1992 (Fig. 2-24a). Mortality reached its high point in 1994, thereafter declining. In 1997 the number of deaths of men was not substantially different from the tendency of 1965–1984 (Fig. 2-24a). For women this occurred earlier, in 1995 (Fig. 2-24b), and the rise in mortality in 1994 was small in comparison to that of men.

It is difficult to estimate the dimensions of alcohol mortality in the short period 1992–1994, despite the very high meaningfulness of the coefficient of regression of mortality to alcohol. This is an example of a situation where statistical significance is meaningless – the calculations give paradoxical results. For this short period of time, for one liter increase in alcohol consumption per year male mortalities increased by 20 times and women's by 16 times as compared with the preceding period (1984–1992). But that is impossible with so small an increase in consumption. This statistical result might be explained by a simultaneous increase in alcohol use in 1992 and an increase in other factors of death, among which distinguishing and quantifying the alcohol constituent is quite difficult. It will be demonstrated later that the alcohol factor assumed new forms at this time which further impede calculations of the desired estimate. However, this is a qualitative way of resolving the problem of whether the increase in consumption in this period affected the increase in mortalities. Now, however, is the time to stop and consider something else.

The Damoclean sword of a possible error in his estimate of alcohol consumption will yet long hang over the head of the investigator of alcohol problems in Russia. The hair by which it hangs became particularly fine after 1992, when the dynamic of mortality in relation to alcohol sharply changed its course (1993–1994; Fig. 2-26) and took alcohol mortalities to a new level. Such a "jump" may reflect the real relationship of the two phenomena, mortalities and alcohol consumption, or it may be the result of error. This possibility must be examined.

Fig. 2-26: Relationship of mortality of men and women who had consumed alcohol (1984–7 and 1992–2001).

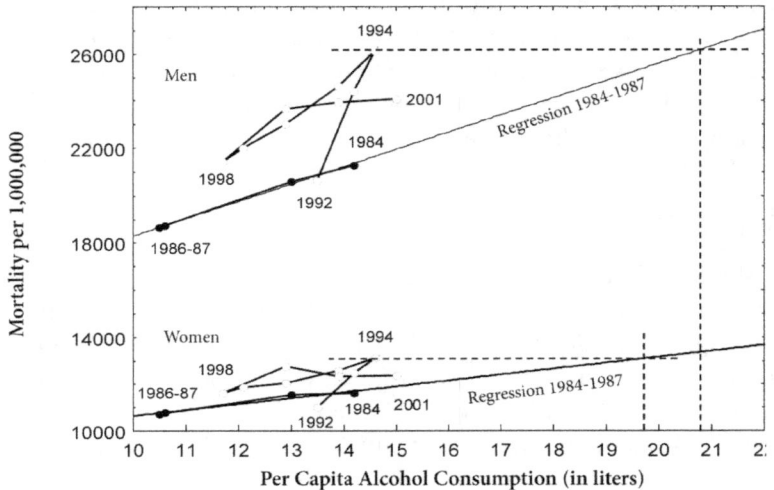

If there is an error in the specification of overall mortalities (the "y" axis of Fig. 2-26), it is not a major one judging by the relatively small share of deaths of people of unspecified age, i.e., bodies found long after death. The error remains small even if it is assumed that there were in fact two or three times as many cases as the stated number. So we acknowledge that by far most deaths are included in the official statistics. These statistics reflect a substantial rise in the number of deaths after 1992 (Fig. 2-19).

The "x" axis of Fig. 2-26 (alcohol consumption) has a different origin. It is no more than an estimate. Moreover, the method of calculating the estimate had to be changed in 1995 (Chapter 2-4) because of the unavailability of data from the Bureaus of Forensic-Medical Expertise, on the basis of which the calculations of consumption for 1980–1994 were based (Nemtsov, 1998b, 2000). Moreover, the basis for the estimate of consumption was the indexes of mortality for 1980–1987, and the possibility of error grows with the distance from these base years. Finally, after 1993 and until 2001, there were no other independent estimates made on the basis of epidemiological research: the State Statistical Committee of the Russian Federation's calculations end in 1990 and Treml's (1997) in 1993. In light of this, it is necessary to study the possibility of errors in the estimate of consumption of alcohol after the anti-alcohol campaign ended.

For the purposes of our investigation, we assume that the estimate of per capita per year alcohol consumption for 1984–1987 is close to actual consumption (it is an average of three independent sources with almost identical dimensions: the State Statistical Committee of the Russian Federation; Treml, 1997, and Nemtsov, 2000). It is also assumed that estimates for succeeding years may skew high or low. But the latter possibility is very unlikely, because in that case one would have to assume a decline in consumption from 1992 until 1994, which in no way agrees with the steep rise at this time in all the alcohol-related effects (for example, Figs. 1-12 and 2-20).

It is harder to resolve the question of the possibility that (the estimate of consumption is low, i.e., that) actual consumption was higher than estimated. This is because we do not know what form the dependence of mortality on consumption takes when consumption is greater than 15 liters. If the dependence remained linear, resolution is simpler. In this case, the test consists of superimposing the mortality indexes for 1993–1994 with the linear regression for 1984–1987, when the dependence of mortality on alcohol was linear (Fig. 2-26). Given such an approach, the possibility of a substantial downward skewing of the estimate disappears. In the opposite case, one would have to assume an unbelievable increase in consumption in two years: from 13.5 liters (1992) to 20–21 liters in 1994 (Fig. 2-26).

The resolution of the problem is made more complex if we assume that the dependence of mortality on consumption when consumption is greater than 15 liters per capita is curvilinear, and this is more than likely. In conditions of such uncertainty, a direct resolution of the problem is impossible. Indirectly, however, we see that there is a very high correlation between the estimate of consumption and the alcohol-related indexes of mortality (Table 14). This means that the estimates are not empty figures but close to the actual consumption. This is further suggested in that one research study (Zaigraev, 2004b), the sole study based on repeated population surveys, found a level of consumption commensurate with the estimates offered here (16 liters of pure alcohol per capita per year in 2001 versus 15 liters).

Having accepted the estimates of alcohol consumption, we can return to the period of 1992–1994. It should be kept in mind, however, that because of the market reforms new socioeconomic conditions emerged, quite different from the conditions of the years before. This might change the character of the relationship between mortality and consumption because alcohol mortalities reflect not only the level and character of consumption but also a whole series of social factors. It has already been demonstrated that factors such as the impoverishment of the population and weaknesses in the public health system in fact did lower the quality of life in Russia. No more however than changes in ecological conditions can be accepted as essential to explaining such a significant increase in mortalities (Leon et al., 1997; Shkolnikov et al., 1998; Shapiro, 1997). What then is the situation? What was alcohol's contribution to the mortalities of this time?

Table 14: Coefficients of linear regression (B) for types of alcohol-related mortality (1980–2001), and their statistical significance level.

	Men		Women		B_M/B_F
	B_M	p	B_F	p	
Alcohol poisoning	84.26	0.00000	21.48	0.00000	3.9
Homicide	51.56	0.00002	14.56	0.00000	3.5
Suicide	73.22	0.00000	6.36	0.00005	11.5
Other external causes	219.07	0.00000	39.34	0.00000	5.6
Liver diseases	22.25	0.00016	9.58	0.00007	2.3
Pancreatic diseases	6.77	0.00000	1.00	0.00317	6.8
Cardiovascular diseases	562.09	0.00008	226.01	0.00377	2.5
Other causes	177.09	0.00067	47.89	0.00198	3.7
Overall mortality	1196.31	0.00000	366.25	0.00049	3.3

The estimates of average per capita consumption for this period are practically identical when compared with the period preceding the anti-alcohol campaign (Table 1). However, mortality in 1993–1995 was substantially greater than the level (linear regression) of 1965–1984, especially among men (Fig. 2-24a). The period 1992–1994 saw a rise in deaths in all the major categories that had fallen during the anti-alcohol campaign (discussed in more detail below). The question arises: Was the almost across-the-board increase in deaths connected with a change in the level of alcohol consumption?

To answer this question, we compare overall mortality with the phenomena tightly dependent on consumption, with, for example, deaths from alcohol poisoning (Fig. 1-12). What is notable, first of all, is the near-synchrony of the changes in the two mortalities (after excluding the linear trend Rs=0.813 for men and Rs=0.701 for women, p=0.0001; 1980–2001). It has already been stated that the small discrepancy in the indexes for 1981–1984 may be explained by the organization in 1976 of narcological and emergency services in the country as well as by the stabilizing of sales of alcohol by state sources (Fig. 1-4). The incidence of alcohol psychoses also showed the same dynamic (Fig. 2-21).

Fig. 1-11 may serve as another illustration of alcohol's contribution to overall mortality in 1992–1994. It is clear that the increase in male mortalities in 1993–1994 affected primarily men of working age, from 20 to 69 years of age, and little affected those of the ages most sensitive to poor living conditions, the elderly and very old; among children mortalities declined slightly in this period. Significant, too, is that the increase in overall male mortalities occurred almost at the same time as the increase in male mortalities from alcohol poisoning. There is a difference, however, for young people (15–29 years), probably because those who die from alcohol-related causes in this age group have not had time to become serious alcoholics, the chief sources of alcohol poisoning deaths (Ugryumov, 1997). Nor can it be ruled out that some part of the difference is attributable to falsification of the cause of death in cases of alcohol poisoning involving young people because of ethical and social considerations that might have more significance for young deaths than for the deaths of elderly alcoholics.

There is yet another point of intersection for these two phenomena, mortality and alcohol consumption: the increased toxicity of surrogate alcohol products. In 1992 the situation in the alcohol market changed radically because of the market reforms and the government's abandonment of its monopoly on alcohol products. Production of samogon using sugar or other products became unprofitable due to the increased prices of these raw materials. As a result new sources of surrogates emerged. The most important in this connection was the appearance on the market of large quantities of surrogates made with technical spirits not subject to excise taxes and thus the beverages were very cheap. Calculations were made on the basis of the production of technical spirits and its declining use by the chemical, rubber and other branches of industry. These calculations showed that technical alcohol accounted for approximately 20 percent of all alcohol consumed (Nemtsov, 1995). There were also other kinds of surrogates. According to data compiled by Roskomtorg from selective reviews of unacceptable products, their percentage in the liquor-products industry rose from

5.6 percent of the volume of acceptable products in 1991 to 30.4 percent in 1994. The quality of imported alcohol products was even worse – rejections were equal to 67.2 percent of the volume of acceptable products in 1994. These and much other data (Chapter 1-7) attest to the fact that the gradually rising share of surrogate alcohol products constituted a significant portion of all consumed alcohol products. This certainly would have an effect on the health and mortality of heavy users.

And, finally, there is one other factor associated with alcohol that is of undoubted importance but hard to quantify: the increase after 1991 of the cohort of individuals with higher risks of an alcohol death. This can be seen in Fig. 1-11: the distribution of deaths in 1992–1994 is not entirely symmetrical with the distribution in 1985–1986: the number of lives saved during the anti-alcohol campaign was significantly fewer than the deaths after it. Yet the lower consumption of 1985–1986 was significantly greater (3.7 liters) than its rise in 1991–1992 (2.1 liters).

The inequality of deaths and saved lives in the two periods is, most likely, connected to the fact that a portion of heavy users of alcohol whose lives were saved during and thanks to the campaign. In the period following 1991 they had a higher risk of dying an alcohol death. The physical form of the risk took the shape of somatic and/or nervous illnesses acquired or worsened by their former (before 1985) drunkenness. It should be borne in mind, too, that consumption of alcohol during the campaign remained very high, at a level of 10–12 liters, and this certainly helped maintain the risk of an alcoholic death.

All these risk-bearers died after 1991 as a result of the increasing availability of alcohol. There was a "transfer of risk" from one historical period (the anti-alcohol campaign) to another (the period of market reforms; the "delayed" deaths of Andreev, 2002, also Shkolnikov et al., 2001). Slightly more than a million lives were saved during the campaign. Another cohort was made up of "new" users, whose deaths "echoed" the rise in consumption. Thus, one may see the steep rise in mortalities in 1993–1994 as, in part, conditioned by the "doubling" of the cohort of persons at high risk by this "mixing" of alcohol deaths.

There is one other kind of evidence of the "transferring of the risk" of alcohol mortality: the doubling of the share of alcohol poisonings at the start of the market reforms as compared with the preceding period (Fig. 2-27). This is expressed in the increase of such deaths per liter of alcohol from 2.3 percent to 5 percent. The relationship returns to the starting point (2.4 percent) in the following period. It appears that the "doubling of the cohort" of alcohol dead at the start of the market reforms is not simply a metaphor but very close to the truth. In connection with this topic, the question arises: how could the doubling of alcohol mortality occur without a substantial increase in consumption beyond the level of the early 1980s? The answer most likely should be related not to heavy drinkers but to moderate consumers, who constitute the majority of alcohol consumers.

Fig. 2-27: Alcohol consumption and mortalities from alcohol poisoning (1980–2001) in percentage terms with 1980 accepted as 100 %. $b_{x/y}$ – coefficients of regression for alcohol mortalities, 1984–1991, 1992–1997 and 1997–2001.

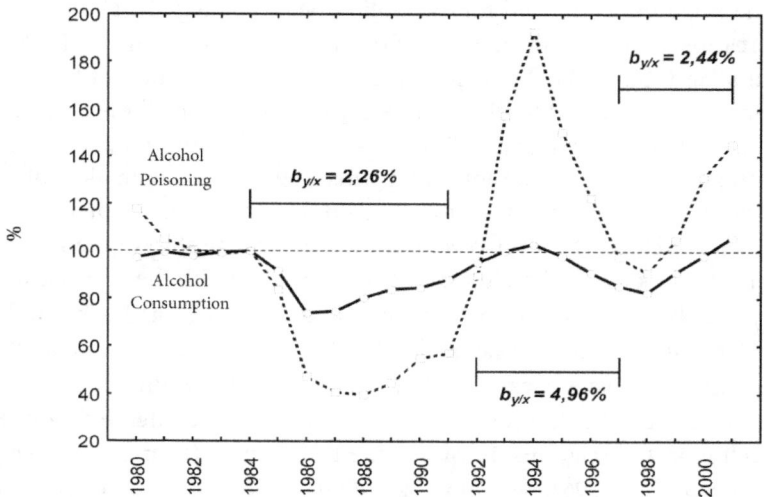

It has now been demonstrated that their contribution to the overall level of consumption is significant (Chapter 2-2). As a consequence of the just ended campaign and "inertia", they may have continued at a level of consumption lower than that of before the campaign, and this would have been reflected in the overall level.

There remains in circulation the idea that the "jump in mortality in the first half of the 90s, the much maligned 'Yeltsin genocide' was a creation; either there was no actual increase of mortality at the time or it was very small" (Vishnevsky, 2000). The author bases his conclusion on his calculation of what he considers the total for the two periods: the anti-alcohol campaign and the beginning of the market reforms (1985–1994). His calculations show that, for deaths in this period, "the 'average' man lived 133 days longer, and women lived 41 days longer". This extended time was a result of the anti-alcohol campaign, and with this as the basis, the jump in mortality in the first half of the 1990s can in no way be termed "an artificial creation" or, even worse, "compensatory". The mortality relation between men and women was that male mortality exceeded female mortality by 2–3 times. Is this not because before 1985 and after 1992, men consumed approximately three times more alcohol than women? Interestingly, the gender relation (sometimes rising to 4) is consistent in all studies of the mortality of men and women in Russia.

Alcohol mortality 1995–1998

For both overall mortality (Fig. 2-19) and mortalities connected to alcohol poisoning (Fig. 2-20), 1994 was a turning point, after which these indexes began to decline. The same dynamic held for alcoholic psychoses (Fig. 2-21) and deaths from pancreatitis. Deaths from cirrhosis of the liver began to decline in 1996, i.e., with a year's lag (Fig. 2-11). These four measures are tightly bound to alcohol consumption. However, in 1995–1996 there began a decline in all the basic kinds of deaths that are not, at first glance, linked to alcohol consumption (see the next section of this chapter). One can infer that, after 1994, a decline in alcohol consumption began in the country, amounting to 11.7 liters per capita in 1998 (Chapter 2-4), i.e., stood at a level lower than the level at the start of the 1980s.

One may also link the decline in alcohol consumption with the increase in life expectancy that began in 1995 for both men and women (Fig. 1-10; the State Statistical Committee of the Russian Federation). It is important to note that this increase occurred against a background of a significant worsening of the quality of life in terms of a decline in caloric intake and the protein content of food (Fig. 1-10), a decline in the relationship of income to expenses (from 8.3 percent in 1993 to 2.2 percent in 1996), an almost doubling of the number of unemployed (between 1992 and 1996) and increases in the amount of unpaid wages (from 0.9 percent of wages in 1992 to 11.7 percent in 1996; Gordon, 1997). It would seem that all this might have led to a shortening of life expectancy. Yet life expectancy rose. The most likely explanation for this is the decline in alcohol consumption that continued right up to 1998. In other words, for life expectancy at this time, lower alcohol consumption was a stronger factor than the substantial decline in the level and quality of life.

One of the possible causes of the decline in alcohol consumption and mortality in 1995–1998 may have been the deaths in 1992–1994 of a significant share of basic users, i.e., alcoholics and heavy drinkers, who, we know, consume a substantial share of the alcoholic beverages consumed in the country (Skog, 1985a). At the beginning of the 1990s, alcoholics, we assume, constituted 7 percent of the population, or 10 million individuals (Entin & Dineeva, 1996), and heavy drinkers were an even larger group (approximately 15, Simpura et al., 1997), which together comes to about 30 million individuals. The number of alcohol deaths in this cohort at the start of the market reforms would account for a drop of approximately 1 liter of per capita consumption. The wave of deaths occurred so rapidly (Fig. 1-11) that it could not be entirely compensated by new cohorts of alcoholics, as the formation of an alcoholic takes on average six (Nemtsov and Pokrovskaya, 1997) or more years of heavy drinking.

Of course, there are other factors involved in the cut in consumption. These include government measures to reduce imports and the domestic sale of surrogates as well as a certain degree of improved order in the alcohol market stemming from new laws (Chapter 1-8). It was probably such government activity that lay behind the small price increase on alcohol products in 1995–1997 relative to prices, for example, on food products (Fig. 1-8). The turning point for prices was 1994–1995, until which time prices for alcohol products were declining relative to other products, although prices on both kinds of products rose before, during and after this period.

An important factor in the decline of alcohol consumption in 1995–1998 might have been the impoverishment of the population and the drop in buying power reflecting unpaid wages, and thus cheap vodka might not have been accessible for a significant portion of consumers, which is even more likely in view of the increase in the relative price of alcohol (Fig. 1-8).

The period in which prices for alcoholic beverages "caught up" with prices on food products and other commodities was not long (1994–1997; Fig. 1-8). A new lag in the prices of spirits began in 1998 and was helped by the default (Chapter 1-8). This may be reflected in the new rise in alcohol consumption of 1999 (Fig. 2-7) and in associated effects (Fig. 2-11). There were other causes, too, for the new increase in consumption, which in 2000–2001 reached the level of 1984. Naturally, one links with this, though only in part, the new rise in human losses after 1998, in consequence of which mortality again reached the level forecast by the regression of 1965–1984 (Fig. 2-19).

Components of alcohol mortality

Up to now in this chapter, we have talked of overall deaths due to alcohol in the country. But it is important to know what diagnoses of death go into overall loss. For this, we look at the dynamics of the various major classes of deaths before, during and after the anti-alcohol campaign.

For men (Fig. 2-28a) in the period 1985–1986, there was a substantial decline in the level of almost all classes of death, which account for 77.8 percent of all deaths (Fig. 2-28a leaves out only "other illnesses", which also declined significantly for men in this period). The substantial decline in mortalities for women in this period occurred in the group of cardiovascular and external, including violent, causes of death (73 percent of all deaths in 1986–1991; Fig. 2-28b). For men and for women, neoplasms and infectious and parasitic diseases were the exception. The unchanged character of their trend during the anti-alcohol campaign indicates that they are not dependent on alcohol consumption or that dependence appears only after a very long lag.

Thus, the overwhelming majority of classes of death "responded" in the same manner; declining in the indexes for alcohol consumption at the start of the anti-alcohol campaign. It follows from this that many other types of deaths with non-alcohol diagnoses are linked to alcohol consumption. The London group of investigators postulated this for Russia earlier (for example, McKee & Britton, 1998; Chapter 2-3). By and large, these are deaths indirectly related to alcohol. At the same time, they can be seen as deaths hidden from the official statistics on the nation's alcohol losses.

Fig. 2-28 (a/b): Number of meaths of men (Fig. 2-28a.) and women (Fig. 2-28b.) from external causes (2), disease of respiratory system (3), cardiovascular system (4), digestive system (5), neoplasms + infections + parasitic diseases (6), and also overall number of deaths (1). «R» and «L» indicate the right and left ordinates, respectively (1965–1995).

Fig. 2-28a

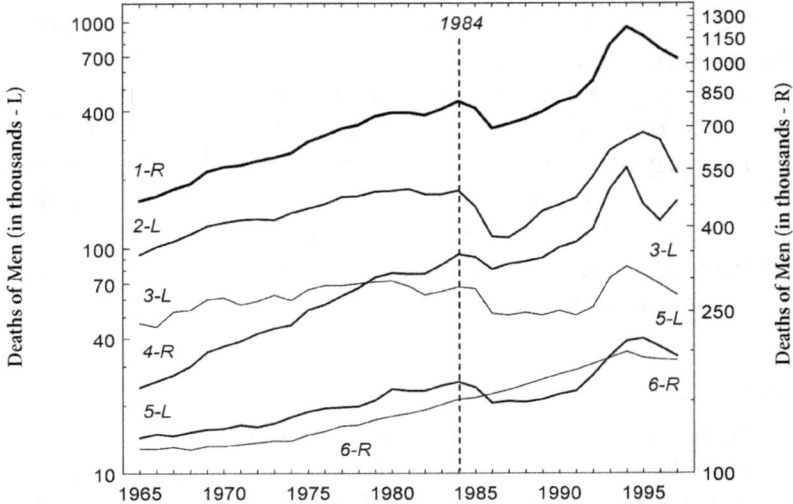

Fig. 2-28b

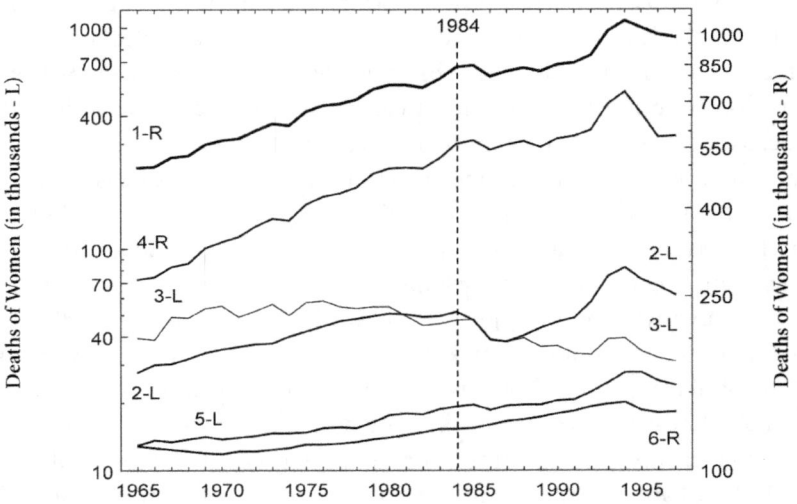

However, the decline in cardiovascular mortalities, for instance, in connection with the decline in the level of alcohol consumption does not mean that alcohol was implicated in all such deaths; more likely the tie is to some portion of them. It remains for us now to determine the portion of alcohol-related deaths that were diagnosed as non-alcohol-related. In other words, it is necessary to develop a quantitative estimate of alcohol's contribution to apparently non-alcohol-related mortalities in Russia.

In developed societies, the estimate of alcohol deaths is arrived at rather simply: the totals for the 10 types of deaths directly linked to alcohol abuse are added together (these types include, for example, alcohol gastritis and cirrhosis of the liver) and another 30 for which alcohol is considered to play a partial role in the cause of death (e.g., arterial hypertension, 8 percent of mortalities from which in the United States are alcohol-related; Schulz J. et al., 1991).

It is not possible in Russia to rely on foreign experience because many of the rubrics, including those pertaining to alcohol, are not included in the list of causes of death: Russian statistics allow for only 188 diagnoses of death, where abroad they number more than 900 and agree with the diagnosis of illness. Moreover, the size of alcohol's share in this or that type of death depends substantially on the level of consumption: higher consumption entails a higher share of responsibility.

There is yet another difficulty in determining the alcohol dependency of mortalities: very imprecise death diagnoses. Thus, deaths from alcohol cirrhosis of the liver rose by 5 times from 1999 to 2005 for men and 8 times for women, most likely because of a change in the criteria for the diagnosis. Even so, however, they constituted only one-third of all cirrhosis deaths, although in Western countries, where alcohol consumption is lower, they make up more than half of the diagnoses (Schulz. et al., 1991; Mäkelä., 1999).

This makes it impossible to come to a direct determination of the dimensions of alcohol mortalities. Therefore it is necessary to use an indirect method. Even here, however, there are uncertainties. While there have been fluctuations, some of them very large (4.5 liters), in alcohol consumption per capita in the past 20 years, they took place at a very high level of consumption, higher than 10 liters (Fig. 2-7). While the character of the link between consumption and mortality in the range of 0–10.5 liters is not known, 10.5 liters is very high per capita consumption and has its own special contribution to make to mortality.

One would have thought that data on the effects of consumption in the range of 0–10.5 liters would have been supplied by countries with low or comparatively low levels of consumption, from Spain (10.5 liters) Iceland (4.4 liters) for Europe and from Paraguay (4.3 liters) to Guatemala (approximately 1 liter) in Latin America (Global Status Report on Alcohol, 2004). But alcohol mortality not only depends on the level of consumption of alcohol, but also on a whole series of other factors which differ from country to country. Thus, foreign data on alcohol consumption and mortality cannot serve to explain the relationship of mortality and alcohol causes in Russia, with its quite different conditions. This is why, in the absence of any other, it has been necessary to work out an original method.

The method is based on the comparison of indexes for various types of mortality with estimates of alcohol consumption. Standardized indexes of mortality per 1 million of population were used (World Health Organization's new standard): for 1956–1964 (Mesle [Mille] et al., 2003), for 1965–1994 (Milleet al., 1996), after 1994 calculations done by E. M. Andreev (personal communication). Separate studies were made of socially significant types of death (alcohol poisonings, homicides and suicides) as well as deaths from pancreatitis. All other external causes of death were grouped separately under "other external causes" (road traffic accidents, drowning, deaths in fires and others), cirrhosis of the liver ("alcohol-related" and "other" as one group because of the very large undercount of alcohol cirrhosis cases). The various cardiovascular causes and all the causes not just listed ("other causes") account for a large number of the deaths. These eight classes (alcohol poisonings, homicides, suicides, other external causes, cirrhosis of the liver – alcohol-related and other – pancreatitis, cardiovascular causes and other causes) cover all mortalities. In addition, overall mortality was itself studied separately. Mortalities of men and women were considered separately. Thus, indexes of nine types of death over 22 years (1980–2001) were used as the basic data for the calculations.

The time limits of the analysis have been determined by the existence of estimates of actual alcohol consumption. As the index for consumption of alcohol for 1980–1994, figures from three sources averaged earlier (Nemtsov, 2000) are used. The estimate of alcohol consumption for 1995–2001 was presented in Chapter 2-4.

Characteristic for Russia in the past two decades have been significant fluctuations in the level of alcohol consumption and mortality caused by the anti-alcohol campaign and the market reforms that followed it. These fluctuations made it possible for us to calculate the contribution of alcohol to various forms of mortality. Every cloud has a silver lining.

Time series analysis presumes exclusion of the trend and other transient components in order that the remainders are, insofar as possible, analogous to "white noise" and can, thus, be comparable. To exclude the time linear trend, regressive dependencies of alcohol consumption and nine types of death on year were calculated, and these were subtracted from the original significances (Box & Jenkins, 1976).

Figure 2-29 gives a sketch of the procedure, showing the starting indexes for alcohol consumption and suicides (Fig. 2-29a) and those same indexes after exclusion of the linear trend (Fig. 2-29b). The result of the changes rids us of the difference in the slopes of the linear regressions, which might have given rise to errors in later calculations.

Fig. 2-29 (a/b): Relationship between suicides and alcohol consumption (1980–2001): Fig. 2-29a. – starting data, Fig 2-29b. – after exclusion of a linear trend.

Fig. 2-29a

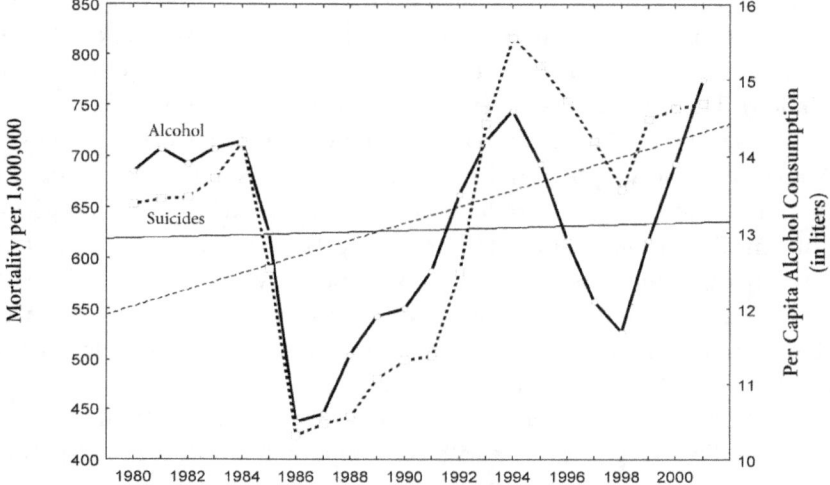

Fig. 2-29b

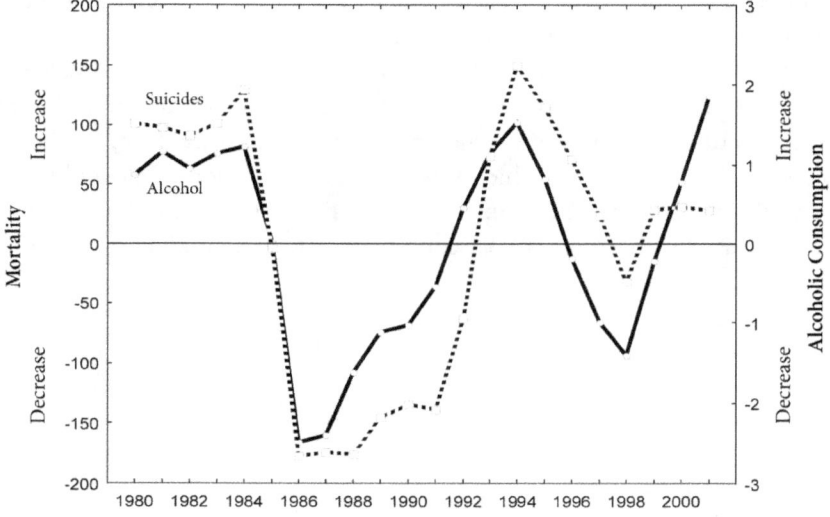

To exclude a time periodic trend in alcohol consumption and mortality, a model of first order "auto-regression – moving average" was constructed (Box & Jenkins,

1976) and, from the remainder after subtracting the linear trend, the estimate for the periodic trend was subtracted.

The choice of the model for further calculations was made on the basis of the correlation of the starting and transformed indexes of mortality with the starting and transformed estimates of alcohol consumption. Figure 2-30 shows the averaged indexes of the correlation of mortality and alcohol consumption. The figure shows that the indexes for various kinds of death correlate weakly with the official data of alcohol consumption (the State Statistical Committee of the Russian Federation). The correlation of overall mortality is generally insignificant.

In all cases, however, the correlation becomes significant when we move on to estimates of consumption and become even more so after exclusion of the linear trend. However, the correlation declines after exclusion of the periodic constituent. This means that this last procedure, typically used in studies of time series analyses, is unnecessary here because periodicity is an essential element of the processes of alcohol consumption and mortality in Russia (Fig. 2-29) in connection with the fluctuations of alcohol effects caused by the anti-alcohol campaign and the market reforms that followed.

A correlation analysis of the remaining types of mortality is presented in Table 15. It is clear that the greatest link with consumption lies with the model that excludes the linear trend. This is why further calculations are based on this model.

Table 14 presents the angular coefficients (B) derived from the regression equations on alcohol after the exclusion of the linear trend for men and women. It is important to emphasize that, in our case, the coefficients of correlation (B) reflect the dimensions linked to alcohol-related mortality per 1 liter of alcohol in the limits of 10.5–15 liters per capita consumption.

On average, the coefficients of regression for women are approximately 3–4 times less than the coefficients of regression for men. At the same time, the relationships to different types of mortalities differ substantially: from 2.3 for liver diseases to 11.5 for suicides, which reflects the contribution of alcohol to these types of deaths for men and women (Table 14). These relationships essentially reflect gender differences in alcohol's contributions to various kinds of mortalities.

Table 15: Correlation of various types of mortality with alcohol consumption (based on Spearman).

Forms of Mortality		Consumption According to Data Issued by the Russian State Statistics Committee		Raw Data		Following the Elimination of the Linear Trend		Following the Elimination of the Periodic Trend	
		R_s	p	R_s	p	R_s	p	R_s	p
Men	Alcohol Poisoning	0.485	0.022	0.844	0.000	0.894	0.000	0.649	0.001
	Homicide	0.008	ns	0.478	0.024	0.825	0.000	0.736	0.000
	Suicide	0.428	0.046	0.694	0.000	0.846	0.000	0.804	0.000
	Other External Causes	0.269	ns	0.654	0.000	0.872	0.000	0.684	0.000
	Liver Diseases	0.429	0.045	0.614	0.002	0.747	0.000	0.645	0.001
	Pancreatic Diseases	0.436	0.042	0.634	0.001	0.835	0.000	0.646	0.001
	Cardiovascular diseases	0.351	ns	0.609	0.002	0.749	0.000	0.629	0.001
	Other Causes	0.422	0.049	0.716	0.000	0.714	0.000	0.513	0.014
	Overall Mortality	0.326	ns	0.665	0.000	0.813	0.000	0.710	0.000
Women	Alcohol Poisoning	0.478	0.024	0.813	0.000	0.879	0.000	0.660	0.000
	Homicide	0.220	ns	0.619	0.002	0.831	0.000	0.731	0.000
	Suicide	0.730	0.000	0.729	0.000	0.741	0.000	0.495	0.019
	Other External causes	0.182	ns	0.586	0.004	0.843	0.000	0.657	0.000
	Liver Diseases	0.267	ns	0.562	0.006	0.743	0.000	0.645	0.001
	Pancreatic Diseases	0.202	ns	0.428	0.046	0.651	0.001	0.226	Ns
	Cardiovascular Diseases	0.297	ns	0.512	0.014	0.680	0.000	0.477	0.024
	Other Causes	0.443	0.038	0.603	0.002	0.616	0.002	0.453	0.034
	Overall Mortality	0.325	ns	0.593	0.003	0.701	0.000	0.506	0.016

ns – non significant

Fig. 2-30: Averaged coefficients of correlation for 9 kinds of mortalities and alcohol consumption according to figures from RussStat and estimates of consumption before and after the elimination of linear and periodic trends. The figures are the significance of differences from the official data (RussStat).

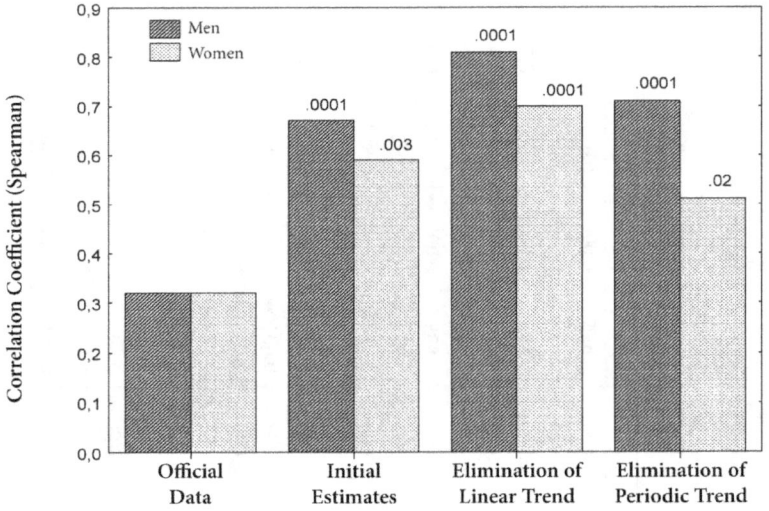

This is evidence that the estimates of consumption accepted for the work are, unlike the statistics of the State Statistical Committee of the Russian Federation, close to the reality. Relying on this feature of the estimates of consumption, the possibility of a substantial error on the low side is excluded (Chapter 2-4).

It may be asserted that mortality caused by an increase in per capita consumption from 10.5 to 15 liters is directly linked to alcohol (Fig. 2-31; triangles abc for alcohol poisonings and a'b'c' for suicides). However, as noted above, 10.5 liters of alcohol also contributes to alcohol mortalities. Determination of this contribution was the main task.

The following characteristics of the starting materials are the basis for the method. First is the linear dependence of all types of mortalities with the level of alcohol consumption within the limits of 10.5–15 liters per capita consumption (Table 14). This made it possible to use rather simply interpreted equations of linear regression. Second, indexes of mortality from alcohol poisoning, which are 100 percent dependent on alcohol abuse, were used as the base. Finally, it is also important for the method that the correlation of types of mortalities with estimates of consumption is of high significance (Table 14). The task is here solved simply for alcohol poisonings, since the rectangle *acde* also conforms to alcohol mortality, as alcohol poisoning obviously cannot take place without alcohol. The contribution of alcohol to deaths from alcohol poisoning is, conditionally, expressed as the relationship *bc/bd* (mortality due to an increase in per capita consumption of

Fig. 2-31: Diagram of calculations of alcohol-related mortality (explanation in text).

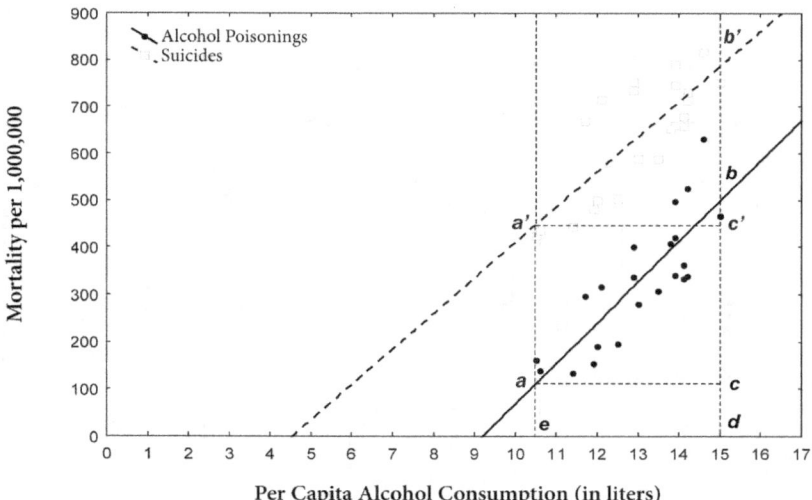

10.5–15 with maximum mortality at 15 liters). This relationship (0.762 for men and 0.789 for women) is accepted for 100 percent alcohol mortality in accord with the nature of this phenomenon. The contribution of alcohol to suicides can be expressed as the relationship $b'c'/b'd$ (Fig. 2-31).

The very same procedure was followed with the remaining types of mortality (Table 16, column 7) on the assumption that with respect to the other types of mortalities the same relationship reflects the share of mortality linked to alcohol. The share expressed in percentages, in turn, made possible calculation of the dimensions of alcohol mortalities in absolute terms (Table 16, column 9). These dimensions as well as the percentage expressions are the average for the period 1980–2001.

The main results (Table 16, columns 7 and 9) are represented in Figures 2-32a and 2-32b. Since direct confirmation of the calculations is not possible, it is important that, in both the percentage relationship (except for alcohol poisoning) and the absolute expression, the alcohol mortality of women is less than for men, which conforms to the gender differences in alcoholization. In share relationship, the alcohol mortality of women by suicide and diseases of the pancreas are half that for men and differs little from cirrhosis of the liver (Fig. 2-32a). The share of cardiovascular mortality linked to alcohol for women is only three fifths of that for men. However, in absolute terms, such deaths among men are in all 13.4 percent more than for women due to the fact that women with cardiovascular diagnoses die 1.5 times more often than men (Fig. 2-32b).

Table 16: Calculations and basic indexes of alcohol-related deaths in Russia, 1980–2001. Mortality change (number of deaths per million persons) by change in alcohol consumption (liter alcohol per capita).

Kinds of mortality	Raw data			Following Elimination of Linear Trend		(5)/(3)	Percent of Alcohol Mortality	Average Amount of Deaths (thousands)	
	Intercept	Coefficient of Linear Regressions	Maximal Mortality at 15 l	Coefficient of Linear Regressions	Accretion of a Mortality with 10.5 l up to 15 l			Total number	Alcohol-related
	1	2	3	4	5	6	7	8	9
Men									
Alcohol Poisoning	-788.5	85.7	497.6	84.26	379.2	0.762	100.0	21.9	21.9
Homicide	-428.1	56.2	414.5	51.56	232.0	0.560	73.5	20.4	15.0
Suicide	-341.0	75.1	786.0	73.22	329.5	0.419	55.0	39.5	21.7
Other External Causes	-1229.7	229.0	2205.0	219.07	985.8	0.447	58.7	112.7	66.1
Liver Diseases	-95.2	23.4	256.4	22.25	100.1	0.390	51.2	10.9	5.6
Pancreatic Diseases	-37.8	7.2	70.7	6.77	30.5	0.431	56.6	3.3	1.8
Cardiovascular Diseases	4082.2	593.1	12979.0	562.09	2529.4	0.195	25.6	404.0	103.3
Other Causes	3948.0	178.3	6623.1	177.09	796.9	0.120	15.8	305.4	48.3
Overall Mortality	5110.0	1248.1	23832.2	1196.31	5383.4	0.226	29.6	918.0	272.1
Women									
Alcohol Poisoning	-206.6	21.9	122.5	21.5	96.7	0.789	100.0	6.2	6.2
Homicide	-111.0	15.6	123.4	14.6	65.5	0.531	67.3	7.1	4.7
Suicide	42.6	6.2	135.4	6.4	28.6	0.211	26.8	9.5	2.6
Other External Causes	-113.8	42.2	519.4	39.3	177.0	0.341	43.2	33.5	14.4
Liver Diseases	-42.0	10.4	114.4	9.6	43.1	0.377	47.8	7.6	3.6
Pancreatic Diseases	11.5	1.1	28.3	1.0	4.5	0.159	20.2	2.1	0.4
Cardiovascular Diseases	4762.0	241.4	8382.6	226.0	1017.0	0.121	15.4	592.6	91.1
Other Causes	2132.2	46.8	2833.7	47.9	215.5	0.076	9.6	245.1	23.5
Overall Mortality	6475.0	385.6	12259.7	366.2	1648.1	0.134	17.0	903.6	153.9

2-5: ALCOHOL MORTALITY

Fig. 2-32 (a/b): Relationship of alcohol's contribution to various kinds of death for men and women in percentage terms; Fig. 2-32b. Relationship of alcohol-related and overall deaths in men and women.

Fig. 2-32a

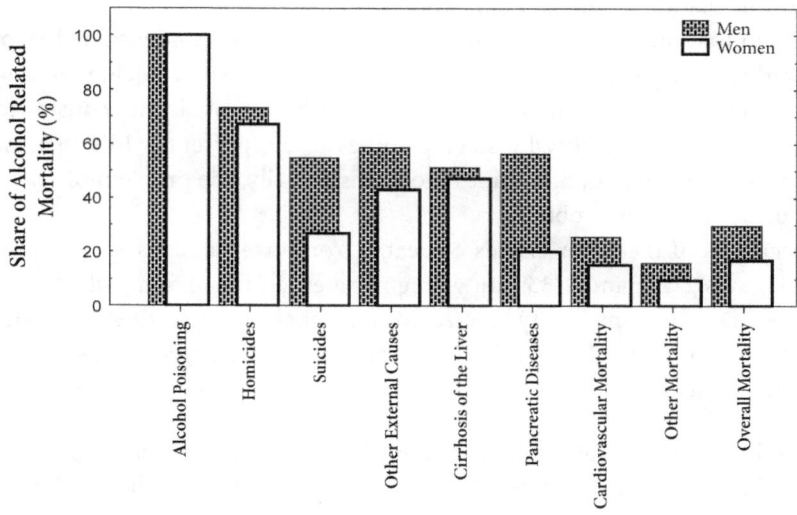

Fig. 2-32b

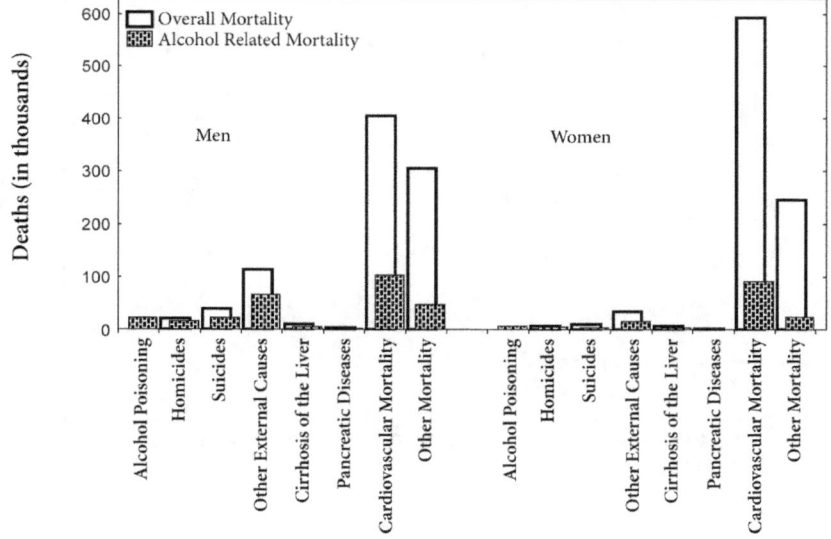

The high share of alcohol mortalities among homicides is striking, especially as the share is barely less for women than for men – in Russia 7 of 10 homicides are linked, one way or another, to alcohol. This is close to the data of the Judicial-Medical Expertise panels on the share of dead with alcohol in their blood (see below).

Suicides in relation to alcohol consumption substantially differ from homicides. First, in that only half of the suicides of women are dependent on alcohol as compared with suicides of men (Fig. 2-32a). The frequency of suicides among women is 25 percent of that among men. The contribution of alcohol consumed by women to overall mortality by suicide comes to 5.5 percent, while that for men comes to 44.3 percent (eight times more). Essentially, the problem of "alcohol and suicide" is a male problem.

The dynamics of the other classes of deaths from external causes are represented in Figures 2-33a and 2-33b. In women and especially in men, all the major forms of this type of mortality reacted with declines to the decline in alcohol consumption at the start of the anti-alcohol campaign and increases at the start of the market reforms.

Fig. 2-33 (a/b): Dynamics of basic types of deaths from external causes in men (Fig. 2-33a.) and women (Fig. 2-33b.), 1956–2003 (WHO new standard). 1 – suicide, 2 – other accidents, 3 – drowning, 4 – automobile injuries, 5 – homicide, 6 – causes unspecified.

Fig. 2-33a

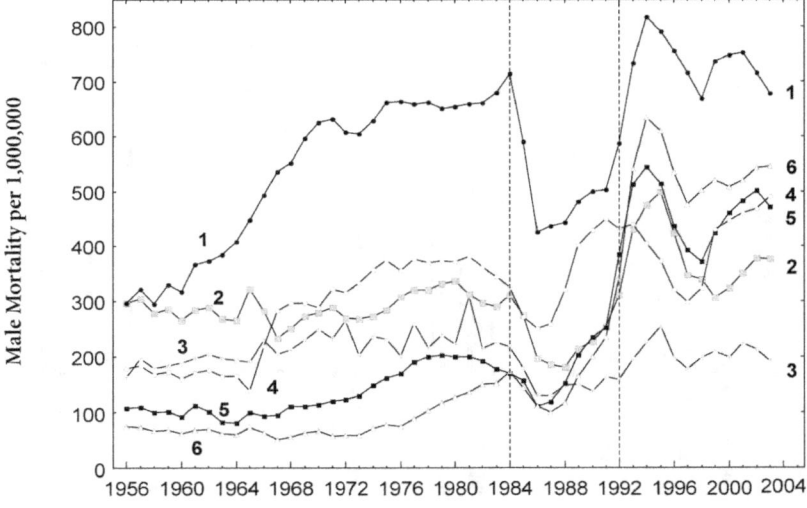

Fig. 2-33b

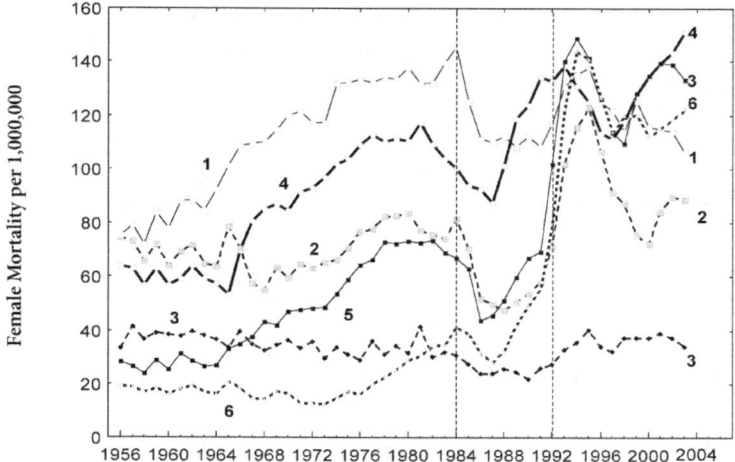

The highest contribution to alcohol mortality is from cardiovascular diseases (or diagnoses) – 194,400 deaths a year, although the share of these deaths in overall cardiovascular mortality is relatively small (19.4 percent). This is more than the contribution of all external causes (152,600) despite the very high share of participation by alcohol in such deaths (60.8 percent). The dependence of particular forms of cardiovascular deaths on alcohol consumption is represented in Figure 2-34.

The only thing that can be considered new is that alcohol's role is so paramount. The first to write about the importance of alcohol was probably Solomatin (1988), who showed, using a great deal of material, a direct link with alcohol of a significant portion of incidents of sudden death from ischemic heart disease. Later, Virganskaya (1991 wrote about the dependence of cardiovascular deaths on alcohol, and later still there were the English researchers (Chenet et al., 1998b; McKee & Britton, 1998). They found that in Moscow most deaths from cardiovascular diseases occur from Saturday through to Monday and linked this with the period of maximum consumption of alcohol. In the view of the English authors, the character of alcohol consumption in binge drinking has a special significance for cardiovascular mortalities in Russia. Now this indirect evidence has been applied to the entire population. The results have additional significance in that, for a long time, alcohol was thought of as a heart-protector. It is now known that this particular characteristic of alcohol manifests itself with very small doses consumed but, with high doses, alcohol emerges as a cardiopathogenetic factor (the so-called J-dependence, review McKee & Britton, 1998).

The main result of the calculations is more dramatic still: overall mortalities linked to alcohol amount to 426,000 a year, or 23.4 percent of all deaths (average for 1980–2001). Of this, 63.9 percent of the alcohol losses are men (272,100).

Fig. 2-34 (a/b): Dynamics of basic types of cardiovascular deaths in men (Fig. 2-34a.) and women (Fig. 2-34b.), (1970–2003) (WHO new standard). 1 – other deaths, 2 – other heart diseases, 3 – strokes with hypertension, 4 – strokes without hypertension, 5 – other types of ischemic heart disease without hypertension, 6 – cardio- and atherosclerosis with hypertension, 7 – general cardiovascular mortalities. Linear trend excluded.

Fig. 2-34a

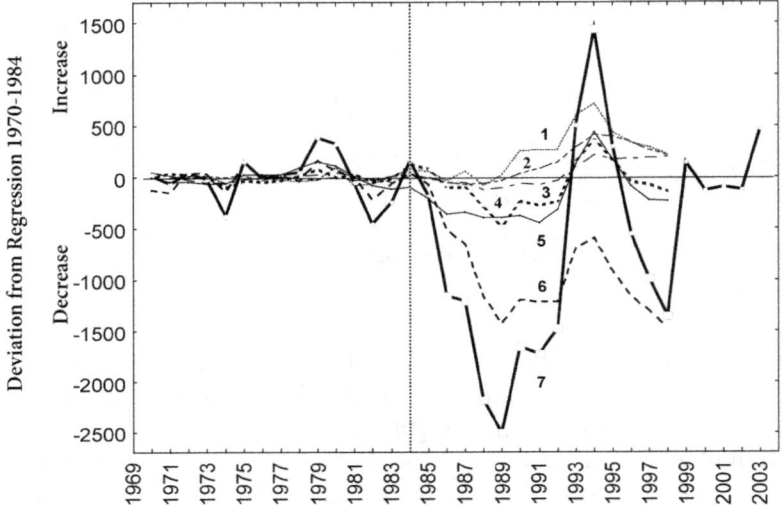

Fig. 2-34b

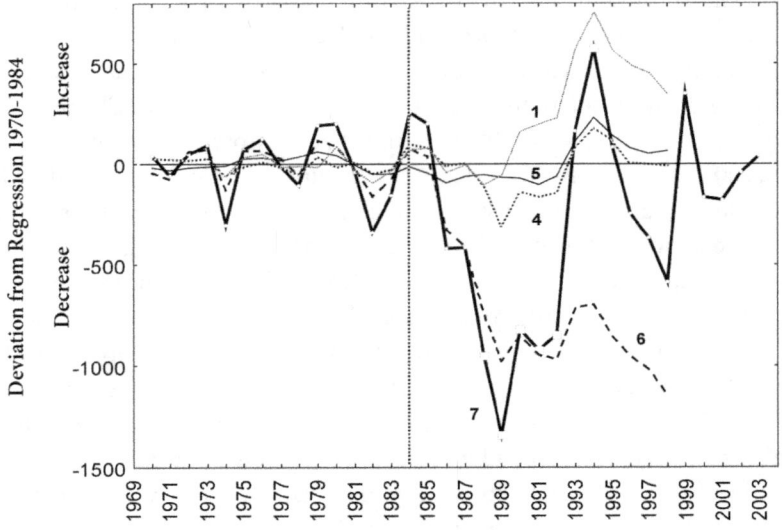

For comparison: 16–17 percent of all deaths in Russia are linked to tobacco smoking (Tkachenko, 1996; Kamardina, 2004; Table 17), which is also terrifyingly many. Official statistics on deaths from "causes associated with consumption of alcohol" in 2001 came to 3.8 percent of deaths, i.e., were a seventh of the estimated actual losses.

It is important once again to note that 426,000 is the sum of direct and indirect losses in which alcohol is either the principal or, as is more often the case, an accompanying cause of death. Strictly speaking, such a division is academic. Most of those who die as a result of alcohol poisoning (direct losses) carry within themselves, as a rule, several illnesses acquired through the abuse of alcohol (Ugryumov, 1997). Such pathologies substantially increase the risk of death from the next, often relatively small, dose of alcohol (Naubatov, 1990; Khotimskaya & Lukash, 1989; Veljkovic et al., 1989). The academic nature of the division is especially clear in terms of individuals. It matters nothing to the victim how one characterizes his early death from alcohol – as "direct" or "indirect".

Table 17: Share of mortalities associated with tobacco-, alcohol and drug use (in percentage of overall mortality) and alcohol consumption (in liters per person per year) in Canada, the United States and Russia.

	Canada		USA	Russia	
	1992^a	1995^b	1995^c	1984–1992	1994–2001
Tobacco	17.1	16.5	18.8	17.0^d (1990)	16.3^e (1994)
Alcohol	3.5	3.1	4.4	22.1	25.6^f
Drugs	0.4	0.4	1.6	–	0.2^f
Alcohol Consumption	6.9	6.5	6.8	12.2	13.4

a Single et al. (1999), b Single et al. (2000), c McGinnis & Foege (1999), d Tkachenko(1996), e Kamardina (2004) and f Data from the Ministry of Home Affairs indicates that there are 3 500 deaths (the recalculation in percentage points was performed by the author)

Recently, a detailed study of the causes of death of all men between the ages of 25 and 54 over a two-year period was conducted in Izhevsk (a total of 1,700 individuals; Leon et al., 2007, Tomkins et al., 2007). It was discovered that 43 percent of the deaths were linked to alcohol abuse. Extrapolation of the Izhevsk results to the entire Russian male population for this age group gives 170,000 deaths linked to alcohol (Leon et al., 2007). It should be noted in this connection, too, that, while 25–54-year-old men are the heaviest drinking part of the Russian male population, they are far from the total number of alcohol abusers (Fig. 1-11). Second, the research focused on city dwellers, but the rural population consumes more alcohol in larger doses (Zaigraev, 2004). With this taken into account, the number of deaths of men of all ages linked to alcohol given by this study (272,000) is in agreement with the findings in Izhevsk.

Besides the summary quantity of deaths linked to alcohol, an important indicator is the share held by alcohol in mortalities. In Russia, every third male and every sixth female death is linked to alcohol (direct and indirect losses).

Homicides and suicides, regional data

It is always desirable to confirm one's calculations using independent methods. This is all the more desirable when the matter concerns human behavior, especially extreme and socially significant behavior such as homicide and suicide. Unfortunately, one cannot always in such situations check one's calculations by a non-mathematical method of any kind. But with respect to homicides and suicides, there is such a possibility.

This arose as a result of the data obtained from the Bureaus of Judicial-Medical Expertise covering eight regions of Russia with a total population of 17.5–18.2 million persons (Amur region, Bashkortostan and Kemerovsk, Novgorod, Orlovsk, Saratov and Sakhalin regions and St Petersburg). In addition to overall numbers of homicide and suicide victims for 1981–1990, the data included information on the presence or absence of alcohol in the blood and other biological information about the victims but lacked, unfortunately, their gender. The information made it possible to study the dynamic of the relationship of the number of homicides and suicides with the amount of alcohol found in the body.

The initial averaged figures for these regions, on the level of homicides and suicides, were practically the same as the all-Russia figures. Only consumption of alcohol in the eight regions had declined slightly more than the average for all of Russia, by 32.5 percent versus 26.1 percent. It is unlikely that so small a difference would make a substantial difference for our purposes.

In the period 1981–1990, 21,930 homicides were recorded in the eight regions. For 1981–1984, homicides with alcohol in their blood came to 64.1 ± 0.5 percent. In these years, in the eight regions as in other regions, there was a decline in the number of homicides, both of those with alcohol in the blood and of sober individuals (Fig. 2-35a; preceding this was a three-year period of stability after an increase). With the start of the campaign, the trend of homicides of sober individuals remained unchanged right up to 1987, and it was only in 1988 that a substantial rise in this indicator began. In contrast with this, the level of homicides with alcohol in the blood deviated downward in 1986–1987 from the linear regression for 1981–1984 and then significantly in the upward direction beginning in 1989. This means that the anti-alcohol campaign substantially influenced the lowered level of intoxicated homicide victims (by 26.8 percent in 1987) in contrast with sober homicide victims. In 1987 the share of homicide victims with alcohol in the blood was 58.8 percent as against 64.1 percent in 1981–1984. The data for the eight regions show that the decrease in homicides during the campaign occurred because of the decline in intoxicated homicide victims.

Fig. 2-35 (a/b): Mortalities by homicide (Fig. 2-35a.) and suicide (Fig. 2-35b) sober (3) and with alcohol in blood (1) in 8 regions of Russia (1981–1990). Alcohol consumption in the same regions (2). Squares represent significant differences from regressions of indexes for 1981–1984.

Fig. 2-35a

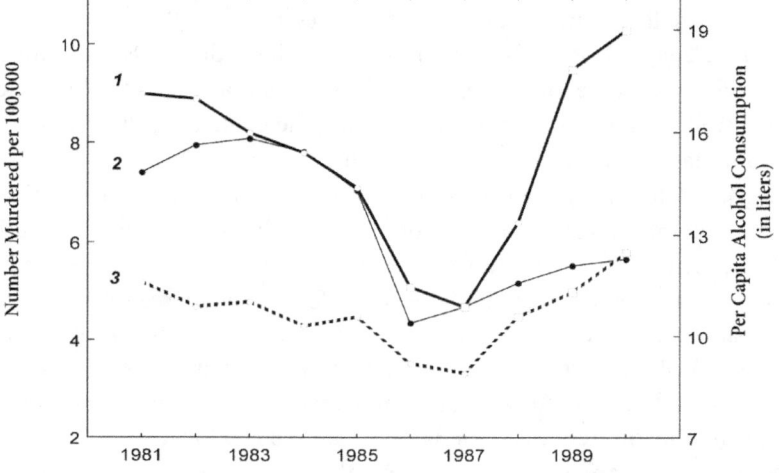

Fig. 2-35b

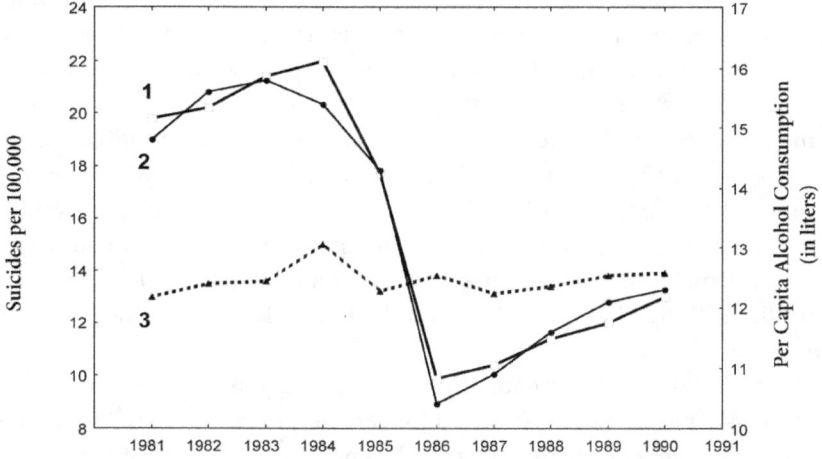

Socioeconomic factors were the main reason for the rise in the level of homicides after 1987, a time of wars between criminal factions and the start of the re-division of property (Chapter 1-6). But the data from the eight regions show that the role of alcohol remained very significant during the period of the first incidents of these wars; the increase in the number of intoxicated homicide victims occurred twice as fast as that for homicides of sober victims (for 1987 to 1989, by 101.3 percent and 52.3 percent, respectively). This example shows that negative social processes, especially such sinister acts as homicides, are very tightly linked to alcohol consumption, which to a significant degree modulates this type of criminality.

It is critical that the decrease in intoxicated homicide victims in 1985–1987 was relatively small (taking account of the regression for 1981–1984, by 23.5 percent, Fig. 2-35a). Most likely, this means that the individuals from among whom such victims can be found were less affected than others by the limitations on the accessibility of alcoholic beverages during the campaign; they were more active about obtaining spirits than other citizens.

Now, using the data for the eight regions, we can compare the calculated (Table 16) and the actual indicators. The share of homicides linked to alcohol in Russia, calculated on the basis of the regression for 1980–2001 for men and women, was on average 71.6 percent, which is higher than for the eight regions (61.4 percent). This difference may be mostly a function of the difference in the periods analyzed: 1981–1990 versus 1980–2001. There was a steep increase in homicides in the latter period and, as shown above, mostly due to intoxicated homicides. For this reason, the difference cannot have substantial significance.

Second, homicides are a two-way process: there is no victim without a killer. The significance of alcohol for the level of homicides reflects not only the homicide victim with alcohol in his blood but killers who were intoxicated (Fig. 2-36, line 3; data for Russia). Their dynamic was in synchronic phase with both alcohol consumption and total number of homicides (Fig. 2-35a, line 1). For Russia, intoxicated killers made up 72.9 percent of those apprehended in this period. At the same time, it should be noted that the risk of apprehension for people who commit the crime while intoxicated is higher than for sober individuals and, thus, their share of apprehended killers may be higher than in the whole cohort of killers. What is important here is that the killer in an intoxicated condition may kill a sober person. This killing will be, therefore, associated with alcohol. Thus the calculated measure of the contribution of alcohol to homicides does not conflict with the data from the Judicial-Medical Expertise panels and criminal practice.

There are no data for homicides from the eight regions for 1990–2001. Moreover all-Russia measures of victims and killers do not help clarify the situation: the number of homicide victims sharply declined, and the share of apprehended intoxicated killers steadily declined beginning in 1992, both against a background of higher and of lower alcohol consumption. Most likely, this is indicative of a decline in the quality of official record-keeping. For this reason, we must rely only on the calculated indexes (Table 16), which show that in Russia the real contribution of alcohol to homicides was very high and close to 70 percent.

Fig. 2-36: Number of dead (1), registered homicides (2), murderers in state of intoxication (3) or sober (4) (1980–1999). Squares represent significant differences from 1980–1984 regressions.

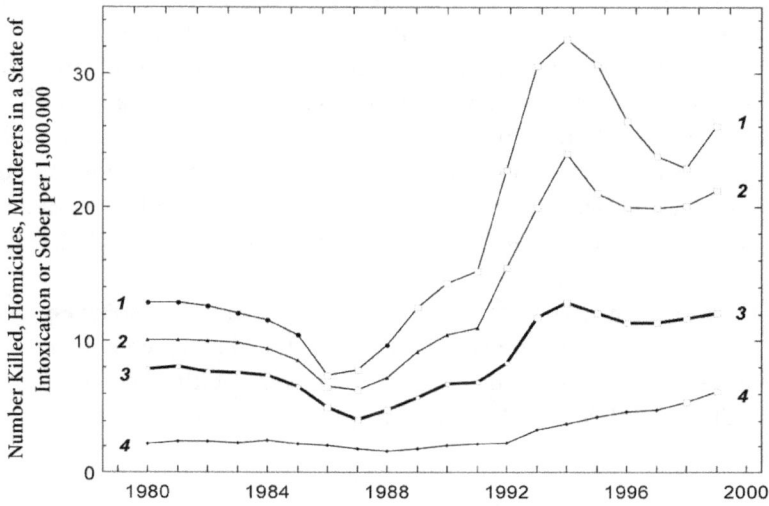

It is possible to compare the calculations of the alcohol component of suicides, done on the basis of the regression (Table 16), with the data for the eight regions. In these regions in 1981–1992 approximately 60,000 fatal suicides were recorded. Before the start of the campaign, in 1981–1984, alcohol was found in the blood of 60.2 percent of the suicides. From the start of the campaign, the number of such suicides changed almost synchronously with change in alcohol consumption and substantially declined from 22 per 100,000 of population in 1984 to 9.9 per 100,000 of population in 1986 (by 55 percent; Fig. 2-35b). In 1985–1990, the average index of suicides with alcohol in their blood was 53.3 percent, which is close to the calculated figure for Russia, if we bring it to a single type for men and women (49.5 percent). The difference can be explained, besides by the difference in the periods analyzed, by the fact that some of the suicides drank alcohol "for courage", thus raising the proportion of suicides with alcohol in the blood.

It is important to note that the level of sober individuals committing suicide in the eight regions during the anti-alcohol campaign went practically unchanged (Fig. 2-35b). This once again attests to the fact that the decline in mortality, specifically from suicide, during perestroika cannot be explained by "social optimism", as has been thought by native researchers (Gilinsky & Rumyantseva, 1998) as well as foreign researchers (Wasserman & Värnik, 1998). Moreover, a national optimism evoked by perestroika remains an entirely unproved presumption; most likely, it is a self fulfilling prophesy by the educated portion of society (including scientists) on the entire Russian population, for whom any perestroika of their accustomed life creates additional tension.

Estimates of the contribution of alcohol to various forms of death were done earlier only by American researchers (Schultz et al., 1990) and in slightly altered form by others (Stinson et al., 1993). Naturally, both forms of research estimated the contribution of alcohol to mortalities from alcohol poisoning identically, as 100 percent. These estimates are lower than the Russian ones. Thus, in the United States, for the population from the age of 15 years, the share of suicides linked to alcohol was 28 percent and for homicides 46 percent. That is though taking account of the fact that alcohol consumption per capita in the United States is significantly lower (8 liters, average for 1979–1989) than in Russia (12.8 liters, average for 1980–1989).

Nor do the relationships agree for alcohol-related homicides and suicides: 1.64 in the U.S. but 0.89 in Russia. In other words, in the U.S. homicides predominate, while in Russia suicides predominate. Most likely, this is linked to differences in socioeconomic and cultural conditions in the two countries.

* * *

The results of the calculation of mortalities in Russia associated with alcohol are so high as to make one wonder – can they be believed? If almost a quarter of deaths (23.4 percent) are linked to alcohol and almost one-fifth with smoking, where is there room for such major categories of deaths as cardiovascular deaths, which make up more than half of all mortalities? Here we must draw a line between deaths of which the sole cause is cardiovascular disease and deaths diagnosed as cardiovascular with a concealed alcohol factor as the sole (in instances of diagnostic falsification) or supplemental but substantial cause of death (Chapter 2-3). It has been shown that chronic alcohol intoxication shortens the life-expectancy of men with diseases of the cardiovascular system by an average of 17 years (Virganskaya, 1991). In exactly the same way, a significant portion of other somatic diagnoses are linked to alcohol abuse. Thus, alcohol mortality "is spread" through various diagnostic groups (Table 16), but, in sum, constitutes a significant part of overall mortality, varying in different periods with changes in the level of alcohol consumption.

This is the way the problem looks through the lens of population. On the individual level, various external dangers and internal diseases often coexist. The result is that internal ailments that arise independently of or as a result of the toxic effects of smoking or alcohol abuse take several years off the life in question. Overall, these years are just those 15–17 years by which Russian men have shorter life expectancies than men in the European countries studied.

To judge the dimensions of alcohol mortality in Russia, one can compare the Russian data on the share of alcohol mortalities with the analogous indexes for the United States (Stinson et al., 1993; McGinnis & Foege, 1999) and for European countries (Ramstedt, 2002). The complete (direct and indirect) alcohol losses in the U.S. at the beginning of the 1980s ranged from 105,000 (Stinson et al., 1993) to 200,000 (Mocher, 1988) by various measures, or from 5 percent to 9 percent of all mortalities, with consumption at 8.2–8.3 liters of alcohol. In the 1990s alcohol losses in the U.S. dropped further (Table 17). The figures are consistent with the Russian figures, if one takes into account both direct and all indirect alcohol losses.

Ramstedt (2002) researched alcohol mortality in European countries, where diagnoses of such mortalities are made significantly more reliably than in Russia. Ramstedt counted only direct alcohol losses, but his list of diagnoses included all somatic diseases linked to alcohol abuse. It is possible that some small portion of indirect losses are not taken into account in this work, but the results are close to the estimate of total alcohol losses for the U.S., where, it is true, consumption is lower than in Europe.

Fig. 2-37: Alcohol-related mortalities in 9 European countries and in Russia (1995) (percentage of alcohol-related deaths in overall mortality of persons aged 15+). Figures over each bar represent life expectancy in each country. For European countries: mortalities based on Ramstedt, M. (2002), alcohol consumption based on Lindberg, J. (1999). For Russia: mortality and consumption, see Chapters 2-4 and 2-5.

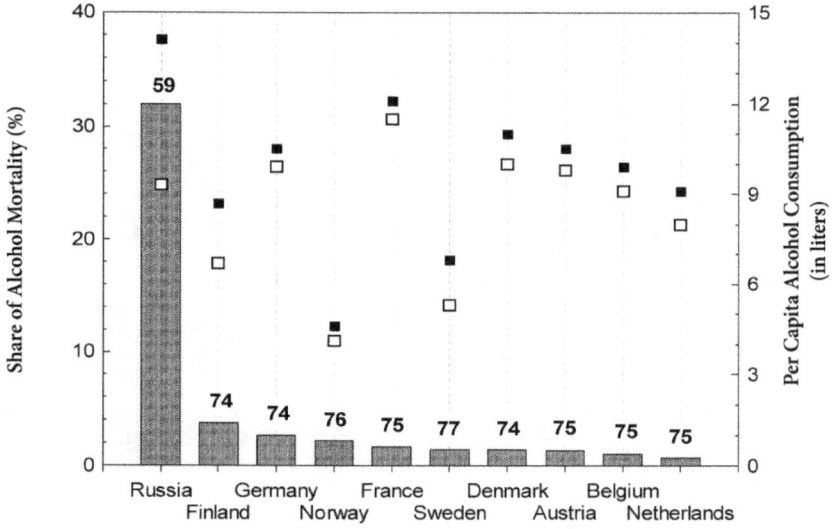

Taking account of these special features, Ramstedt's figures may be compared with the Russian (Fig. 2-37; the Russian indexes are recalculated for the population from the age of 15 years and older, the population used in Ramstedt's work): Russia, 32.2 percent, next, and with the highest index in Europe, Finland,

3.7 percent. Is it possible that alcohol mortalities in the two countries can differ by almost 10 times with a 1.5 times difference in consumption? To show that the estimate of alcohol mortalities in Russia is, nonetheless, meaningful, as we can compare the figures on life-expectancy for men in Russia (59 years), in the European countries (74–77 years) and also in the U.S. (74 years): the difference comes to 15–18 years, i.e., almost one-third taken from the lives of Russian men. However, the difference in alcohol mortality between Russia, the U.S. and the countries of Europe is not just a function of average per capita consumption. It also reflects the conditions and quality of life, including the quality of nutrition, medical services and much else that works to counter the toxic effects of alcohol. The heavy character of consumption in Russia, which differs from the character of consumption in Europe, the greater toxicity of illegal alcoholic beverages and the very large share of hard liquor among beverages consumed all contribute to this difference. Finally, the population of Russia is sharply distinguished by its lack of concern for its own health. There is a gloomy saying on this point: The American senses his illness five years before it begins, but the Russian starts treatment five days before death. This, essentially, is what Fyodor Abramov was writing about when he said (1972): "the historic trouble of Russia is that we learn to die before we learn to live".

Conclusion

One must give our history since 1985 its due. At no other time has the alcohol fate of Russia and the alcohol history of the country been so crammed, tense and contradictory. Never in its entire history did our state derive so little income from so much consumed in drinking. In 1992 the government separated itself from the monopoly on wines and liquors for the first time since 1894. It did so, on the basis of a badly misconstrued concept of liberalism. The cost was millions lost from the budget and tens of thousands added to the death toll.

Under any circumstances, a government must take into account the specific role and harmful aspects of a commodity like alcoholic beverages. The Soviet government forgot this when it relied on a quintupling of vodka sales over 30 years to solve its postwar and later economic problems. In 1979 average per capita alcohol consumption of alcohol from government sources reached its maximum (10.6 liters a year). Consumption of samogon increased that figure by one-third. In 1984, on the eve of the anti-alcohol campaign, alcohol consumption was at a record high for Russia, and the country surpassed France as Europe's leading consumer of alcohol. The chief culpability for the seriousness of today's alcohol situation in Russia lies with the Soviet government.

A significant portion of responsibility also lies with the "architects of perestroika" and the leaders after the dismantling of the Soviet Union. In 1985 and in 1992 the government ignored what was known about alcohol and its unique features. The voluntaristic and amateur alcohol policy of these years set in motion the wavelike fluctuations in consumption that will be a long time yet in finding a point of balance at some high or, more precisely, very high level.

The alcohol situation is a basic element of the economic and political life of the country. Accordingly, the country's alcohol history cannot be isolated from its general history. Processes taking place in the spheres of alcohol production, the alcohol market and alcohol consumption are a particular reflection of general processes taking place in the country, they are a particular manifestation of the moving forces in its history.

The words on the milestones marking the path of Russian history since 1985 read: *uskorenie* (speeding-up), *perestroika, glasnost', razryadka* (relaxation of tensions), and the collapse of the USSR, market reforms and privatization. The first in the series – uskoreniye (1985–1987) – was a typically Soviet attempt to mobilize the population. But in December 1999 Boris Yeltsin handed over to

Vladimir Putin a nation with a new economic (oligarchic capitalism) and political (bureaucratic oligarchy) system.

Both before and after, the development of the country proceeded on a path of ever-increasing bureaucratization and corruption of the government. Contemporary Russia has twice the number of state employees of the Soviet period. Government is increasingly closed in upon itself, occupied with the resolution of corporate tasks, competition between groups of influence, redistribution of state and now, increasingly, private property. Those in power live in another Russia, in their own "special economic zone", behind high fences and far from the people. The misdoings of the Russian political elite and its games of tug o' war (with a rope of gold, we observe) have been weakening the central government and, consequently, freeing centrifugal forces and separatist tendencies and even the nation's potential for protest. To oppose and control this, "managed democracy", "vertical power" and a revival of imperial traditions have been found necessary. This unusually large concentration of power was already burdensome for the country. On top of this came the confusion of petrodollars out of the blue, the accumulation of which brought a shift from a broad economic policy to a narrowly financial one and legalization of the export of capital abroad.

We have reached the point where "the state is the private property of the bureaucrats" (Karl Marx). At the end of the 1990s, oligarchic-bureaucratic capitalism was aware of its ability to survive and its independence from the population of the country. "No one needs the people", as an anonymous Pskov peasant justly said in a radio interview in 2002. Once again people joked, as they had a century before, that "at the bottom is the power of darkness but at the top is the darkness of power", although neither time was a time for jokes.

The inner concerns and clan struggles of the ruling elite distract it from its principal function – professional management of the state for the good of the people and, first of all, for the largest number of them. This has always been the basis for the strength and prosperity of the nation. But "managed democracy" and "vertical power" turned out to be ineffective in this regard. Few of the people have benefited: 36 million of our citizens do not have running water at home and 42 million are without indoor toilets. In a nation with the richest reserves and production of natural gas, half of all homes are not equipped for gas. Compared with 10 years ago, "the statistically average citizen of Russia eats 30 percent worse" (A. Gordeev, Russia's Minister of Agriculture, 2002).

Some 20 percent of the population live in terrible poverty, below the official poverty line, and most of these people (70 percent) are in families with children. Another 40 percent also lives in poverty; their incomes are less than what is actually needed to live. In total, that is 70–80 million people. And for many of these people, "poverty" has become "chronic", with all the psychological health issues that it entails. Especially frightening is the chronic poverty of working people whose labor goes uncompensated. In recent years the population has been told that life is steadily improving, stability has been achieved, the economy is growing and poverty is retreating. The trump card is a rising GNP. But the share of wages in GNP is declining: 32 percent in 2003, 30.4 percent in 2004 and 28.5 percent in 2005 on average. Furthermore, the additions to income that are based on GNP for the top and bottom 10 percent of the population differ by a factor of 40 but their incomes by a factor of 36 (Shevyakov, 2007).

With respect to alcohol, it is not only important how people live but how they perceive their lives.

> The main thing that has entered our lives in the past 10–15 years is persistent fear... Russians fear tomorrow. In early 2000, 57 percent said so, in June 2004, 63 percent and in December 67 percent. Instability is the chief phobia of our society. People also fear arbitrary action on the part of the government. (Levada, 2004)

These fears and poverty cause additional tension and a desire to drink in order to temporarily relieve the tension. Need we be surprised by the increasing nostalgia for Soviet times? The heightened feeling for the past is the other side of dissatisfaction with the present and lack of trust in the future.

The following observations may be added:

> Respondents feel a sense of shame more often than a sense of national pride. Reasons for pride in their country among Russians are mostly found 'outside' and mostly in the heroic-victorious sphere of the past (victory in the war, space flight). But reasons for shame are found mostly in daily life (material difficulties, obvious social ulcers), i.e., the lowest sphere of daily existence. As long as Russians find their reasons for pride in their country far-off and remember them only on holidays and see the causes of their shame in front of them every day, they will live with a dominant feeling of shame". (Foundation for Public Opinion, P. Bavin, Feb. 14, 2002)

And with that they find yet more reason to drink.

During two periods in recent history – in 1992–1994 and in 1999–2001 – Russia experienced unusually steep increases in deaths from alcohol poisoning (Fig. 1-12). This is the one index of the negative aspects of the alcohol situation that has been noted in the peripheral vision of the government. That would have been the time, in 1993 or 1999, for stepped-up government action to stop these deaths from drink. The government however was otherwise occupied – in 1993 a desperate struggle for power and wealth was underway, and 1999 was a time of leapfrog among prime ministers as President Yeltsin sought a successor. If not in 1993, then 1999 was the time to launch an alcohol policy that would at a minimum:

- limit sales of spirits by time (e.g., from 10 a.m. to 10 p.m.), by age (from 18) and by place (e.g., no more than one sales point per square kilometer in cities and no closer than 1 kilometer to educational institutions and, in rural areas, no closer than 5 kilometers by road to the nearest settlement);
- impose severe fines for violations of these rules, and especially severe for the sale of spirits to children and adolescents;
- introduce more severe legal sanctions on the illegal production and sale of spirits with mandatory full or partial confiscation of property;
- introduce administrative sanctions on local organs of the Interior Ministry and police that permit underground production and sale of spirits in their areas;
- introduce more severe fines and administrative and juridical sanctions for driving while intoxicated;
- increase the number and widen the distribution of emergency and intensive-care units;
- revive institutions of a closed type for alcoholics who disturb the peace with mandatory treatment for alcoholism;
- increase the number and widen the distribution of dispensaries for the anonymous and free treatment of alcoholics;
- create institutions for the rehabilitation of alcoholics after their mandatory or voluntary treatment at the dispensaries;
- train primary-care doctors and nurses in the detection of alcohol-related somatic pathologies; upon repeated appearances of such patients in connection with alcohol excesses, they would be sent to the narcological dispensaries;
- create at the regional dispensaries units to collect information on those who abuse alcohol;
- develop an anti-alcohol curriculum for school, vocational schools and institutes;
- develop an educational program for the general population using the media, especially television;
- ban advertising of all alcoholic beverages on television.

Not one item from this very narrowly focused and incomplete list of measures was acted upon. The government demonstrated that it served the narrow group of the "successful", the "club of millionaires", the "golden thousand", for whom democracy and capitalism had succeeded. That was true then, and it is still true now. Will it continue to be? There are reasons to fear that it will be. Using the idea and words of Max Weber, one can put it this way: the "royal bourgeoisie", under the wing of the government, is ineffective on behalf of, and alien to, the national interests. Moreover, the "royal bourgeoisie" has no financial stake in essential changes in the country; "stability" has become its watchword in the sense of preserving what has been obtained through privatization. It is not the nation but the "royal bourgeoisie" that is the foundation of the contemporary Russian government. And the government repays the "foundation" many times over, with its flat (non-progressive) income tax, for example. The extremes of our society bear the same tax burden, those who live below the line of oppressive poverty and those with incomes above the line of munificence face the same 13 percent. And so a citizen of Russia who makes 1 million USD a year pays in taxes (if he pays) 130,000 USD, while his U.S. counterpart pays 270,000 USD, or twice as much.

To this must be added the reduction of the period in which suits challenging privatization deals may be filed – from 10 years to 3 years (it was in that intermediate space of time that the plundering of the basic part of the economy took place). The result of this orientation of domestic policy on the interests of the elite is the growing income disparity between poor and rich in Russia: in 1998 the proportion was 1 to 13.8; in 2004, it was already 1 to 15.

The economic doctrine of "primitive capital accumulation" was the basis for the privatization of property, and the idea was to have shut the door on any restoration of Soviet power. But the door was not shut but only covered, and the task of achieving "general well-being" was pushed a long way off. That distance is suggested by our holding 115th place in the world in quality of life for the population and by our standing on many of the most important social measures: 142nd place in life expectancy (between Iraq and Belize), 115th place in economic freedom (between Niger and Burundi), 97th place in GNP per capita (between Brazil and Salvador), 79th place on self-evaluations of "level of happiness" (between Moldova and Ukraine). The fact that Russia holds 3rd place in the world in its number of dollar billionaires (27) – between Germany (57) and Japan (24) – is a serious obstacle on the long road to general well-being.

The doctrine of "primitive capital accumulation" went hand-in-hand with the doctrine of a "free market", which it was assumed would serve dependably to regulate the economic life of the country. A free market is truly needed for the balancing of supply and demand. But a balance that endangers the health and lives of the population of the country demands administrative anti-market measures, whether for commerce in nuclear hazardous materials or weapons, the predatory felling of forests or the sale of tobacco or alcohol products. The market in such commodities must have built-in negative feedback controls, and there was no thought of such a feedback mechanism when market reforms were put into place – and the government monopoly on alcohol products was ended. Controls on the alcohol market are not in place to this day.

These comments on the internal political and social situation of the country may seem to have diverted us from our principal theme, alcohol. In fact, the link is direct and may be fundamental to explaining that coarse defect in our life as a society that is almost universal heavy drinking.

A survey by the Foundation for Public Opinion (July 20, 2006) showed the population to be of the same opinion. In answer to the question, "what specific measures might contribute to lowering the level of drunkenness in Russia", a large portion of Russians (43 percent) spoke of social problems (guarantees of jobs, improved working and living conditions, raising the level of culture and morality in the country). A small portion of respondents (18 percent) saw ways to lower the level of drinking in the country in anti-alcohol measures (limits on the sale of alcoholic beverages, stepped-up control over sales, a fight against samogon distilling, more severe punishments for drunkenness and others). Of the respondents, 75 percent thought that the level of drinking in the country had increased since 10 years before.

The government and those in power do not believe it is their place to act against the nation drinking so much resulting in lost human potential. Although it is no longer chiefly the government that nurtures drinking, as in the Soviet period, there are new capitalists of various stripes – from rural samogon distillers to the "vodka kings".

Whilst it is true that declarations were made and laws signed, what should not be forgotten is the chaos caused by the laws in the alcohol market in 2006. That chaos and the virtual collapse of trade in spirits is an example of how badly coordinated is the work of the post-Soviet bureaucracy as it employs Soviet-style command-administrative methods.

Of course, the alcoholic answers for his own drunken life and for the lives of those close to him, but the government answers for the sum of these lives. Is this a paradox? No, it is dialectical, the unhappy interaction of opposites, of personal drunkenness and the state. The responsibility of the government is especially great if there are many such drunken lives, and such lives do multiply if it is not just so much faults of individual psychology but social ills that drive people to drunkenness. It is not the state, which it should be, but the wife who has become the chief and almost the only anti-alcohol factor in our country. It is rare for a married woman in Russia to have a husband who does not drink.

An important feature of life in Russia in the past 10–15 years has been the dangerous melding of power and capital. The key and dominant word in this economy has been and remains the word "oligarch". Under the influence of the "pseudo-boyars", the meaning of the word has shifted slightly from "rule of a few" toward "wealth", although the basic idea remains power. Earlier, under Russia's first president, the oligarchs were in the first instance big businessmen and secondarily oligarchs. Under the second president a dwindling number of "pseudo-boyars" stepped aside and were disarmed politically. Now the oligarchy is made up of different people – the highest-ranking bureaucrats and governors, who own large amounts of stock in big companies or have become members of the boards of directors of large corporations. Today there can be no question – the state and the oligarchs are twin brothers.

Smaller capital, the alcohol business, for example, is not connected, we hope, to the very highest level of the pyramid of power; its principal level of assimilation with power is regional. Regional budgets and local bureaucrats depend on the capital of these producers. This is why regional authority defers to vodka capital and closes its eyes to its criminal or semi-criminal activities. The huge means accumulated by the producers of alcoholic beverages during and after the anti-alcohol campaign make it possible to lobby for their interests through the media and at the highest levels of corrupted authority. As a result, the economic side of the alcohol situation has stabilized, and there remains large-scale underground production of hard liquors. Medium and small illegal production and sale of spirits also maintains itself by corruption.

In the main text of this book, the object has been to stick to obvious facts and calculations made on their basis, to emphasize science, i.e., what can be proved. Thus, the unacceptably high level of alcohol consumption has been linked with its illegal production, cheapness and accessibility for even the poorest strata of the population. But this is only half the truth or the truth of only one side of the alcohol counter, the side of the seller. In this concluding section of the book, one can go beyond the limits of the exactitude required of research and of the analytic style. This will allow us to look at the problem from a wider perspective.

As a start, we must place ourselves among those on the other side of the counter, among the consumers of spirits, preferably in some remote area of Russia, somewhere in a small city, perhaps with just a single working factory paying wages at the level of unemployment compensation. This is no exaggeration. According to material compiled by the research company ROMIR-monitoring (Dec. 23, 2004), the portrait of the statistically average drinking Russian looks like this: lives in a rural area or small city, has had little schooling, often does not work. Paraphrasing Oscar Wilde, one can say that poverty and joblessness is "The curse of the drinking classes".

Grouped on this side of the counter are not the 'best' people of our homeland; these are people it is hard to respect, let alone love. One can only feel for them. However, we must not forget that they are numerous, that they are, first of all, humans, and only then, that they are not the 'best'. The reason is perhaps that they have met with more injustice than others.

First of all, most of them were born into poor families, often to drinking parents. Although supposedly "the son does not answer for the father", in a country of "universal literacy" these people are uneducated. From childhood, then, they were turned off the road that leads to success, herded onto the path, taken by millions, surrounded by the remains of binges and carousals. Uneducated, they start work at an early age earning low wages, live in sparse and gray conditions among drunken adults who are already confirmed losers. For people on this path, aged 25–30 the dramatic finale of their lives at 50–60 is visible, a fate that awaits one-third of men and one-sixth of women. It takes an enormous strength of spirit to turn off the path, to climb out of the drunken bog and emerge onto the road! Have we any right to demand heroism of people? Of course not! But what is to be done? Again, wait upon a hasty initiative from "above"? There have been three of these in the most recent alcohol history of Russia – in 1985, 1992 and 2001–2002 (the anti-beer campaign). All were disasters.

The fourth, the follow-up to the presidential initiatives, is now (in 2005–2006) being realized. On July 1, 2005, the president expressed at a meeting of the State Council a desire for a transition "to a state monopoly on spirits". On July 21, 2005, he signed two federal laws (Nos. 102-F3 and 114-F3) on consolidating enterprises engaged in the production and sale of alcohol products, a new stamp system and other innovations. Appropriate government resolutions on these federal laws were published on December 27–31, 2005, and began to go into force, following the timing deadlines laid out in the laws, on January 1, 2006. The end result of the laws and resolutions was a farce: the first stamps – and these were only for vodka in half-liter containers – were printed at the end of January 2006 and reached producers in February. Production of alcoholic beverages was halted for one, two or three months. Naturally, the underground producers did not fail to supply the population with drink while the bureaucrats fussed to hastily correct the errors of the start of the new anti-alcohol campaign.

And although for nine months of 2006 the number of fatal alcohol poisonings decreased by 5,000 as compared with the same period of 2005 (from 27,000 to 22,000), the media began proclaiming that "a massive wave of poisonings is sweeping the country". And that was the case, but only because as of July 1, 2006, the industry producing liquid household products containing alcohol were required to replace the denatured additives in them that caused acute toxic hepatitis and jaundice. The minister of health and social development (M. Zurabov), declared in an interview:

> This is a planned action. Its purpose is to convince society that the government cannot resolve problems in the alcohol market with the measures it has adopted. These acts are directed at getting the government to set aside the normative measures it has adopted. (RIA Novosti)

The rambunctious campaign ended in October, although the poisonings continued. Declarations by the chairmen of the Duma and the Federation Council about the need for a state monopoly may have been the signal for the end. But was that what was needed as a first step?

What is required, first of all, of government is that it clamp down on the corruption that keeps the underground production of strong alcoholic beverages alive, that it step up its activities in the struggle with illegal production and make it impossible to use industrial liquids containing alcohol for "internal consumption" and halt the sale of beer and other alcoholic beverages to adolescents. The government should not attack the non-criminal desires of the population; it must learn to manage them by political, economic and other means. To put it more broadly, the government must care about the people and, in the first place, about its well-being so that, even if it takes 40 years, the people can exit the desert of poverty. And we are talking about 56 million people (40 percent of the population) coming out of poverty, if we include as poor those whose income is less than 60 percent of the average for the country (N. Krichevsky, 2008). This would be the best kind of anti-alcohol campaign.

But, no, it is cheap, illegal alcohol that "marches" to greet the poor. The question arises: Why does the government not, with the vast material resources at its command, the powerful structures of the *siloviki*, a subordinate judiciary and a rigorously "vertical" system, clamp down on the underground production of hard liquor? Is corruption in the alcohol sphere the only barrier to doing so? Perhaps the government looks at underground production of spirits through closed fingers because it cannot, or does not want to, improve the well-being of the poorer part of the population or, in other words, the chief consumers of cheap surrogates? If such consumers could turn their backs on home-brewed vodka and, without harm to the family budget, buy a "bottle" at a store for 75–100 rubles, they would thereby slam shut the door on underground production: no demand means no production. But for this impoverished segment of the population, which spends 60–70 percent, if not 80 percent, of its income on food, the most that can be spent on a "bottle" is 30 rubles. It may well be simpler to suppose this as a "solution" to the problem of poverty in the country.

Throughout this book, the author has stubbornly taken the position that our main problem is the underground production of hard liquor and consumption in incredibly large quantities of cheap hard drinks. Nor does the preceding paragraph stop me from so thinking, although it complicates the problem of drunkenness in Russia by tying it to the poverty of a large portion of the population.

Solution of this problem is further complicated by the fact that the leadership of the country underestimates its importance. This is clear from the Conception of a Demographic Policy for the Russian Federation for the period up to 2025, where the task of "lowering the quantity of consumed alcohol" is listed along with many other problems and is not designated as a top priority, nor are specific aims formulated for achievement by 2025, nor the means for achieving them. "The authors of the Conception were more concerned not to forget anything (or anyone) than to indicate the most important" (Andreev, 2008).

Is the author asking too much of the government chosen by the people? By that same people, half of whom are drinkers? The author would not have demanded that the government turn its attention to alcohol problems in the mid-1980s, when he began his epidemiological work on alcohol, but he is now obligated to do so by his knowledge of the seriousness of Russian drunkenness and the depths of degradation linked to it that have been matters of national dimension for the span of two generations. Finally, he is obliged to do so by the knowledge that the drunkenness of our population is "the most significant cause of the extremely critical indexes of mortality in Russia" (World Bank, 2005).

With such knowledge and great pleasure, the author would appeal to the public, but one person cannot conquer such a large field. The field of power is smaller. Moreover, the players on it are in debt to the people for electing them, have great material resources gathered for their use, and they have the powerful structures of the *siloviki* and courts. We expect action from these people, but in the first place we expect them to be informed. Yet the president in a direct television interview in December 2001 stated that, "when calculated in terms of pure alcohol per person, [Russian] consumption is lower than France's." And that is true, but only by the official figures, which do not take into account underground production and consumption. He said further:

> In order to attract a person away from the bottle, it is necessary to create and steadily to raise the material well-being of the people, to develop interests that the individual can realize, that give him hope for the future.

After this, unfortunately, nothing was done for the "formation of interests and perspectives", let alone for "the raising the material well-being of the people".

When, a year later, President Putin received the draft "Conception of a State Alcohol Policy" for a session of the State Council, he said: "Do you want me to become a second Ligachev?" and canceled the session planned on the alcohol problem (Zaigraev, 2004a). But canceling the meeting did not cancel the problem. It had grown to such an extent that the president, in fact, had to say this in his annual Message to the Federal Assembly in 2005: "I must speak particularly about another complex topic facing our society – the consequences of alcoholism and drug addiction." And again there were fine words: "the result of our work must be a young generation conscious of the need for a healthy style of life, for physical culture and sport." Do you hear an echo of a declaration made four years earlier and of Soviet propaganda at the time of the anti-alcohol campaign?

Development of the president's message took the form of the two already mentioned laws (Nos. 102-F3 and 114-F3, of July 21, 2005). Their main feature was consolidation of enterprises producing ethyl alcohol and alcohol products with more than 15 percent ABV and trading in these products. This was done by raising the minimum capitalization to 10 million rubles (for vodka producers to 50 million). Conditions of retail trade were changed by excluding individual entrepreneurs from the alcohol market and increasing capitalization requirements, to be set by local governments. As of July 1, 2006, Law No. 102-F3 tightened the rules on alcohol sales and limited places of sale.

May we assume that the situation in the alcohol market and regarding consumption will now change for the better? One can hope so, of course, but there is little basis for hope. This is largely because the alcohol market does not exist in isolation from the general socioeconomic situation, which is entangled with corruption from top to bottom. Moreover, the problems of alcohol have deep roots in the criminal economy. Finally, changing the alcohol situation in the country is impossible without substantial improvement in the quality of life of the population.

The consolidation prescribed by the laws of 2005 for manufacturing and trading enterprises would seem to be a good initiative in that it would make it easier to control these enterprises. But consolidation may turn into monopolization of the market and strengthened lobbying on behalf of these enterprises at the expense of the national health.

A new Russian question arises – Did they want to make things better? It is hard to say, but as always the answer is muddled.

With the highest alcohol consumption in all of Russian history (Chapter 2-4), the portion of federal income coming from alcoholic beverages is tiny – 5–7 percent – as contrasted with the Soviet period, when such income came to, by various estimates, 12–27 percent (Zaigraev, 2004b), although average consumption in the postwar period was half what it now is. The basic explanation for this disgracefully small tax share is the illegal production of 40–60 percent of all hard liquor (by various estimates; Chapter 1-8). The low market price of alcoholic beverages derives from this and their accessibility.

According to official figures (2003), spending by the population on alcoholic beverages, despite their cheapness, constitute 10 percent of all expenses and is comparable only with spending on meat products (spending on bakery products, which is next in order of magnitude, comes to 2.8 percent). The State Statistical Committee of the Russian Federation (now Rosstat) maintains that the figure on alcohol spending includes "hidden volumes". But this is doubtful. Those same "volumes" were included in the calculations of alcohol consumption in 2003 as they were in 1984 (9.7 and 13.5 liters, respectively, of pure alcohol per capita per year), while the figures on mortality show an inverse relationship (252 and 180.4 per 1 million). This is why one thinks that spending on alcohol was significantly more than 10 percent, i.e., it is the main item in the family budget of those who live in Russia.

Here as in many other situations described in the text, we run up against the fact that the alcohol situation in the country is not reflected to any significant degree in official indexes. This distorts the real picture and makes it less alarming than it in fact is. Of course, Rosstat is responsible for its failure to properly "account for the volume of hidden activity" in the production and sale of alcoholic beverages, for spending on alcoholic beverages, for alcohol-related disease and mortality and for many other aspects of the alcohol situation. However, in the face of the collapse of government institutions, of all-penetrating corruption, the decline of culture, the general indifference to the lives of citizens and now more administrative reforms, we can only say thank-you for doing something.

The principal trouble with Russian alcohol statistics lies in the carelessness, the sloppiness and sometimes the deliberate falsification in the compiling of initial information on this and many other negative processes underway in the country. And this is the basis for Rosstat's relatively moderate finding on alcohol consumption in the country (8.3 liters in 2001).

But what, after all, is the significance of an estimate of real alcohol consumption of 15 liters of pure alcohol per capita per year (2001)? Is that a lot or a little? It will be simpler to answer if we translate the index of average per capita consumption of alcohol into vodka, Russia's most widely consumed alcoholic beverage, in its typical half-liter bottle form.

15 liters of alcohol are the equivalent of 37.5 liters of vodka or 75 bottles per capita for the entire population. It has been demonstrated (for example, Bekhtel, 1986) that Russian men consume alcohol four times as often as women. So that makes 120 bottles per man. Taking into account the male-female ratio in the country (1:1.15), the ages of the basic consumers (15–65 years) and the male share of the population, the figure now comes to 155 bottles of vodka a year or 3 bottles a week. So in answer to the question about whether 15 liters of pure alcohol (per annum), per average person, is to be considered much, one can say it is not simply much, but a great deal more than much! "Dosage" of this kind leads us to believe that the average Russian man is an alcoholic or a near-alcoholic.

There is yet another important implication in the heavy burden of drunkenness in Russia. Heavy drinking is less a matter of the cheapness and accessibility of alcohol than of a felt need for it (Chapter 2-1). This need is a function of the poverty and disorder of the lives of a great portion of the population. Many people have to make great spiritual and physical efforts just to subsist: half of the population (54 percent) only earns enough to feed their family. Then there is the uncertainty about the future and the low level of education and cultural decline. It is also important that honest striving by citizens is thwarted. For countless individuals, all their energy has to be directed towards scraping out a living and not realizing themselves or their own ideas, as almost "everything is taken" by rich appointees or "protection"-offering criminals.

These and many other examples of disorder give rise to a desire to escape, to "turn off" and run away from the dingy reality and to drink so as, for a time, to forget one's self or achieve an artificial lifting of mood. This is not to romanticize drunkenness, but to take into consideration that the drinker's "Do you respect me?" or his hung over "But we had a good time!" express the spirit's need for a little lift. Russia's cheap alcohol moves to meet that need. To simplify a bit, one might say that a ruble spent on alcohol buys three times the satisfaction that the same ruble might buy in food (Fig. 1-8).

There is yet another reason behind alcohol consumption – the population's loss of its moral compass and spiritual well-being.

The Great Fatherland War (the Eastern Front of World War II) was a turning point in the spiritual life of the people of the USSR. Before the war an artificial and almost seamless dimension for a utopian consciousness had been created. The lies of official propaganda were inspired and elevating. The project of creating a new man inspired many people. The faith in a bright future was, for the majority, sincere, and their consciousness was whole and intact. For such a consciousness, even such a phenomenon as the Moscow trials of 1936-1938 found little space. The war, along with the grief for what had been lost and its psychological and physical tensions, brought unity and spiritual renewal – Russia finally had a real and dangerous enemy.

But the nation emerged from the war in terrible poverty and ruin. The enormous cost of victory and the difficulties of the postwar era pushed aside the hope to realize a communist utopia. "The Communist religion died first in the souls of the priests and only later in the souls of the parishioners" (Piontkovsky, 2005). The official lies had lost their flavor, and gone stale. The "faith, hope and love" toward the government began to ebb away.

Especially destructive for the mind of Soviet man was that the 20-year worship of Josef Stalin as a god were followed by his abrupt expulsion from the pantheon and denunciation. This was accompanied by the execution of one and the separation from power of other top-level state leaders and those closest to Stalin. For the politically naive people, it was hard to understand and accept that all of them – the executed Lavrenty Beria and the victorious Nikita Khrushchev – had all been among "Stalin's falcons". Before another 10 years had passed, Khrushchev was deposed. The historically brief period from Stalin to Khrushchev to Brezhnev (1953–1964) was a time of intense drama for the national consciousness.

The contrast between the official ideology and actual life was especially great for the peasants, who had not yet forgotten collectivization and their forced labor for the collective farms (the state), for which they received nothing or almost nothing; they did not even have passports. The collective values that so many people had absorbed and that were reinforced by propaganda were increasingly in conflict with the peasant's personal interests, which were focused on the little home garden plot that, badly and insufficiently, still fed the family.

That was when and where Soviet society began to distance itself from many former norms and values, the collapse of which has been termed anomie (Durkheim, 1897; cited from Durkheim, 1998), and understood here as a social phenomenon. This process was abetted by chronic shortages and consumer crises that spread it to more and more social groups. In the Brezhnev era, society was already deeply anomic. For the topic of alcohol, it is important that social anomie leads on the individual level to frustration and frustration leads to drinking. Perhaps the rapid rise in alcohol consumption that began in the USSR in the mid-1950s and continued into the early 1980s (Fig. 1-4) was a kind of index of the broadening and deepening of anomie. It has reached its high point and point of most tension in the past two decades.

Defeat in the Cold War along with Russia's loss of superpower status was a blow to the Russian people, not just Russia's politicians. And then on top of all that came privatization, which has left the public with a strong sense that it has been robbed and fervent anger against the robbers. And this is but a factor feeding the need for alcohol (Chapter 2-1), one more reason "to drown the insult" and "pick up a bottle".

One can, in a variety of ways, judge the authoritarian, imperial mind-set that is firmly rooted in the Russian consciousness, but in any case it was dealt a powerful blow with the disintegration of the USSR. That collapse and the accompanying emergence of a few with immodest wealth only added to the grim experience of Soviet poverty being transformed into post-Soviet poverty. And there was another transformation – from a shortage-plagued consumers' market to a consumers' market replete with choice confronting a population, a large portion of which had very little buying power. All this and much else multiplied the negative potentials in the consciousness of the former Soviet individual and, like an image in a curved mirror, magnified the felt need for alcohol.

This is not a justification of Russian drunkenness. It is an attempt to find one's way through the realities of the very complex alcohol situation in our country. In such a context, the lack of substance in the president's words became evident when he proposed to solve the problems of alcohol through "the awareness by the younger generation of the necessity… for being active in physical culture and sport". The president's words reflect the formal, bureaucratic understanding of our alcohol situation held by the presidential administration that prepared the president's message. And it is now these individuals who comprise the supreme leadership of the country. But can we expect of the bureaucracy any other conception of the catastrophic changes in the social existence of the population?

Unhappily for post-Soviet Russia, the country has been without individuals and institutions determined to support the people and capable of fashioning new and understandable values. Liberalization of the country has proceeded without the people and has passed them by. They have not starved, but they have paid the price of hyperinflation, nullification of savings, voucher privatization and "fixed" property auctions.

The artificial quest for a national idea is either obscene or absurd. Such ideas are not sought; they grow of themselves as soon as the citizens of the country become a nation, i.e., a community. The wholeness of the nation, barely "glued together" after the civil war and the Great Fatherland War, soon began to come apart along the line of city versus country. But the fault line in the post-perestroika period was the line between rich and poor or government and people. There remains a community of language and, for the time being, a territorial community, although a part of it has had to be held together by war. One does not want to praise the Soviet government, but that was a time of cultural community, although it was imposed from above. Now economic stratification is increasingly accompanied by a division into "our" and "their" culture. We cannot even say any longer that we enjoy the community of government, when the government increasingly serves the interests of the rich, i.e., acts against the majority. It is this that especially undermines national wholeness. It is unclear what the idea of "preserving the people" (Count Shuvalov as retranslated by Alexander Solzhenitsyn) might now attach itself to, although it would be good, and timely, for it to become the national idea and be developed into care for the health of children and the elderly, in the "preservation" of the Russian peasantry, now almost totally made up of drinkers. "Drink less, live longer – there is your preservation of the people" (Vasilyev, writer).

No national idea can be born among the people of a country that has lost its spiritual communality. None can appear in a populace that has ceased to be the backbone of the country. That "backbone" is now made up of an "elite" deficient of many elite qualities, such as superior intellect and finer spirit, and whose interests are far removed from the national interests. What is now (in 2005) going on in the country is a movement away from any national idea toward social breakdown. How could it be different when there is no faith in the future, no respect for the present and no trust in the government? Our "social" government and its leaders have only in the most recent period begun to notice and, then, only in words the degraded state of the population. Our country is not only experiencing a decline in population, but it is experiencing a catastrophic decline in the "quality" of the population. This is due, to a significant degree, to the heavy drinking that is the population's response to the hopelessness and despair of everyday life, to the mass alienation of citizens from any real power. Without a spiritual basis for unity, drink has become almost the only tie binding the nation. Hopes for unity under the wings of the church have been unavailing. Surveys suggest that the image of the president is working in this direction, but it is only an image, a picture, the relationship to which is more emotional than meaningful.

As long ago as 2001, the Duma approved the concept of a law "On the Russian People", but the deputies later forgot both the conception and the Russian people. It was not until 2005 that the president took note (Message to the Federal Assembly of the Russian Federation) of the serious demographic problems facing the nation and listed them by priority: first, he touched on problems of the high level of mortality, then on the low birth rate and then on policies concerning migration. Tasks were accordingly assigned to the government. But how quickly can an unwieldy bureaucratic machine sift out, if not gut, the president's wishes and then give some life to what is left? And by then how many tragedies connected with alcohol will have occurred and how many early deaths from alcohol?

All this and poverty have given rise to the bewilderment of the majority and the loosening of social ties, one result of which is massive drinking, especially among men. The call to "save the men" was heard in the 1900s (Urlanis, 1968). But now it is obvious that the Russian man – drinker and heavy smoker, poorly fed – will soon be entered on to the list of Endangered Species (IUCN); as early as 1999 he no longer was reaching pension age, and by 2002 the gap between his death and pension eligibility had widened to 18 months. In addition Russian man had begun going to the grave 13.5 years earlier than Russian woman, who lived in as poor conditions. The gap in life expectancy between Russian men and their counterparts in Western European countries was even wider – 16.5 years (the life expectancy for males in Western European countries is 74–78 years).

One need not read the newspapers, listen to the radio or watch television. One need know nothing about the intrigues at the top rungs of power. One need know only those three figures – 58.5, 13.5 and 16.5 – to surmise that government has long been unconcerned with the plight of the people of the nation. Knowing nothing but these three figures, one can easily infer the seriousness of the consequences of Russian drinking. Without any further knowledge we are forced recognize that the alcohol situation in the country is catastrophic. Furthermore the government has yet to do much to address it.

They may refer in rebuttal about the post-Soviet period to the anti-beer campaign led by Onishchenko, our chief political figure in matters of health (2001-2002), to the meeting of the State Council in Kaliningrad on the alcohol problem, and the Presidential addresses of 2005 and 2006, which broach the topic. Finally, there were the federal laws specifically aimed at regulating alcohol production and the alcohol market (2005). Yes, all this happened, but with what result? The bacchanalia in the beer industry of 2001–2002, the crisis in the alcohol market in the first half of 2006, and massive poisonings by surrogate liquors in the second half, spring to mind. The words of the president set off a wave of mindless bureaucratic activity, which this author had occasion to observe firsthand and that still continues. There were committee meetings, larger gatherings and conferences at which little or nothing was said about the main item: the underground production of alcohol and the corruption on which it depends. These fundamental topics were not touched on even at the conference "Conception of a Russian Alcohol Policy and Problems of Effective State Regulation", which took place in May 2006 under the aegis of the Protection of Health Committee of the Duma of the Federation Council of the Russian Federation.

An alcohol policy, like any other policy, can be effective only when the existing state of the problem is known and appropriate goals are set, i.e., achievement of a desirable and realistically possible situation within 5 or 10 years. In this view, policy represents the optimal trajectory between two points – the starting point and the situation to be achieved by the sequenced execution of the actions seen as necessary. This is why, before choosing the proper course for an alcohol policy, it is necessary, first, to assess the real alcohol situation in the country and, second, to define the goals of the policy and, third, to choose criteria for judging the effectiveness of the policy. Yet the main constituent elements of the alcohol situation in our country remain unknown. First of all, we do not know for certain the actual level of alcohol consumption, nor do we know the dimensions of alcohol mortalities and, finally, the overall loss to the country linked to consumption of alcoholic beverages – economic, social and psychological – is unclear. If we are to begin to move toward a serious alcohol policy, we must know which groups in the population are at highest risk from alcohol and the mechanisms of the illegal production of alcohol products and how to force them from the market. Improvements in these areas could serve as criteria of the effectiveness of the chosen policy. We did not, however, have these figures 20 years ago, and we do not have them now.

With respect to goals, the situation is even worse. In this regard, the anti-alcohol campaign of 1985 was as an alcohol policy a coarse profanation, in terms of goals, and shameful in terms of methods. We have yet to hear anyone in Russia talk about an aim of reducing consumption to a relatively safe level. Such a level has long been in place, defined by specialists of the World Health Organization as 8 liters per capita of alcohol per year on average (as against the 14, 15 or 16 liters that is Russia's estimated current level; Chapter 2-4).

It is now clear that the first order of business should be to lower the human cost of alcohol by lowering the level of alcohol consumption, and illegal alcohol, first of all. But by what means and by how many liters and by what date? By what means can it be done in a seriously compromised industry? Until the unknowns of the alcohol situation are filled in and questions of aims and means resolved, one cannot speak of a sensible alcohol policy. Moreover, it is not just these questions that need answers. The answers must be arranged by priority and practicality for the nation and for the individual regions.

Lowering mortalities linked to alcohol should be the very first, rather simple step to take in the face of our demographic crisis. But first it is necessary to know the dimensions of this type of mortality. We only have estimates, specifically those provided in Chapter 2-5. They are sufficient for outlining the task, but for a policy they need to be made more concrete as to groups at risk and the specific causes of heavy drinking. We do not know enough about these things. And without such knowledge, a rational policy is impossible. In other words, for the time being, solution of the alcohol problem of Russia is not possible.

This is the place, in conclusion, for a graph of the life expectancy for men in relation to alcohol consumption (Fig. 2-38). It is obvious that alcohol is not only the principal factor in the fluctuations of life expectancy for men but absolutely critical to its downward motion (the "scissors" of the linear regression shown).

The mass media are full of talk about drug addicts in our country. And this is quite right; among other negative effects of drug use, 3,500 individuals lost their lives from drug overdoses in 2003 (Interior Ministry figures; 0.2 percent of all deaths). Unfortunately, the media have had much less to say and have printed almost nothing about the country's losses caused by alcohol.

Fig. 2-38: Alcohol consumption and life expectancy for men in Russia (1980–2002). Straight lines – lines of regression for alcohol consumption (dotted line) and life expectancy (solid line).

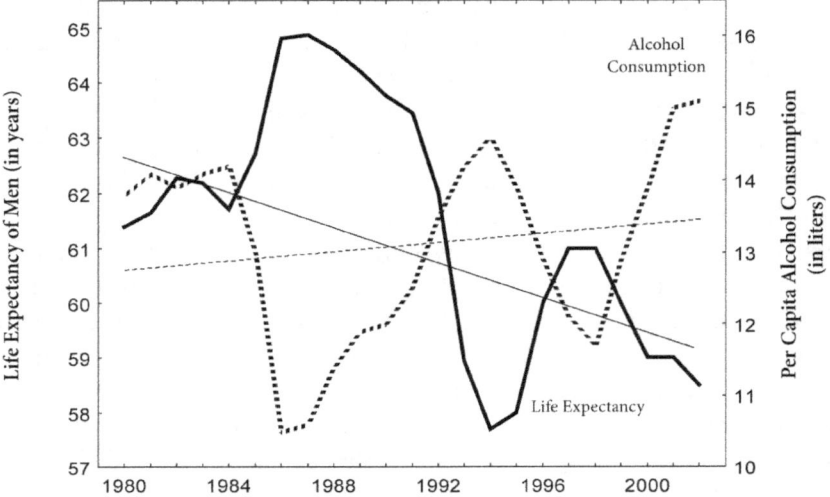

This distorts the picture as to the seriousness of these two problems and places the emphasis unjustly; in that same year, 63,000 Russians (official figures) died of causes linked to alcohol, which was 3.8 percent of all deaths. 63,000 was the official figure and referred only to deaths directly related to alcohol, i.e., only deaths recorded as having alcohol as the main cause of death. There are other, still direct but unrecorded alcohol deaths. These are mostly of alcohol poisonings where the diagnosis is deliberately falsified or otherwise incorrect. These are not rare instances either. They account for thousands of deaths.

Yet the principal loss of life for Russia comes in the form of indirect losses, cases in which alcohol is not the sole cause of death but a substantial contributor to an early death. Losses of this kind are far greater than direct losses. Fig. 2-27 is indicative: almost all the main categories of death, including cardiovascular, echoed the decline in alcohol consumption at the start of the anti-alcohol campaign and the increase at the start of the market reforms and the sharp rise in consumption that then took place. Looked at this way, total (direct and indirect) alcohol losses for Russia amounted to one-quarter of all mortalities (Chapter 2-5), which is 6–10 times higher than the analogous rate for European countries (Finland, less than 4 percent; Germany, 3 percent, and the remainder, less still; Chapter 2-5).

Russia's alcohol losses in recent years amount to more than 400,000 early deaths, most of which occur at working ages (Fig. 1-11). Alcohol holds first place in Russia in number of years of work lost, ahead of deaths from high blood pressure and smoking (Table 18, World Bank, 2006). This is the price of Russia's heavy drinking. It means that the exceedingly high level of alcohol consumption is an essential factor in the decreasing population of the country and, especially, of Russian men.

The low birthrate in our country is insufficient to reproduce the population (127 children per 100 women). By this index, Russia little differs from the countries of Western Europe. But the crux here is not only the birth of a child, it is the raising and, more importantly, nurturing of it. How well can this be done by a drinking father or, more importantly, a drinking mother? They are more likely to doom him. Parental drunkenness is a significant, if not the basic, source of social orphans, children who are essentially orphaned but have at least one parent alive. In Russia the majority of the country's 710,000 orphans (*Argumenty i Fakty*, 2004) are social orphans. How many more are hidden orphans of drunken parents?

Table 18: Loss of disability-adjusted life years ("DALYs") from 10 basic risk factors in Russia (2002).

Rank	Cause	Total DALYs %
1	Alcohol	16.5
2	High Blood pressure	16.3
3	Tobacco	13.4
4	High Cholesterol	12.3
5	High BMI	8.5
6	Low Fruit and Vegetable Intake	7.0
7	Physical Inactivity	4.6
8	Illicit Drugs	2.2
9	Lead	1.1
10	Unprotected Sex	1.0
All 10 factors		82.9

* Source: The World Bank "Dying Too Young", 2005, table 4.1, page 35

Government statistics count 2.2 million persons sick as a result of alcoholism (2003), but the actual number is two or three times higher. There are even more heavy drinkers or alcoholics. They make up approximately one-third of the population of adult males.

It is necessary to mention yet one more important attribute of the alcohol situation in our country: many of the most primitive behaviors in our country are "bound up" with alcohol, more than 70 percent of homicides, for example, more than 50 percent of deaths from external causes and of male suicides (Table 16). Eighteen percent of deaths with diagnoses of somatic diseases, including the very large group of cardiovascular diagnoses, are brought on earlier because of the abuse of alcohol.

These findings and 25 years of experience in the study of alcohol problems do not encourage in the author a sense of social optimism and do not make him hopeful of solutions in the near future. This is especially true because of the economic and political processes that started earlier and which are still actively at work and moving away from the real needs of the population. But absence of optimism is no reason to sit with hands folded and hope for the alcohol situation in our country to suddenly heal. If nothing is done, spontaneous processes are more likely to lead to the further abasement of the population in connection with alcohol. Great efforts over a long period will be needed to resist these destructive forces. And such efforts are vitally needed!

* * *

But for all that is made, there must be an end. As the boundary for this book, I chose the meeting of two millennia. That was only provisional. As I was writing the book, new, important alcohol "events" continued to occur, and it was hard not to try to include them in the book. It is clear that the alcohol history of Russia has not ended with this book. We leave the alcohol situation in the country with a mass of unresolved problems. Earlier (Chapter 2-5) much was said about alcohol mortalities, the most serious manifestation of the dire alcohol situation. But the effects of heavy drinking are a crucial factor in lowered human potential, in the growth of crime, alcohol-related illness and injury, the dissolution of families, the wrecked lives of children, lost work-days. And on and on!

Unfortunately, one must recognize that neither the government nor the public is really aware of the dimensions of the loss of life in connection with massive drinking and of the seriousness of the other Russian alcohol problems. Moreover, 83 percent of Russians "do not believe in the ability of the government to somehow make changes in this sphere" (www.strana.ru/stories/02/01/14).

The inebriated country has long forgotten how to count its dead. The great frequency of early deaths linked to alcohol has so twisted the psychology of the people that these losses are accepted as natural. In Russia the social presumption of sobriety and, more widely, of concern for health are absent. The value placed on human life is very low. It awaits us to come to understand that every individual life is of the highest value and part of our general wealth and, thus, our concern. "No man is an island, entire of itself; every man is a piece of the continent, a part of the main; if a clod be washed away by the sea, Europe is the less" (John Donne, 1625). And Russia, too, we add. Paraphrasing Andrei Platonov, one can say that even one death to alcohol leaves "a people incomplete". Will a majority of our people soon take this to heart and force the leadership seriously and not just in words concern itself with the problems associated with alcohol?

Sometime in the future perhaps this may occur, but not soon. Understanding is coming however. The whole course of our much-troubled history, with its great heights and fallings back, like those of today, is proof of this. If one measures history in 20-year chunks, the result can be nothing but despair. Yet our "bad" of today would have been a splendid existence for the majority of Russians 200–300 years ago. Progress is relentless. That, of course, is little consolation for the living – the human span is much briefer than the historical. This is, however, the best that the author can suggest to his readers.

This book has been devoted to a very dark side of Russian life – to the heavy drinking and drunkenness that is so widely present and so deeply entwined with our everyday existence. But, in all honesty, this shadowy side of our life is not all of Russian life. One cannot but be amazed – after a single century of two world wars and one civil war, of revolution, collectivization and state terror – that the population still preserves its incredible optimism. How much nature has invested in Russian man, and how much has he been taught by centuries of history that "to live" is to persevere "in patience"? Yet one is worried by the question: Is Russian optimism not also somewhat warmed by alcohol, which cheers us, certainly, and dissolves ugliness, but also keeps us from thinking deeply and confronting our lives?

Bibliography

Accounting Chamber of the Russian Federation (2003) Conclusions of the Accounting Chamber of the Russian Federation with respect to results of the topical review of questions on the development of the tax base, fullness and timeliness of payment of excises on alcohol products in 2002 and for the period to date of 2003. (In Russian. Vyvody Schetnoĭ palaty RF po rezul'tatam proverki voprosov razvitiya nalogovoĭ bazy, polnoty i svoevremennosti postupleniya aktsizov na alkogol'nuyu produktsiyu v 2002 godu i za istekshiĭ period 2003 goda). *Russkaya Vodka Plus.* 6. 48–53.

Afanasyev A. L. (1997) Trezvennoe dvizhenie v Rossii, Evrope, SShA kak dvizhenie za samosokhranenie chelovechestva (XIX v. - 1914) (In English. The sobriety movement in Russia, Europe and the USA as a movement for the preservation of mankind (1800–1914). *Sotsiologicheskie Issledovaniya.* 9. 117–122.

Afanasyev V., Gilinsky Ya., Sokolov V. (1995) Peterburgskie bezdomnye: sotsiologicheskoe issledovanie. *Ezhegodnik: Aktual'nye Problemy Deviantnogo Povedeniya (Bor'ba s Sotsial'nymi Boleznyami).* (In English. Petersburg homeless: a sociological study. *Annual: Topical Problems of Deviant Behavior (The Struggle Against Social Diseases)).* Moskva: IS RAN. 117–133.

Anderson P. (1995) Alcohol and risk of physical harm. In: H.D.Holder & G.Edwards (eds.) *Alcohol and Public Policy: Evidence and Issues.* Oxford: Oxford University Press. 82–113.

Anderson S., Hibis V. (1992) Alcoholism in the Soviet Union. *International Social Work.* 35. 441–453.

Andreev eE. M. (2002) Vozmozhnye prichiny kolebaniya prodolzhitel'nosti zhizni v Rossii v 90-e. (In English. Possible reasons for the swings in life expectancy in Russia in the 1990s). *Voprosy Statistiki.* 11. 3–15.

Andreev E. (2008) Kakoĭ budet prodolzhitelnost' zhizni rossiyan. (In English. What is the life expectancy of Russians?). http://demoscope.ru/weekly/2008/0321/tema01.php

Andrienko Y., Nemtsov A. (2005) Estimation of individual demand for alcohol. Economics Education and Research Consortium. Working Paper Series 05/10. http://www.eerc.ru/details/download.aspx?file_id=9459

Anikst A. (1964) *Shekspir.* Seria ZhZL (In English. Shakespeare. In the series: Lives of Remarkable People). Moskva: Molodaya Gvardiya

Artemyev I. A., Minevich V. B. (1989) Migratsiya naseleniya i alkogolizm v Zapadnoĭ Sibiri. (In English. Population migration and alcoholism in Western Siberia). *Voprosy Narkologii.* 3. 38–41.

Ashley M.J., Rankin J.G. (1988) A public health approach to the prevention of alcohol-related health problems. *Annual Review of Public Health.* 9. 233–271.

Audigier J-C., Coppéré H., Barthélémy C. (1984) Alcohol consumption and cirrhosis: epidemiology aspects. *Gastroenterology and Clinical Biology.* 8. 925–933.

Avksentyuk A.V., Kurilovich S.A., Duffy L.K., Segal B., Voevoda M.I., Nikitin Y.P. (1995) Alcohol consumption and flushing response in natives of Chukotka, Siberia. *Journal of Studies on Alcohol.* 56. 194–201.

Babor T.F. (1995) The social and public health significance of individually directed interventions. In: H.D.Holder & G.Edwards (eds.) *Alcohol and Public Policy: Evidence and Issues*. Oxford: Oxford University Press. 164–189.

Babor T.F., Kranzler H.R., Lauerman R.J. (1987) Social drinking as a health and psychosocial risk factor: Anstie's limit revisited. *Recent Developments in Alcoholism*. 5. 373–402.

Babor Th., Caetano R., Casswell S., Edwards G., Giesbrecht N., Graham K., Grube J., Gruenwald P., Hill L., Holder H., Homel R., Österberg E., Rehm J., Room R., Rossow I. (2003) *Alcohol: no ordinary commodity. Research and public policy*. Oxford-N.Y: Oxford University Press.

Balkau B. (1999) All the evidence points to alcohol being implicated in the recent changes in mortality in Russia. *Annals of Epidemiology*. 9. 339–340.

Barker D.J.F. (1973) *Practical epidemiology*. Edinburgh: Churchill Livingstone

Bekhtel E. (1986) *Donozologicheskie formy alkogolizma*. (In English. Pre-nosological forms of alcohol abuse). Moskva: Meditsina

Bezrukikh M. M. (2000) *Problemnye deti*. (In English. Problem Children). Moskva: Izdatel'stvo URAO

Bjarnason T., Andersson B., Choquet M., Elekes Z., Morgan M., Rapinett G. (2003) Alcohol culture, family structure and adolescent alcohol use: multilevel modeling of frequency of heavy drinking among 15–16 year old students in 11 European countries. *Journal of Studies on Alcohol*. 64. 200–208.

Bobak M., Marmot M. (1999) Alcohol and mortality in Russia: is it different than elsewhere? *Annals of Epidemiology*. 9. 335–338.

Bobak M., McKee M., Rose R., Marmot M. (1999) Alcohol consumption in national sample of the Russian population. *Addiction*. 94. 857–866.

Bobak M., Murphy M., Rose R., Marmot M. (2003) Determinants of adult mortality in Russia. A study based on sibling' survival. *Epidemiology*. 14. 603–611.

Bobak M., Room R., Pikhart H., Kubinova R., Malyutina S., Pajak A., Kurilovitch S., Topor R., Nikitin Y. (2004) Contribution of drinking patterns to differences in rates of alcohol related problems between three urban populations. *Journal of Epidemiology and Community Health*. 58. 238–242.

Bokhan N. A., Zalevsky G. V., Semke V. Ya., Galaktionov O. K., Kolosov A. V. (1991) Regional'nye osobennosti alkogolizma v Sibiri. (In English. Regional characteristics of alcoholism in Siberia). *Byulleten' Tomskogo nauchnogo tsentra AMN SSSR* (In English. *Bulletin of the USSR Academy of Medicine's Tomsk Research Center*). 3. 80–84.

Boks G.E.P., Jenkins G.M. (1976) *Time Series Analysis: forecasting and control*. San Francisco: Holden-Day.

Borinskaya S.F., Gesemianrodsari F., Kal'ina N.R., Sokolov M.V., Yankovsky N.K. (2005) Polimorfizm gena ADH1B vostochno-slavyanskikh i irano-govoryashchikh populyatsiĭ. (In English. Polymorphism of a gene ADH1B of East-Slavic and Iran-lingual populations). *Genetics*. 41. 1563–1566.

Britton A., McKee M. (2000) The relationship between alcohol and cardiovascular disease in Eastern Europe: explaining the paradox. *Journal of Epidemiology and Community Health*. 54. 328–332.

Brunn K. et al. (1975) *Alcohol control policies in public health perspective*. 25. Helsinki: Finnish Foundation for Alcohol Studies.

Carlson P. (2001) Risk behaviours and self related health in Russia 1998. *Journal of Epidemiology and Community Health*. 55. 806–827.

Carlson P., Vågerö D. (1998) The Social pattern of heavy drinking in Russia during transition: Evidence from Taganrog 1993. *European Journal of Public Health*. 8. 280–285.

Chenet L., Leon D., McKee M., Vasin S. (1998a) Deaths from alcohol and violence in Moscow: socio-economic determinants. *European Journal of Population*. 14. 19–37.
Chenet L., McKee M., Leon D., Shkolnikov V., Vasin S. (1998b) Alcohol and cardiovascular mortality in Moscow; new evidence of a causal association. *Epidemiology and Community Health*. 52. 772–774.
CINDI (Countrywide Integrated Noncommunicable Disease Intervention). Izuchenie povedencheskikh faktorov riska NIZ[neinfektsionnykh zabolevaniĭ] sredi naseleniya Moskvy v 2000-2001 g.g. (In English. The study of the behavioral risk factors of non-infectious diseases). http://cindi.gnicpm.ru/m2.htm
Clark W.G., Hilton M.E. (1991) (eds.) *Alcohol in America*. Albany, NY: State University of New York Press.
Cockerham W.C., Snead M.C., Dewaal D.F. (2002) Health lifestyles in Russia and socialist heritage. *Journal of Health and Social Behavior*. 43. 42–55.
Connolly G.M., Casswell S., Zhang J.F., Silva P.A. (1994) Alcohol in mass media and drinking by adolescents: a longitudinal study. *Addiction*. 89. 1255–1263.
Cornelius J.R., Lynch K., Martin C.S., Cornelius M.D., Clark D.B. (2001) Clinical correlates of heavy tobacco use among adolescents. *Addictive Behaviors*. 26. 273–277.
Crime and delinquency in the USSR. Statistical Collection 1989 (1990) (In Russian. Prestupnost' i pravonarusheniya v SSSR. Statisticheskiĭ sbornik 1989 (1990). A.I.Smirnov (ed.) Moskva: Yuridicheskaya Literatura.
Davis Ch. (2006) Commentary: The health crisis in the USSR: reflections on the Nicholas Eberstadt 1981 review of Rising Infant Mortality in the USSR in the 1970s. *International Journal of Epidemiology*. 35. 1400–1405.
Deev A., Shestov D., Abernathy J., Kapustina A., Mahina N., Irving S. (1998) Association of alcohol consumption to mortality in middle-aged U.S. and Russian men and women. *Annals of Epidemiology*. 8. 147–153.
De Lint J., Schmidt W. (1968) The distribution of alcohol consumption in Ontario. *Quarterly Journal of Studies on Alcohol*. 29. 968–973.
Duffy J. (1991) *Trends in alcohol consumption patterns, 1978–1989*. Henley-on-Thames: NTC Publications Ltd.
Duffy J., Cohen G. (1978) Total consumption and excessive drinking. *British Journal of Addiction*. 73. 259–264.
Durkheim, E. (1897) *Suicide: A study in sociology*. New York: Free Press. 1997. Russian Translated from French Published in 1998. Sankt-Petersburg: Soyuz
Dutton J. (1979) Changes in Soviet mortality patterns, 1959–77. *Population and Development Review*. 5. 267–291.
Edwards G. et al. (1994) *Alcohol policy and the public good*. Oxford Univ. Press. Oxford-N.Y.-Tokyo: Oxford University Press
Egorov A. E. (2002) Rano nachinayushchiĭsya alkogolizm: sovremennoe sostoyanie problemy (In English. Early-starting alcoholism: contemporary state of the problem). *Voprosy Narkologii*. 2. 50–54.
Elgarov A. A., Elgarova L. V. (1994) Otnoshenie shkol'nikov Nal'chika k vrednym privychkam (In English. The attitude of Nal'chik schoolchildren to harmful habits). *Terapevticheskiĭ Arkhiv*. 66. 45–48.
Engelsman E.L. (1990) Alcohol policies in the Netherlands: a three-pronged attack. *World Health Forum*. 11. 257–263.
Entin G. M., Dineeva N. R. (1996) Formal'naya otsenka rasprostranennosti alkogolizma po sotsial'nym kriteriyam (In English. A formal assessment of the distribution of alcoholism by social criteria). *Voprosy Narkologii*. 3. 77–80.
Ermakov S. P., Ivanova A. E., Semyonova V. G. (1998) *Regional'nyĭ analiz poter' DALY ot smertnosti i invalidnosti. Rossiya, 1993–1995 g.g.* (In English. A region-

al analysis of DALY losses from death and invaliding injury. Russia, 1993-1995). MZ RF Nauchno-proizvodstvennoe ob"edinenie mediko-sotsial'nykh issledovaniĭ (In English. Science-Industry Collective for Medical-Social Research of the Ministry of Health of the Russian Federation).

Fahrenkrug H. (1990) Neue Drogen – neue Mдrkte – neue Sьchte? Oder: Bekommt die Schweiz den amerikanischen Schnupfen? *Drogalkphol.* 14. 83–92.

Filatov A. T. (1986) *Alkogolizm, vyzvannyĭ upotrebleniem samogona* (In English. Alcoholism caused by consumption of samogon). Kiev: Zdorov'e.

Fillmore K.M., Golding J.M., Leino E.V., Ager C.R., Ferrer H.P. (1994) Societal level predictors of groups' drinking patterns: a research synthesis from the collaborative alcohol-related longitudinal project. *American Journal of Public Health.* 84. 247–253.

Floyd K. et al. (2006) Health-systems efficiency in the Russian Federation: tuberculosis control. *Bulletin of the World Health Organization.* 84. 43–51.

FOM (Fond Obshchestvennogo Mneniya) (2002) Alkogol' i rossiyane (In English. Alcohol and Russians). http://www.bd.fom.ru/report.

Food and Agiculture Organization of the United Nations, FAOSTAT (2001) http://faostat.fao.org/.

Frankl V.E. (1985) *Man's Search for Meaning.* New York: Washington Square Press

Fromm E. (1973) *The anatomy of human destructiveness.* New York: Holt, Rinehart and Winston.

Gadalina I. D., Ryazanova R. A., Malysheva M. V., Pavlenko S. M. (1986) Eksperimental'noe issledovanie toksichnosti gidroliznogo spirta (In English. Experimental Study of the Toxicity of Hydrolyzed Alcohol). *Gigiena i Sanitariya.* 7. 32–34.

Gadard J. (1990) Mais au fait, qu' est ce que l'alcoologie? *Alcool ou santé.* 4. 6–7.

Galkin V. A. (1988) (Ed). Narkologicheskaya pomoshch' naseleniyu RSFSR, 1976–1986 (In English. Narcological help for the population of the RSFSR, 1976–1986). Moskva: Ministerstvo Zdravookhraneniya RSFSR.

Gilinsky Ya., Rumyantseva G. (1998). Samoubiistva v Rossii (In English. Suicide in Russia). *Naselenie i Obshchestvo. Informatsionnyĭ byulleten' Tsentra Demografii i ekologii cheloveka Instituta narodnokhozyaĭstvennogo prognozirovaniya RAN (In English. People and Society. Information bulletin of the Center for Human Demography and Ecology of the Russian Academy of Sciences' Institute for Economic Forecasting).* 25.

Ginneken van S, van Iwaarden T. (1989) Alcohol control policy in The Netherlands. *Health Policy.* 13.109–113.

Global Status Report on Alcohol (1999) Geneva: World Health Organization

Global Status Report on Alcohol (2004) Geneva: World Health Organization

Global Status Report: Alcohol and Young People (2001) Geneva: World Health Organization

Godfrey C. (1989) Factors influencing the consumption of alcohol and tobacco: the use and abuse of economic model. *British Journal of Addiction.* 84. 1123–1138.

Godfrey C., Maynard A. (1992) A health strategy for alcohol: Setting targets and choosing policies. YARTIC Occasional Paper 1. York: Centre for Health Economics. University of York & Leeds Addiction Unit.

Godfrey C., Maynard A. (1995) The economic evaluation of alcohol policies. In: Holder H.D. & Edwards G. (eds.) *Alcohol and Public Policy. Evidence and Issues.* Oxford: Oxford University Press. 238–259.

Gorbachev M. S. (1995) Perestroĭka. Desyat' let spustya. (In English. Perestroika. Ten years later). [Transcript of speech] Moskva: Aprel'-85.

Gordon L. (1997) Nevyplachennye zarabotki (In English. Unpaid wages). *Naselenie i Obshchestvo. Informatsionnyĭ byulleten' Tsentra Demografii i ekologii cheloveka*

Instituta narodnokhozyaĭstvennogo prognozirovaniya RAN (In English. People and Society. Informational bulletin of the Center for Human Demography and Ecology of the Russian Academy of Sciences' Institute for Economic Forecasting). 24.

Grechanaya Ye. B., Romanova O. L. (1997) Rasprostranennost' upotrebleniya psikhoaktivnykh veshchestv podrostkami v Moskve. Nauchnyĭ otchet issledovaniya 1996 (reprint) (In English. Distribution of use of psychoactive substances by adolescents in Moscow. Summation of scientific accomplishment for 1996 (offprint)). Nauchno-issledovatel'skiĭ institut profilaktiki narkomanii.(In English. Research Institute for the Prevention of Drug Addiction).

Griffith E., Anderson P., Babor T., Casswell S. et al. (1994) *Alcohol policy and the public good*. Oxford-NY-Tokyo: Oxford University Press.

Gual A., Colom J. (1997) Why has alcohol consumption declined in countries of southern Europe? *Addiction*. 92. Suppl 1. S21–31.

Gukovsky V. N., Kolomin A. R. (1989) Effektivnost' antialkogol'nogo zakonodatel'stva po dannym raboty meditsinskogo vytrezvitelya (In English. Effectiveness of anti-alcohol legislation based on data on the work of a medical sobering-up station). *Aktual'nye Voprosy Psikhiatrii*. Publication 4. 172–174.

Haberman P.W., Baden M.M. (1978) *Alcohol, other drugs and violent death*. N.Y.: Oxford University Press.

Hasin D., Rahav G., Meydan J., Neumark Y. (1999) The drinking of earlier and more recent Russian immigrants to Israel: comparison to other Israelis. *Journal of Substance Abuse*. 10. 341–353.

Haugerud A. (1995) *The culture of politics in modern Kenya*. Cambridge: Cambridge University Press.

Hugo H. (1990) Geschlechtskrankheiten und Alcohol. *Wien Zietschrift Suchtfookschung*. 13. 45-57.

Interior Affairs Ministry, Research Institute (1995) 19 January. Rotaprinte publication.

Jaroszewski Z., Dzibuszko T., Muszyńska-Kutner A. (1989) Spożycie alkoholu a zapadalność napsychozy alkoholowe w Polsce w latach 1956–1986. *Psychiatria Polska*. 23. 97–103.

Johnson J.A., Oksanen E.H. (1974) Socio-economic determinants of the consumption of alcoholic beverages. *Applied Economics*. 6. 293–301.

Kalinina A. M., Chazova L. V. (1991) Prognosticheskoe znachenie povedencheskikh privychek (kurenie, potreblenie alkogolya, fizicheskikh uprazhneniĭ) v populyatsii muzhchin 40–59 let v Moskve (In English. Predictive significance of behavioral habits (smoking, alcohol use, physical exercise) for men ages 40–59 in Moscow)). *Terapevticheskiĭ Arkhiv*. 63. 20–24.

Kamardina T. V. (2004) Smertnost', obuslovlennaya kureniem, v Rossii (In English. Mortalities from smoking in Russia). *Obshchestvennoye Zdorov'e i Profilaktika Zabolevaniĭ*. 2. 29–35.

Kariis T. (1994) Reply to a questionnaire on the alcohol situation in Estonia from the WHO Regional Office for Europe. Copenhagen.

Katcher B.S. (1993) Benjamin Rush's educational campaign against hard drinking. *American Journal of Public Health*. 83. 273-281.

Kendell R.E. (1987) The First Benno Pollak lecture. Drinking sensibly. *British Journal of Addiction*. 82. 1279-1288.

Khotimskaya M. F., Lukash A. A. (1989) Kharakteristika ostrykh smertel'nykh otravleniĭ alkogolem (In English. Description of acute and fatal cases of alcohol poisoning). *Aktual'niye Problemy Meditsinskoĭ Toksikologii v ESSR*. Tallinn. 151–154.

Knibbe R., Drop M., van Reek J., Saenger G. (1985) The development of alcohol consumption in the Netherlands: 1958-1981. *British Journal of Addiction.* 80. 411-419.

Korolenko C.P., Botchkareva N.L. (1990) A review of the problem of alcohol in Siberia. *Drugs and Society.* 4. 5-14.

Korolenko C.P., Kensin D.V. (2001) The quality world change as a cause of addiction development in conditions of the North. *International Journal of Circumpolar Health.* 60. 294-299.

Koshkina Ye. A., Korchagina G. A., Shamota A. Z. (2000) *Zabolevaemost' i boleznennost' alkogolizmom i narkomaniyami v Rossiĭskoĭ Federatsii. Posobie dlya vrachei psikhiatrov-narkologov* (In English. Case rate and morbidity of alcoholism and drug addiction in the Russian Federation. A reference work of psychiatrist-drug specialists). Moskva: Ministerstvo Zdravookhraneniya RF.

Koshkina Ye. A., Vyshinsky K. V., Shamota A. Z., Gurtovenko V. M. (2004) Monitoring rasprostranennosti potrebleniya psikhoaktivnykh veshchestv sredi uchashchikhsya g. Moskvy (In English. Monitoring of the distribution of the use of psychoactive substances among pupils in the city of Moscow). Pul's. Obshchestvennoe Mnenie, Sotsiologicheskie Issledovaniya. 2. 38.

Kozlov A.I., Vkshubskaya G.G. (2001). Vliyanie "modernizatsii" na zdorov'e aborigenov Severa Rossii. (In English. Influence of the "modernization" on health of the aborigines in the North of Russia). In: *Ekologiya cheloveka: ot proshlogo k budushchemu. Nauchnye trudy MNEPU.* (In English. Human ecology: from the past to the future. Scientific works MNEPU). Moskva. 237-243.

Krasik Ye. D., Moskvitin P. N. (1988) Sravnitel'naya rasprostranennost' p'yanstva i alkogolizma sredi naseleniya krupnogo promyshlennogo goroda Zapadnoĭ Sibiri (In English. Comparative distribution of drunkenness and alcoholism in the populations of the largest industrial city of Western Siberia)). *Voprosy Narkologii.* 4. 21-24.

Krichevsky N. (2008) Khorosho zhivem? (In English. We live well, don't we?). *Argumenty i Fakty.* 43.16.

Kurilovich S. A. (1994) Nekotorye epidemiologicheskie i kliniko-biokhimicheskie aspekty somaticheskoĭ patologii, svyazannoĭ s potrebleniem alkogolya. Dissertatsiya doktora meditsinskikh nauk. Aftoreferat. (In English. Several epidemiological and clinical-biochemical aspects of somatic pathology associated with alcohol consumption. Dissertation for doctorate in medical sciences. Author's summary). Novosibirsk.

Kurilovich S.A., Jakuschenko I.A., Egorova N.G., Avksentyuk A.V., Trusov V.B. (1998) Flushing response and its role in alcohol disease in Siberian populations. *International Journal of Circumpolar Health.* 57. Suppl. 454-458.

Kurts B. T. (1937) *Sochinenie Kil'burgera o russkoĭ torgovle v tsarstvovanie Alekseya Mikhaĭlovicha* (In English. Kilburger's essay on Russian commerce in the reign of Aleksei Mikhaĭlovich). Leningrad.

Kurukin I. (1998). Gosudarevo kabatskoe delo. (In English. The Tsar's tavern business). *Itogi.* 1 (136). 36-34.

Laatikainen T., Alho H., Vartiainen E., Jousilahti P., Sillanaukee P., Puska P. (2002) Self-reported alcohol consumption and association to carbohydrate-deficient transferrin and gamma-glutamyl transferase in a random sample of the general population in the Republic of Karelia, Russia and in North Karelia, Finland. *Alcohol and Alcoholism.* 37. 282-288.

Labys W.C. (1976) An international comparison of price and income elasticities for wine consumption. *Australian Journal of Agricultural Economics.* 20. 33-36.

Lau H.H. (1975) Cost of alcoholic beverages as a determinant of alcohol consumption. In: R. J. Gibbins, Y. Israel, H.Kalant (eds.) *Research advances in alcohol and drug problems*. N.Y.: John Wiley and Sons Inc. 211–245.
Ledermann S. (1956) *Alcool, alcoolisme, alcoolisation*. Paris: Presse Universitaires de France.
Ledermann S. (1964) Can one reduce alcoholism without changing total consumption in a population? In: 27th International Congress on Alcohol and Alcoholism. Frankfurt-am-Main, Germany.
Leifman H. (2001) Estimation of unrecorded alcohol consumption levels and trends in 14 European countries. *Nordisk Alkohol & Narkotikatidskrift*. (English supplement) 18. 54–69.
Lemmens P. (1991) Measurement and distribution of alcohol consumption. Dissertation. University of Limburg.
Lemmens P., Tan E., Knibbe R. (1990) Comparing distributions of alcohol consumption: empirical probability plots. *British Journal of Addiction*. 85. 751–758.
Leon D., Chenet L., Shkolnikov V.M., Zakharov S., Shapiro J., Rakhmanova G., Vassin S., McKee M. (1997) Huge variation in Russian mortality rates 1984–94: artifact, alcohol, or what? *Lancet*. 350. 383–388.
Leon D., Saburova L., Tomkins S., Andreev E., Kiryanov N., McKee M., Shkolnikov V. (2007) Hazardous alcohol drinking and premature mortality in Russia: a population-based case control study. *Lancet*. 369. 2001–2009.
Levada Yu. (2004) Interview. *Argumenty i Fakty*. 51. 10.
Lindberg J. (1999) Alcohol sales and estimated alcohol consumption in EU 1997. Saariselkä Seminar.
Lisitsyn Yu. P. (1985) Alkogol' – faktor riska (In English. Alcohol – Risk Factor). *Terapevticheskiĭ Arkhiv*. 57. 3–8.
Lundborg P. (2002) Young people and alcohol: an econometric analysis. *Addiction*. 97. 1573–1582.
Luzhnikov Ye. A., Nemtsov A. V., Nechayev A. K. (1989) Dinamika otravleniĭ psikhotropnymi veshchestvami v Moskve v 1984–1987 g.g. (In English. Dynamics of poisonings with psychotropic substances in Moscow, 1984–1987). *Voprosy Narkologii*. 4. 40–41.
Lyalikov D. N. (1987) *Gosudarstvennoe regulirovanie potrebleniya alkogolya v Finlyandii. Nauchno-analiticheskiĭ obzor* (In English. State regulation of alcohol use in Finland. A Scientific-Analytical Review). Moskva: Institut nauchnoĭ informatsii po obshchestvennym naukam AN SSSR.
Mäkelä K., Room R., Single E., Sulkunen P., Walsh B. (1981) Alcohol, society and the state. Vol. 1.Toronto: Addiction Research Foundation
Mäkelä P. (1999) Alcohol-related mortality as a function of socio-economic status. *Addiction*. 94. 867–886.
Mäkinen I.H. (2000) Eastern European transition and suicide mortality. *Social Science and Medicine*. 51. 1405–1420.
Malyutina S., Bobak M., Kurilovitch S., Ruizova E., Nikitin Y., Marmot M. (2001) Alcohol consumption and binge drinking in Novosibirsk, Russia, 1985–95. *Addiction*. 96. 987–995.
Malyutina S., Bobak M., Kurilovitch S., Gafarov V., Simonovs G., Nikitin Y., Marmot M. (2002) Relationship between heavy and binge drinking and all-cause and cardiovascular mortality in Novosibirsk, Russia: a perspective cohort study. *Lancet*. 360. 1448–1454.
Markov K. V., Britov A. N., Vedeneeva I. A. (1990) Rasprostranenie p'yanstva i struktura prichin smertnosti muzhchin 40–54 let (In English. Distribution of

drunkenness and causes of death in men 40–54 years of age). *Sovetskoe Zdravookhranenie.* 4. 15–18.

Marusin A. V., Stepanov V. A., Spiridonova M. G., Puzyryov V. P. (2004) Polimorfizm genov ADH1B i ADH7 v russkikh populyatsiyah sibirskogo regiona (In English. Polymorphism of the genes ADH1B and ADH7 in Russian populations of the Siberian Region). *Molekulyarnaya Biologiya.* 38. 652–631.

McGinnis J., Foege W.H. (1999) Mortality and morbidity attributable to use of addictive substances in the United States. *Proceedings of the Association of American Physicians.* 111. 109–118.

McKee M., Britton A. (1998) The positive relationship between alcohol and heart disease in eastern Europe: potential physiological mechanisms. *Journal of the Royal Society of Medicine.* 91. 402–407.

McKee M., Sanderson C., Chenet L., Vassin S., Shkolnikov V. (1998) Seasonal variation in mortality in Moscow. *Journal of Public Health Medicine.* 20. 268–274.

McKee M., Leon D.A. (2005) Social transition and substance abuse. *Addiction.* 100. 1205–1209.

Mendelson A. (1916) *Itogi prinuditel'noĭ trezvosti i novye formy p'yanstva* (In English. Results of forced sobriety and new forms of drunkenness). Petrograd

Menninger K.A. (1938) Man against himself. N.Y: Harcout, Brace and Co.

Menzhulin V. (2002) *Raskoldovyvaya Yunga. Ot apologetiki k kritike* (In English. Demystifying Jung. From Apologetics to Criticism). Kiev: Sfera.

Mesle F., Vallin J., Hertrich V., Andreev E., Shkolnikov V. (2003) Causes of death in Russia: assessing trends since the 50s. In I. Kotowska and J. Jozwiak (eds.) *Population of Central and Eastern Europe. Challenges and Opportunities.* Warsaw: Statistical Publishing Establishment. 389–414.

Midanik L. (1982) The validity of self-reported alcohol consumption and alcohol problems: A literature review. *British Journal of Addiction.* 77. 357–382.

Midanik L. (1988) Validity of self-reported alcohol use: a literature review and assessment. *British Journal of Addiction.* 83. 1019–1039.

Mille F., Shkolnikov V. M., Ertrish V., Vallen Zh. (1996) *Sovremennye tendentsii smertnosti po prichinam smerti v Rossii: 1965–199.* Prilozhenie na dvukh disketakh (In English. Contemporary trends in mortality by cause of death in Russia: 1965–1994 Supplement on two diskettes). Paris: INE.

Mocher J.F. (1988) Public action and awareness to reduce alcohol related problems: a plan of action. *Journal of Public Health Policy.* 9. 17–41.

Moiseev V. S., Ogurtsov P. P. (1997) Alkogol'naya bolezn': patogeneticheskie, diagnosticheskie i klinicheskie aspekty (In English. Alcohol disease: pathogenetic, diagnostic and clinical aspects). *Terapevticheskiĭ Arkhiv.* 12. 5–12.

Morozov L. T. (1988) Samootsenka zloupotrebleniya alkogolem u bol'nyh i zdorovyh: rol' situatsii obsledovaniya i vozrasta (In English. Self-appraisal of alcohol abuse by ill and healthy persons: the role of the examination situation and age). In collection: *Alkogolism.* Mokva. 27–29.

Moskalewicz J., Rabczenko D., Wojtyniak B. (1997) Alcohol factor in mortality in societies under rapid transitions first draft. Reprint: UNU/WIDER Project Meeting on "Economic Shocks, Social Stress and the Demographic Impact". Helsinki.

Moscow's Health Inspection Services (SES) (1993) Annual Report. Rotaprinte publication.

Mukomel V. (2005; latest updating) Demograficheskie posledstviya etnicheskikh i regional'nykh konfliktov v postsovetskom prostranstve (In English. Demographic consequences of ethnic and regional conflicts in the territory of the Former Soviet Union). www.demoscope.ru Document No. 16884.

Nace E. (1984) Epidemiology of alcoholism and prospects for treatment. *Annual Review of Medicine*. 35. 293–309.
Nalpas B, Pol S, Thepot V, Zylberberg H, Berthelot P, Brechot C. (1998) Relationship between excessive alcohol drinking and viral infections. *Alcohol and Alcoholism*. 33. 202–206.
National Health and Medical Research Council (1987*) Is there a safe level of daily consumption of alcohol for men and women? Recommendations regarding responsible drinking behaviour*. Canberra, Australia: Australian Publishing Service
Naubatov T. Kh. (1990) Analiz ostrykh otravleniĭ etilovym spirtom zhiteleĭ g. Ashhabada (itogi za 10 let) (In English. Analysis of acute ethyl alcohol poisonings among residents of the city of Ashkhabad (Results after 10 Years)). *Aktualnye Voprosy Alkogolisma i Narkomaniĭ Turkmenskoi SSR*. Ashkhabad. 38–39.
Naveillan P., Vargas S. (1989) Pravalencia del alcoholismo durante tres dňen Chile (1952–1982). *Revista de Saude Publica*. 23. 128–135.
Negrete J.C. (1980) Sociocultural and economic change in relation to alcohol problems. In J. Moser (Ed.) *Prevention of Alcohol-related Problems*. Toronto: Addiction Research Foundation. 159–170
Nemtsov A. V. (1992a) Uroven' real'nogo potrebleniya alkogolya v Rossiĭskoĭ Federatsii (1981–1990) (In English. Actual consumption level of alcohol in the Russian Federation (1981–1990)). *Psikhiatriya*. 2. 46–53.
Nemtsov A. V. (1992b) Nasil'stvennaya smert' kak pokazatel' urovnya samogonovareniya (In English. Violent death as an indicator of level of samogon production). *Voprosy Narkologii*. 5. 102–106.
Nemtsov A.V. (1992c) The actual consumption of alcohol in Russia and Latvia (1981–1991). The report at the conference on alcohol statistics. June, 15–17. Riga, Latvia.
Nemtsov A. V. (1995) *Alkogol'naya situatsiya v Rossii* (In English. The Alcohol Situation in Russia). Moskva: Assotsiatsiya obshchestvennogo zdorov'ya.
Nemtsov A. V. (1997) Potreblenie alkogolya i zavisimye ot alkogolya meditsinskie yavleniya v Moskve (1983–1993) (In English. Alcohol Consumption and alcohol-related medical phenomena in Moscow (1983–1993)). *Sotsialnaya i Klinicheskaya Psikhiatriya*. 7. 80–87.
Nemtsov A. V. (1998a) Tendentsii potrebleniya alkogolya i obuslovlennye alkogolem poteri zdorov'ya i zhizni v Rossii v 1946–1996 g.g .(In English. Trends in alcohol consumption and alcohol-related losses of health and lives in Russia, 1946–1996). In: A. K. Demin (ed.) *Alkogol' i zdorov'e naseleniya Rossii.1900-2000* (In English. *Alcohol and the Health of the Population of Russia. 1900–2000*). Rossiĭskaya Assotsiatsiya Obshchestvennogo Zdorov'ya. 98–107.
Nemtsov A.V. (1998b) Alcohol-related harm alcohol consumption in Moscow before, during and after a major anti-alcohol campaign. *Addiction*. 93. 1501–1510.
Nemtsov A.V. (2000) Estimates of total alcohol consumption in Russia, 1980–1994. *Drug and Alcohol Dependence*. 58. 133–142.
Nemtsov A. V. (2001a) *Alkogol'naya smertnost' v Rossii, 1980–90-e gody* (In English. Alcohol Mortality in Russia, 1980s–1990s). Moskva.
Nemtsov A. V. (2001b) Potreblenie alkogolya v Rossii vo vtoroĭ polovine 1990-h godov (In English. Alcohol consumption in Russia in the second half of the 1990s). *Voprosy Narkologii*. 2. 59–64.
Nemtsov A. V. (2002) Alcohol-related harm losses in Russia in the 1980s and 1990s. *Addiction*. 97. 1413–1425.
Nemtsov A. V. (2003a) Alcohol consumption in Russia: Is monitoring health in the Russia Federation (RLMS) trustworthy? *Addiction*. 98. 386–388.

Nemtsov A. V. (2003b) *Alkogol'nyĭ uron regionov Rossii* (In English. Alcohol losses of Russia's regions). Moskva: NALEX.
Nemtsov A. V. (2003c) Alcohol consumption level in Russia: a viewpoint on monitoring Health Conditions In the Russian Federation (RLMS). *Addiction.* 98. 369–370.
Nemtsov A. V., Nechaev A. K. (1991) Potreblenie alkogolya i nasil'stvennye smerti (In English. Alcohol consumption and violent death). *Voprosy Narkologii.* 1. 34–36.
Nemtsov A. V., Nechaev A. K. (1996) Faktory zabolevaemosti alkogol'nymi psikhozami (In English. Factors in the incidence of alcoholic psychoses). *Sotsialnaya i Klinicheskaya Psikhiatriya.* 6. 68–77.
Nemtsov A. V., Pokrovskaya I. A. (1997) Primenenie statisticheskikh metodov. Soobshchenie 1. Srednie velichiny (In English. Application of statistical methods. Communication No. 1. Average Dimensions). *Sotsialnaya i Klinicheskaya Psikhiatriya.* 4. 94–96.
Nemtsov A. V., Shkolnikov V. M. (1994)Zhit' ili pit' (In English. To live or to drink). *Izvestia.* July 19. 4.
Nielsen J. (1965) Delirium tremens in Copenhagen. *Acta Psychiatrica Scandinavica. Suppl.* 187. 1–92.
NOBUS – http://www.worldbank.org.ru/ECA/Russia.nsf-
Nordum I., Eide T.J., Jorgenson L. (2000) Alcohol in a series of medico-legally autopsied deaths in northern Norway 1973–1992. *Forensic Science International.* 110. 127–137.
Norström T. (1987) The abolition of the Swedish rationing system: effect of consumption distribution and cirrhosis mortality. *British Journal of Addiction.* 82. 633–641.
Norström T. (1996) Per capita alcohol consumption and total mortality: an analysis of historical data. *Addiction.* 91. 339–344.
Norström T. (2001) Per capita alcohol consumption and all-cause mortality in 14 European countries. *Addiction.* 96 (Suppl. 1). S113–S128.
Norström T., Skog O.-J. (2001) Alcohol and mortality: methodological and analytical issue in aggregate analysis. *Addiction.* 96 (Suppl.). S5–S17.
Nuzhny V. P. (1995) Toksikologicheskaya kharakteristika etilovogo spirta, alkogol'nykh napitkov i soderzhashchikhsya v nikh primeseĭ (In English. A toxicological description of ethyl alcohol, alcoholic beverages and additives found in them). *Voprosy Narkologii.* 3. 65–74.
Nuzhny V. P., Savchuk S. A., Kayumov R. I. (2002a) Khimiko-toksikologicheskoe issledovanie krepkikh alkogol'nykh napitkov domashnego izgotovleniya (samogon) iz raznykh regionov Rossii (In English. A chemic-toxicological study of homemade strong alcoholic beverages (samogon) from various regions of Russia). *Narkologiya.* 5. 43–48.
Nuzhny V. P., Savchuk S. A., Kayumov R. I. (2002b) Issledovanie toksichnosti spirta etilovogo sinteticheskogo rektifikovannogo (A study of the toxicity of synthetic rectified alcohol). *Toksikologicheskiĭ Vestnik.* 5. 13–22.
Obbo C. (1980) African women. Their struggle for economic independence. London: Zed Books.
Ogurtsov P. P. (1997) Raspoznavanie khronicheskoĭ alkogol'noĭ intoksikatsii u somaticheskikh bol'nykh (In English. Diagnosis of chronic alcohol intoxication among the somatically ill). *Medical Market.* 27. 38–41.
Ogurtsov P. P. (2002) Rol' khronicheskoĭ alkogol'noĭ intoksikatsii i geneticheskogo polimorfizma alkogol'degidrogenazy v formirovanii patologii vnutrennikh organov. Dissertatsiya doktora meditsinskikh nauk (In English. The role of chron-

ic alcohol intoxication and the genetic polymorphism of alcoholdehydrogenase in the formation of pathologies of the Inner organs. Dissertation for a doctorate in the medical sciences). Moskva.

Ogurtsov P.P., Nuzny V.P., Garmash I.V., Moiseev V.S. (2001) Mortality in Russia. *The Lancet*. 358. 669–670.

Ohta Y., Horiike N., Michitaka K. (1988) Effect of alcohol on the replication of HBV and the integration of HBV-DNA into the liver cell of nuclei of patients with chronic hepatitis and hepatocarcinoma. In: K. Kuriyama, A.Takada, H. Ishii (eds.) *Biomedical and social aspects of alcohol and alcoholism*. Amsterdam: Elsevier. 827–835.

Österberg E. (1987) Recorded and unrecorded alcohol consumption. In: J. Simpura (ed.) *Finnish drinking habits*. Helsinki:The Finnish Foundation for Alcohol Studies. 35. 17–36.

Österberg E. (1995) Do alcohol prices affect consumption and related problems? H.D.Holder and G.Edwards (eds.) *Alcohol and Public Policy: Evidence and Issues*. 145–163.

Ostroumov S. (1914) *Iz istorii p'yanstva na Rusi* (From the History of Drunkenness in Rus') Sankt- Peterburg

Palosuo H. (2000) Health-related lifestyles and alienation in Moscow and Helsinki. *Social Science and Medicine*. 51. 1325–1341.

Partanen J. (1991) *Sociality and Intoxication: Alcohol and drinking in Kenya, Africa, and the modern world*. Helsinki.

Partanen J., Montonen M. (1991) *Alcohol and the mass media*. Euro Reports and Studies 108. Copenhagen: World Health Organization.

Pessione F., Degos F., Marcellin P., Duchatelle V., Njapoum C., Martinot-Peignoux M., Degott C., Valla D., Erlinger S., Rueff B. (1998) Effect of Alcohol Consumption on Serum Hepatitis C Virus RNA and Histological Lesions in Chronic Hepatitis C. *Hepatology*. 27. 1717–1722.

Petrov V. N., Dovgii A. V. (1989) Sotsial'no-psikhologicheskie aspekty p'yanstva sredi rabochikh i sluzhashchikh promyshlennogo predpriyatiya (In English. Socio-psychological aspects of drunkenness among factory workers and clerks in industrial enterprises). *Voprosy Narkologii*. 1. 43–46.

Piontkovsky A. (2005) *Za Rodinu! Za Abramovicha! Ogon'!* (In English. For the Homeland! For Abramovich! Fire!). Moscow: EPIcenter

Plant M. (1991) The Epidemiology of alcohol use and misuse. In M. Plant (ed.) *Alcohol-related problems in high risk-groups*. Copenhagen: World Health Organization. 1–48.

Plant M. (1992) Alcohol, tobacco and illicit drug use in Scotland. In M. Plant, B. Ritson and R. Robertson (eds.) *Alcohol and Drugs. The Scottish Experience*. Edinburgh: Edinburgh Univ. Press. 3–9.

Plavinski S.L., Plavinskaya S.I., Klimov A.N. (2003) Social factors and increase in mortality in Russia in the 1990s: prospective cohort study. *British Medical Journal*. 326. 1240–1242.

Polyakov I. V., Petrov N. G. (1989) Smertnost' v svyazi s potrebleniem alkogolya (In English. Mortality in connection with alcohol consumption). *Zdravookhranenie Rossiĭskoĭ Federatsii*. 11. 24–27.

Putin V. V. (2006) Poslanie Federal'nomu Sobraniyu Rossiĭskoĭ Federatsii (In English. Message to the Federal Assembly of the Russian Federation). htp://kremlin.ru/text/appears/2006/05/105546.shtml.

Rahav G., Hasin D., Paykin A. (1999) Drinking patterns of recent Russian immigrants and other Israelis. *American Journal of Public Health*. 89. 1212–1216.

Ramstedt M. (2002) Alcohol-related mortality in 15 European countries in postwar period. *European Journal of Population*. 18. 307–323.
Red'ko A. N., Sakharova P. B. (2006) Alkogol'nyĭ faktor v probleme prezhdevremennoĭ smertnosti naseleniya (In English. The factor of alcohol in the problem of early mortality in the population). In: V. I. Starodubov (ed.) *Prezhdevremennaya i predotvratimaya smertnost' v Rossii – kriterii poteri zdorov'ya naseleniya* (In English. Early and Preventable Mortality in Russia – Criteria for Health Losses in the Population). Moskva. 223–228.
Rehm J., Gmel G. (2001) Alcohol per capita consumption, pattern of drinking and abstention worldwide after 1995. *European Addiction Research*. 7. 155–157.
Rehn N., Room R., Edwards G. (2001) *Alcohol in the European Region – consumption, harm and policies*. World Health Organization, Regional Office for Europe.
Reisch M.S. (1987) Major chemical producers toughen stance on drug abuse. *Chemical English News*. 65. 7–12.
RLMS – http://www.cpc.unc.edu/rlms
Robinson D. (1986) Alcohol, education and action: shifting emphases. *Health Education and Research: Theory and Practice*. 1. 325–331.
Romelsjö A. (1987) Epidemiological studies on the relationship between a decline in alcohol consumption, social factors and alcohol-related disabilities in Stockholm county and the whole of Sweden. Dissertation. Sundbyberg. Sweden.
ROMIR-monitoring http://romir.ru/.
Ronellenfitsch U. (2003) Time of risk factor assessment is of special importance. *British Medical Journal*. 327. 751.
Room R. (1984) Alcohol control and public health. *Annual Review of Public Health*. Volume 5. Palo Alto. California. 293–317.
Room R. (1991) Cultural changes in drinking and trends in alcohol problems indicators: recent U.S. experience. In: W. G. Clark and M. E. Hilton (eds.). *Alcohol and America*. 149–162. Albany. NY.: SUNY Press.
Rumyantseva L. A. (1999) Toksikologo-gigienicheskie issledovaniya spirtov, proizvodimykh gidroliznymi zavodami (In English. Toxic-hygienic studies of spirits produced by hydrolyze factories). *Gigiena i Sanitariya*. 1. 46–48.
Ryan M. (1995) Alcoholism and rising mortality in the Russian Federation. *British Medical Journal*. 310. 646–648.
Schmidt W. (1977) The epidemiology of cirrhosis of the liver: a statistical study of mortality data with special reference to Canada. In: M. M. Fisher and J. G. Rankin (eds.) *Alcohol and the Liver*. New York: Plenum Press. 1–26.
Schultz J.M., Rice D.P., Parker D.L. (1990) Alcohol-related mortality and years of potential life lost —United States, 1987. *Morbidity and Mortality Weekly Report*. 39. 173–178.
Schultz J., Rice D., Parker D., Goodman R., Stroh G., Chalmers N. (1991) Quantifying the disease impact of alcohol with ARDI software. *Public Health Reports*. 106. 443–450.
Segal, B.M. (1990) The drunken society: alcohol abuse and alcoholism in the Soviet Union. A comparative study. New York: Hippocrene books.
Segal B., Duffy L.K., Kurilovitch S.A., Avksentyuk A.V. (1991) Alaskan and Siberian studies on alcoholic behavior and genetic predisposition. *Arctic Medical Research*. (Suppl.) 474–477.
Seixas FA., Eggleston S. (1976) Alcoholism around the world. In: F.A. Seixas, S. Eggleston (eds.) *Work in Progress in Alcoholism*. Part I. 4–78. N.Y.: New York Academy of Sciences.
Shamota A.Z., Egorov E.F., Koshkina E.A., Korchagina G.F. (1998) Narkologicheskaya situatsiya v Rossii po dannym ofitsial'noĭ statistiki (In English.

Drug situation in Russia according to official statistics). *Russian Medical Journal.* 98. 2. 109-114

Shapiro J. (1997) Health care policy and Russian health. In: S. White, A. Pravda, Z. Gitelman (eds.) *Developments in Russian politics.* London: Macmillan.

Sheregi F. E. (1986) Prichiny i sotsial'nye posledstviya p'yanstva (In English. Causes and social consequences of drunkenness). *Sotsiologicheskie Issledovaniya.* 2. 144–152.

Shevyakov A. (2007) Pochemu rost ekonomiki v Rossii vygoden bogatym (In English. Why the growth in the economy of Russia is good for the rich). *Argumenty i Fakty.* 16. 11.

Shkolnikov V., Leon D., Adamets S., Andreev E., Deev A. (1998) Educational level and adult mortality in Russia: an analysis of routine data 1979 to 1994. *Social Science in Medicine.* 47. 357–369.

Shkolnikov V., McKee M., Leon D.A. (2001) Changes in life expectancy in Russia in the mid-1990s. *The Lancet.* 357. 917–921.

Shkolnikov V.M., McKee M., Chervyakov V.V., Kyrianov N.A. (2002) Is the link between alcohol and cardiovascular death among young Russian men attributable to misclassification of acute alcohol intoxication? Evidence from the city of Izhevsk. *Journal of Epidemiology and Community Health.* 56. 171–175.

Shkolnikov,V.M., Nemtsov, A.V. (1997) The anti-alcohol campaign and variations in Russian mortality. In: J. L. Bobadilla,C. A. Costello & F. Mitchel (eds.) *Premature death in the new independent states.* Washington: National Academy Press

Simpura J. (1995) Trends in alcohol consumption and drinking patterns: lessons from world-wide development. In: Holder H.D. & Edwards G. (eds.) *Alcohol and Public Policy. Evidence and Issues.* Oxford: Oxford University Press. 9–37.

Simpura J., Levin B.M., Mustonen H. (1997) Russian drinking in the 1990's: patterns and trends in international comparison. In: J. Simpura & B. M. Levin (eds.) *Demystifying Russian Drinking.* Research Report. National Research and Development Centre for Welfare and Health. 85. 79–107.

Single E., Giesbrecht N., Eakins B. (1981) *Alcohol, society and the state. Vol.2. A social history of control policy in seven countries.* Toronto: Addiction Research Foundation

Single E., Robson L., Rehm J., Xie X. (1999) Morbidity and mortality attributable to alcohol, tobacco, and illicit drug use in Canada. *American Journal of Public Health.* 89. 385–390

Single. E., Rehm J., Robson L., Truong M. (2000) The relative risks and etiologic fractions of different causes of death and disease attributable to alcohol, tobacco and illicit drug use in Canada. *CM AJ.* 162. 1669-1675

Skog, O.-J. (1980) Liver cirrhosis epidemiology: some methodological problems. *British Journal of Addiction.*75. 227–243.

Skog, O.-J. (1984) The risk function for liver cirrhosis from lifetime alcohol consumption. *Journal of Studies of Alcohol.* 45. 199–208.

Skog O.-J. (1985a) The collectivity of drinking cultures: A theory of the distribution of alcohol consumption. *British Journal of Addiction.* 80. 83–99.

Skog, O.-J. (1985b) The wetness of drinking cultures: a key variable in epidemiology of alcoholic liver cirrhosis. *Acta of Medical Scandinavica.* Suppl. 703. 157–184.

Skog, O.-J. (1986) Trends in alcohol consumption and violent deaths. *British Journal of Addiction.* 81. 365–379.

Skog, O-J. (1993) Alcohol and suicide in Denmark 1911-24 – experiences from a 'natural experiment'. *Addiction.* 88. 1189–1193.

Skvortsova E. S. (1997) Sotsial'no-gigienicheskie aspekty potrebleniya alkogolya, narkoticheski deīstvuyushchikh veshchestv, kureniya sredi gorodskikh podrostkov-shkol'nikov Rossiĭskoĭ Federatsii. Dissertatsiya doktora meditsinskikh nauk (In English. Socio- hygenetic aspects of the use of alcohol, actively addictive substances and smoking among urban adolescents-pupils of the Russian Federation. Dissertation for doctorate in medical sciences).

Smart R.G. (1989) Is the postwar drinking binge ending? Cross-national trends in per capita alcohol consumption. *British Journal of Addiction.* 84. 743-748.

Smart R.G. (1991) World trend in alcohol consumption. *World Health Forum.* 12. 99-103.

Smart R.G. (1995) Do some types of alcohol beverages lead to more problems for adolescents? *Journal of Studies on Alcohol.* 56. 35-38.

Smart R.G., Mann R.E. (1992) Alcohol and the epidemiology of liver cirrhosis. *Alcohol Health and Research World.* 1992. 16. 217-222.

Smart R.G., Murray G.F. (1983) Drug abuse and affluence in five countries: a study of economic and health conditions, 1960-1975. *Drug and Alcohol Dependence.* 11. 297-307.

Smart R.G., Schmidt W. (1970) Blood alcohol levels in drivers not involved in accidents. *Quarterly Journal of Studies on Alcohol.* 31. 968-971.

Smart R.G., Walsh G.W. (1995) Do some types of alcoholic beverages lead to more problems for adolescents? *Journal of Studies on Alcohol.* 56. 35-38.

Smith G.S., Kraus J.F. (1988) Alcohol and residential and occupational: A Review of the epidemiologic evidence. *Annual Review of Public Health.* 9. 99-121.

Solomatin A. P. (1988) Alkogolizm i ego rol' v geneze vnezapnoĭ smerti (In English. Alcoholism and its role in the genesis of sudden death). *Nauchnye Trudy Novosibirskogo Medintsinskogo Instituta.* 132. 93-94.

State Statistical Committee of the RSFSR (1989) Potreblenie alkogol'nykh napitkov v raschete na dushu naseleniya iz gosudarstvennykh resursov RSFSR. (In English. Alcohol consumption per capita from the state resources of the RSFSR). Reprint.

State Statistical Committee of the USSR (1991) *Potreblenie alkogolya i sotsial'nye posledstviya p'yanstva i alkogolizma* (In English. Alcohol consumption and the social consequences of drunkenness and alcoholism, 1986-1990). Reprint.

Stinson F. S., Dufor M. C., Steffens R. A., DeBakey S. F. (1993) Alcohol-related mortality in the United States, 1979-1989. *Alcohol Health & Research World.* 18. 251-260.

Strzdins J. (1994) Opportunities for an effective alcohol control policy in Latvia. Baltic Meeting on Alcohol Policy. Riga. 31 August-2 September.

Strzdins J., Caunītis J., Resins A. (1995a) Absolūtā alkohola patēņa vērtējums Latvijā. *Latvijs Ārsts.* 1. 32-34.

Strzdins J., Caunītis J., Jakosone D., Resins A (1995b) Straujšalkohola psihozes gadīskaita pieaugums Latvijā. *Latvijs Ārsts.* 7/8. 535-536.

Subata E., Grimaluskienne O. (1994). Reply to a questionnaire on the alcohol situation in Lithuania from the WHO Regional Office for Europe. Copenhagen

Sulkunen P. (1989) Drinking in France 1965-1979. An analysis of household consumption data. *British Journal of Addiction.* 84. 61-72.

Sumida T. (1990) Problem of alcoholism in Japan. *Journal of the Kyorin Medical Society.* 21. 529-531.

Takagi S. et al. (1986) Alcohol and alcohol-related disease. *Asian Medical Journal.* 29. 398-405.

Tarter R., Kirisci L., Hegedus A., Mezzich A., Vanyukov M. (1994) Heterogeneity of adolescent alcoholism. *Annual of New-York Academy of Science.* 708. 172-180.

Tishuk Ye. A. (1997) Mediko-statisticheskie aspekty deĭstviya alkogolya kak prichiny smertnosti naseleniya (In English. Medico-statistical aspects of the ef-

fect of alcohol as a cause of death in the population) *Zdravookhranenie Rossiĭskoĭ Federatsii.* 2. 34-36.
Tkachenko G. B. (1996) Kurenie tabaka i zdorov'e naseleniya Rossii (In English. Tobacco smoking and the health of the population of Russia). In: A. K. Demin (ed.) *Kurenie ili zdorov'e v Rossii?* (In English. Smoking or Health in Russia?). Moskva: Zdorov'e i Okruzhayushchaya Sreda Foundation. 28-155.
Tomkins S., Saburova L., Kiryanov N., Andreev E., McKee M., Shkolnikov V., Leon D.A. (2007) Prevalence and socio-economic distribution of hazardous patterns of alcohol drinking: study of alcohol consumption in men aged 25–54 years in Izhevsk, Russia. *Addiction.* 102(4). 544–53.
Treml,V.G. (1982) *Alcohol in the USSR. A Statistical Study.* Durham. N.C.: Duke Press Policy Studies.
Treml,V. G. (1985) Interview. *Times.* September 23.47.
Treml,V. G. (1997) Soviet and Russian statistics on alcohol consumption and abuse. In: L. Bobadilla, C. A. Costello & F. Mitchell (eds.). *Premature Death in the New Independent States* Washington: National Academy Press. 220–238.
Ugryumov A. I. (1997) Organnaya patologiya i prichiny smerti bol'nykh, zloupotreblyavshikh alkogolem (In English. Organ pathology and causes of death in sick alcohol abusers). *Voprosy Narkologii.* 3. 47–50.
Urakov I. G., Miroshnichenko L. D. (1989) Tendentsii v zabolevaemosti alkogolizmom i slozhivshayasya alkogol'naya situatsiya (In English. Trends in the incidence of alcoholism and the alcohol situation). *Zdravookhranenie Rossiĭskoĭ Federatsii.* 1. 35–39.
Urakov I. G., Miroshnichenko L. D. (1991) The Union of Soviet Socialist Republics. In : M.Plant (ed.) *Problems Associated with Alcohol Consumption in Groups at High Risk.* World Health Organization. European Bureau. Report and Studies 109. 144–164.
Urlanis B. Ts. (1968) Beregite muzhchin (In English. Save the men). *Literaturnaya Gazeta.* July 26 . Reprinted in *Population. Research. Journalism.* (1976) Moskva: Statistika. 326–332.
U.S. Apparent Consumption of Alcohol Beverages based on State Sales, Taxation, or Receipt Data. U.S. Alcohol Epidemiologic Data Reference Manual. V. 1. (1985)
Värnik A., Wasserman D., Dankowicz M., Eklund G.(1998) Marked decrease in suicide among in the former USSR during perestroika. *Acta Psychiatrica Scandinavica.* 98. Suppl. 394. 34–39.
Veljkovic S, Uzelac Z, Vukovic B, Strundzalic M, Denic N, Savic S, Mikovic M. (1989) Deaths from acute alcohol poisoning. *Acta Medicinae Legalis et Socialis.* 39. 513–514.
Virganskaya I. M. (1991) Vnezapnaya smert' i alkogol' (In English. Sudden death and alcohol). *Zdravookhranenie Rossiĭskoĭ Federatsii.* 6. 18–20.
Vishnevsky A. (2000) Pod"em smertnosti v 90-e gody: fakt ili artefakt? (In English. Swift rise in mortality in the 90s: fact or artefact?) *Naselenie i Obshchestvo. Informatsionnyĭ byulleten' Tsentra demografii i ekologii cheloveka Instituta narodnokhozyaĭstvennogo prognozirovaniya RAN (In English. Information bulletin of the Center for Human Demography and Ecology of the Russian Academy of Sciences' Institute for Economic Forecasting).* 45.
Vishnevsky A., Shkolnikov V. (1997a) Smertnost' v Rossii: glavnye gruppy riska i prioritety deĭstviya (In English. Mortality in Russia: main groups at risk and priorities for action). Publication 19. Moskva: Moscow Carnegie Center.
Vishnevsky A., Shkolnikov V. (1997b) *Smertnost' v Rossii: glavnye prioritety deĭstviya* (In English. Mortality in Russia: main priorities for action). Moskva.
Vlasov V., Gafarov V. (2001) Mortality in Russia. *The Lancet.* 358. 669.

Vlassak R. (1928) *Alkogolizm* (In English. Alcoholism). Translated from German. Moskva-Leningrad: Gosudarstvennoe izdatel'stvo.

Voinova L. V. (1999) Statisticheskiĭ analiz zabolevaniĭ pecheni na osnove dannykh vskrytiĭ umershikh v klinikakh Moskovskoĭ Meditsinskoĭ Akademii im. I. M. Sechenova v 1978–1987 gg. (In English. Statistical analysis of liver diseases based on autopsies performed in clinics of the I. M. Sechenov Moscow Medical Academy, 1978–1987). *Arkhiv Patologii.* 61. 45–47.

Vorobyev M. I., Khudyakov A. V. (1988) Dinamika alkogol'nykh psikhozov za poslednie gody v usloviyakh bor'by protiv p'yanstva i alkogolizma (In English. Dynamics of alcohol psychoses in the recent years of the struggle against drunkenness and alcoholism). *Zhurnal Nevropatologii i Psikhiatrii.* 88. 105–107.

Vyazmina N. A., Savchuk S. A. (2002) Issledovanie primesnogo sostava etilovogo spirta i produktov ego rektifikatsii (In English. A Study of admixtures in ethyl alcohol and its products after purification). *Partnyory i Konkurenty.* 2. 30–40.

Walberg P., McKee M., Shkolnikiv V., Chenet L., Leon D. (1998) Economic change, crime, and mortality crisis in Russia: regional analysis. *British Medical Journal.* 317. 312–318.

Wald I., Jaroszewski Z. (1983) Alcohol consumption and alcoholic psychoses in Poland. *Journal of Studies on Alcohol.* 44. 1040–1048.

Walsh D. (1985) Medico-social problems associated with alcohol use and their prevention. World Health Organization. European Regional Bureau. Public health services in Europe 17.

Walsh, B., Grant,M. (1985) International trend in alcohol production and consumption: implications for public health. *World Health Statistics Quarterly.* 38. 130–141.

Wasserman D., Värnik A. (2001) Changes in life expectancy in Russia. *The Lancet.* 357. 2058.

Wasserman D, Värnik A, Eklund G. (1994) Male suicides and alcohol consumption in the former USSR. *Acta Psychiatrica Scandinavica.* 89. 306–313.

Wasserman D, Värnik A, Eklund G. (1998) Female suicides and alcohol consumption during perestroika in the former USSR. *Acta Psychiatrica Scandinavica.* 98. 26–33.

Whitlock F.A. (1974) Liver cirrhosis, alcoholism, and alcohol consumption. *Quarterly Journal of Studies on Alcohol.* 35. 586–605.

WHO (2004) Regional Office for Europe. Health for All database.

Williams C.L., Grechanaia T., Romanova O., Komro., Perry C.L., Farbakhsh K. (2001) Russian-American patterns for prevention. Adaptation of a school-based parent-child programme for alcohol use prevention. *European Journal of Public Health.* 11. 314–321.

Willis J. (2000) "The only money a woman cam claim": a history of distilling in Buryoro. *Uganda Journal.* 46. 1–16.

Willis J. (2001) Unrecorded alcohol consumption in East Africa, 1960–2000: a critical review of the estimates. Printed report on workshop *Assessment of Alcohol as a Risk Factor for the Global Burden of Disease-Unrecorded Alcohol Consumption.* Geneva, Switzerland: World Health Organization

World Bank (2005) Dying too young. Addressing Premature Mortality and Ill Health Due to Non-Communicable Diseases and Injuries in the Russian Federation. http://siteresources.worldbank.org/INTECA/Resources/DTY-Final.pdf

World Drink Trends (1991). Edition Oxfordshire: NTC Publications

World Drink Trends (1994). Edition Oxfordshire: NTC Publications

World Drink Trends (1999) Henley-on-Thames:NTC Publications

World Drink Trends (2003) Country Profiles of the United Nations. http://who.int/substance_abuse/publications/en/1_all_profiles_amro.pdf

Wyllie A., Zhang J.F., Casswell S. (1998) Responses to televised alcohol advertisements associated with drinking behaviour of 10–17-year-olds. *Addiction*. 93. 361–371.

Yu J., Perrine M.W. (1997) The transmission of parent/adult-child drinking patterns: testing a gender-specific structural model. *American Journal of Drug and Alcohol Abuse*. 23. 143–165.

Zaigraev G. G. (1992) *Obshchestvo i alkogol'* (In English. Society and Alcohol). Nauchno-issledovatel'skiĭ institut MVD RF (In English. Research Institute of the Ministry of Internal Affairs of the Russian Federation).

Zaigraev G. G. (2004a) Chernoe protiv "beloĭ" (In English. Black against "White"). *Profil'*. 1. 24–25.

Zaigraev G. G. (2004b) The Russian model of noncommercial alcohol consumption. Moonshine Markets. In: A.Haworth & R. Simpson (eds.) *Unrecorded Alcohol Beverage Production and Consumption*. New York, Hove: Brunner-Routledge. 31–40.

Zaigraev G. G., Murashov A. V. (1990) *Aktual'nye voprosy bor'by s samogonovareniem* (In English. Current Issues in the Struggle with samogon production). Moskva: *Znanie*.

Zamborov Kh. Kh. (1999) Analiz smertnosti sredi patsientov s legochnym tuberkulezom (In English. Analysis of mortality among patients with tuberculosis of the lungs). *Problemy Tuberkuleza*. 4. 12–13.

Zaratyants O. V. (2001) Analiz smertel'nykh iskhodov na osnove dannykh moskovskoĭ patalogo-anatomicheskoĭ sluzhby (1996–2000 g.g.) (In English. Analysis of mortal outcomes on the basis of data from the Moscow Pathological-Anatomical Service (1996–2000)). *Arkhiv Patologii*. 63. 9–13.

Zaridze D., Borisova E., Maximovitch D., Chkhikvadze V. (2000) Alcohol consumption? Smoking and risk of gastric cancer: case-control study from Moscow, Russia. *Cancer Causes and Control*. 11. 363–371.

Zaridze D., Lifanova Y., Maximovitch D., Day N.E., Duffy S.W. (1991) Diet, alcohol consumption and reproductive factors in a case-control study of breast cancer in Moscow. *International Journal of Cancer*. 48. 493–501.

Zhirov N. P., Petrova F. N. (1998) *Antialkogol'noe zakonodatel'stvo Rossiĭskoĭ Imperii: istoricheskiĭ opyt formirovaniya* (In English. Anti-alcohol legislation of the Russian Empire: historical experience of formation). Sankt-Peterburg: Sankt-Peterburgskiĭ Universitet.

Zohoori N., Kline L., Popkin B., Kohlmeier L. (1997a) *Report submitted to the U.S. Agency for International Development*. Carolina Population Center, University of North Carolina at Chapel Hill, North Carolina.

Zohoori N., Kline L., Popkin B., Kohlmeir L. (1997b) *Monitoring health conditions in the Russian Federation: the Russian Longitudinal monitoring survey 1992–1996. Report submitted to the U.S. Agency for International Development*. Carolina Population Center, University of North Carolina at Chapel Hill, North Carolina.

Zohoori N., Kline L., Popkin B., Kohlmeir L. http://www.cpc.unc.edu/rlms

Södertörn Academic Studies

1. Helmut Müssener & Frank-Michael Kirsch (eds.), *Nachbarn im Ostseeraum unter sich. Vorurteile, Klischees und Stereotypen in Texten*, 2000.
2. Jan Ekecrantz & Kerstin Olofsson (eds.), *Russian Reports: Studies in Post-Communist Transformation of Media and Journalism*, 2000.
3. Kekke Stadin (ed.), *Society, Towns and Masculinity: Aspects on Early Modern Society in the Baltic Area*, 2000.
4. Bernd Henningsen et al. (eds.), *Die Inszenierte Stadt. Zur Praxis und Theorie kultureller Konstruktionen*, 2001.
5. Michal Bron (ed.), *Jews and Christians in Dialogue II: Identity, Tolerance, Understanding*, 2001
6. Frank-Michael Kirsch et al. (eds.), *Nachbarn im Ostseeraum über einander. Wandel der Bilder, Vorurteile und Stereotypen?*, 2001.
7. Birgitta Almgren, *Illusion und Wirklichkeit. Individuelle und kollektive Denkmustern nationalsozialistischer Kulturpolitik und Germanistik in Schweden 1928–1945*, 2001.
8. Denny Vågerö (ed.), *The Unknown Sorokin: His Life in Russia and the Essay on Suicide*, 2002.
9. Kerstin W. Shands (ed.), *Collusion and Resistance: Women Writing in English*, 2002.
10. Elfar Loftsson & Yonhyok Choe (eds.), *Political Representation and Participation in Transitional Democracies: Estonia, Latvia and Lithuania*, 2003.
11. Birgitta Almgren (Hrsg.), *Bilder des Nordens in der Germanistik 1929–1945: Wissenschaftliche Integrität oder politische Anpassung?*, 2002.
12. Christine Frisch, *Von Powerfrauen und Superweibern: Frauenpopulärliteratur der 90er Jahre in Deutschland und Schweden*, 2003.
13. Hans Ruin & Nicholas Smith (eds.), *Hermeneutik och tradition. Gadamer och den grekiska filosofin*, 2003.
14. Mikael Lönnborg et al. (eds.), *Money and Finance in Transition: Research in Contemporary and Historical Finance*, 2003.
15. Kerstin Shands et al. (eds.), *Notions of America: Swedish Perspectives*, 2004.
16. Karl-Olov Arnstberg & Thomas Borén (eds.), *Everyday Economy in Russia, Poland and Latvia*, 2003.
17. Johan Rönnby (ed.), *By the Water. Archeological Perspectives on Human Strategies around the Baltic Sea*, 2003.
18. Baiba Metuzale-Kangere (ed.), *The Ethnic Dimension in Politics and Culture in the Baltic Countries 1920–1945*, 2004.
19. Ulla Birgegård & Irina Sandomirskaja (eds.), *In Search of an Order: Mutual Representations in Sweden and Russia during the Early Age of Reason*, 2004.
20. Ebba Witt-Brattström (ed.), *The New Woman and the Aesthetic Opening: Unlocking Gender in Twentieth-Century Texts*, 2004.
21. Michael Karlsson, *Transnational Relations in the Baltic Sea Region*, 2004.
22. Ali Hajighasemi, *The Transformation of the Swedish Welfare System: Fact or Fiction?: Globalisation, Institutions and Welfare State Change in a Social Democratic Regime*, 2004.

23. Erik A. Borg (ed.), *Globalization, Nations and Markets: Challenging Issues in Current Research on Globalization*, 2005.
24. Stina Bengtsson & Lars Lundgren, *The Don Quixote of Youth Culture: Media Use and Cultural Preferences Among Students in Estonia and Sweden*, 2005
25. Hans Ruin, *Kommentar till Heideggers Varat och tiden*, 2005.
26. Ludmila Ferm, *Variativnoe bespredložnoe glagol'noe upravlenie v russkom jazyke XVIII veka* [Variation in non-prepositional verbal government in eighteenth-century Russian], 2005.
27. Christine Frisch, *Modernes Aschenputtel und Anti-James-Bond: Gender-Konzepte in deutschsprachigen Rezeptionstexten zu Liza Marklund und Henning Mankell*, 2005.
28. Ursula Naeve-Bucher, *Die Neue Frau tanzt: Die Rolle der tanzenden Frau in deutschen und schwedischen literarischen Texten aus der ersten Hälfte des 20. Jahrhunderts*, 2005.
29. Göran Bolin et al. (eds.), *The Challenge of the Baltic Sea Region: Culture, Ecosystems, Democracy*, 2005.
30. Marcia Sá Cavalcante Schuback & Hans Ruin (eds.), *The Past's Presence: Essays on the Historicity of Philosophical Thought*, 2006.
31. María Borgström och Katrin Goldstein-Kyaga (eds.), *Gränsöverskridande identiteter i globaliseringens tid: Ungdomar, migration och kampen för fred*, 2006.
32. Janusz Korek (ed.), *From Sovietology to Postcoloniality: Poland and Ukraine from a Postcolonial Perspective*, 2007.
33. Jonna Bornemark (eds.), *Det främmande i det egna: filosofiska essäer om bildning och person*, 2007.
34. Sofia Johansson, *Reading Tabloids: Tabloid Newspapers and Their Readers*, 2007.
35. Patrik Åker, *Symboliska platser i kunskapssamhället: Internet, högre lärosäten och den gynnade geografin*, 2008.
36. Kerstin W. Shands (ed.), *Neither East Nor West: Postcolonial Essays on Literature, Culture and Religion*, 2008.
37. Rebecka Lettevall and My Klockar Linder (eds.), *The Idea of Kosmopolis: History, philosophy and politics of world citizenship*, 2008.
38. Karl Gratzer and Dieter Stiefel (eds.), *History of Insolvency and Bankruptcy from an International Perspective*, 2008.
39. Katrin Goldstein-Kyaga och María Borgström, *Den tredje identiteten: Ungdomar och deras familjer i det mångkulturella, globala rummet*, 2009.
40. Christine Farhan, *Frühling für Mütter in der Literatur?: Mutterschaftskonzepte in deutschsprachiger und schwedischer Gegenwartsliteratur*, 2009.
41. Marcia Sá Cavalacante Schuback (ed.), *Att tänka smärtan*, 2009.
42. Heiko Droste (ed.), *Connecting the Baltic Area: The Swedish Postal System in the Seventeenth Century*, 2011.
43. Alexandr Nemtsov, *A Contemporary History of Alcohol in Russia*, 2011.

www.ingramcontent.com/pod-product-compliance
Lightning Source LLC
Chambersburg PA
CBHW080407230426
43662CB00016B/2338